Psycho-Social Perspectives on Mental Health and Well-Being

Srinivasan Padmanaban
Central University of Tamil Nadu, India

Chittaranjan Subudhi
Central University of Tamil Nadu, India

A volume in the Advances in Psychology, Mental Health, and Behavioral Studies (APMHBS) Book Series

IGI Global
DISSEMINATOR OF KNOWLEDGE

Published in the United States of America by
IGI Global
Medical Information Science Reference (an imprint of IGI Global)
701 E. Chocolate Avenue
Hershey PA, USA 17033
Tel: 717-533-8845
Fax: 717-533-8661
E-mail: cust@igi-global.com
Web site: http://www.igi-global.com

Library of Congress Cataloging-in-Publication Data

Names: Padmanaban, Srinivasan, 1971- editor. | Subudhi, Chittaranjan, 1989- editor.
Title: Psycho-social perspectives on mental health and well-being / Srinivasan Padmanaban, Chittaranjan Subudhi, editors.
Description: Hershey, PA : Medical Information Science Reference, [2020] | Includes bibliographical references and index. | Summary: "This book examines the physical, social, and emotional aspects of mental health and well-being"--Provided by publisher.
Identifiers: LCCN 2019025737 (print) | LCCN 2019025738 (ebook) | ISBN 9781799811855 (hardcover) | ISBN 9781799811862 (ebook)
Subjects: MESH: Mental Health | Population Health | Quality of Life | Sociological Factors | Spirituality
Classification: LCC RA790 (print) | LCC RA790 (ebook) | NLM WM 101 | DDC 616.89--dc23
LC record available at https://lccn.loc.gov/2019025737
LC ebook record available at https://lccn.loc.gov/2019025738

This book is published in the IGI Global book series Advances in Psychology, Mental Health, and Behavioral Studies (APMHBS) (ISSN: 2475-6660; eISSN: 2475-6679)

British Cataloguing in Publication Data
A Cataloguing in Publication record for this book is available from the British Library.

All work contributed to this book is new, previously-unpublished material.
The views expressed in this book are those of the authors, but not necessarily of the publisher.

For electronic access to this publication, please contact: eresources@igi-global.com.

Advances in Psychology, Mental Health, and Behavioral Studies (APMHBS) Book Series

ISSN:2475-6660
EISSN:2475-6679

MISSION

The complexity of the human mind has puzzled researchers and physicians for centuries. While widely studied, the brain still remains largely misunderstood.

The **Advances in Psychology, Mental Health, and Behavioral Studies (APMHBS)** book series presents comprehensive research publications focusing on topics relating to the human psyche, cognition, psychiatric care, mental and developmental disorders, as well as human behavior and interaction. Featuring diverse and innovative research, publications within APMHBS are ideally designed for use by mental health professionals, academicians, researchers, and upper-level students.

COVERAGE

- Addiction
- Human Behavior
- Socialization
- Personality Disorders
- Emotional Health
- Cognition
- Eating Disorders
- Trauma & Stress
- Mental Health & Disorders
- Neurological Disorders

IGI Global is currently accepting manuscripts for publication within this series. To submit a proposal for a volume in this series, please contact our Acquisition Editors at Acquisitions@igi-global.com or visit: http://www.igi-global.com/publish/.

The Advances in Psychology, Mental Health, and Behavioral Studies (APMHBS) Book Series (ISSN 2475-6660) is published by IGI Global, 701 E. Chocolate Avenue, Hershey, PA 17033-1240, USA, www.igi-global.com. This series is composed of titles available for purchase individually; each title is edited to be contextually exclusive from any other title within the series. For pricing and ordering information please visit http://www.igi-global.com/book-series/advances-psychology-mental-health-behavioral/110200. Postmaster: Send all address changes to above address.

Titles in this Series

For a list of additional titles in this series, please visit:
https://www.igi-global.com/book-series/advances-psychology-mental-health-behavioral/110200

Evaluating Mental Workload for Improved Workplace Performance
Arturo Realyvásquez-Vargas (Instituto Tecnológico de Tijuana, Mexico) Karina Cecilia Arredondo-Soto (Universidad Autónoma de Baja California, Mexico) Guadalupe Hernández-Escobedo (Instituto Tecnológico de Tijuana, Mexico) and Jorge González-Reséndiz (Instituto Tecnológico de Tijuana Mexico)
Medical Information Science Reference • © 2020 • 334pp • H/C (ISBN: 9781799810520) • US $265.00

Mental Health Intervention and Treatment of First Responders and Emergency Workers
Clint A. Bowers (University of Central Florida, USA) Deborah C. Beidel (University of Central Florida, USA) and Madeline R. Marks (University of Central Florida, USA)
Medical Information Science Reference • © 2020 • 372pp • H/C (ISBN: 9781522598039) • US $255.00

The Psychology and Dynamics Behind Social Media Interactions
Malinda Desjarlais (Mount Royal University, Canada)
Information Science Reference • © 2020 • 477pp • H/C (ISBN: 9781522594123) • US $195.00

Multifaceted Approach to Digital Addiction and Its Treatment
Bahadir Bozoglan (IF Weinheim Institute for Systemic Education and Development, Germany)
Information Science Reference • © 2019 • 388pp • H/C (ISBN: 9781522584490) • US $225.00

Media Models to Foster Collective Human Coherence in the PSYCHecology
Stephen Brock Schafer (Pacific Rim Enterprises, USA)
Information Science Reference • © 2019 • 307pp • H/C (ISBN: 9781522590651) • US $195.00

Developing and Sustaining Play Therapy Clinics
Erin M. Dugan (LSU Health New Orleans, USA) Krystal Vaughn (LSU Health New Orleans, USA) and Kellie Camelford (LSU Health New Orleans, USA)

IGI Global
DISSEMINATOR OF KNOWLEDGE

701 East Chocolate Avenue, Hershey, PA 17033, USA
Tel: 717-533-8845 x100 • Fax: 717-533-8661
E-Mail: cust@igi-global.com • www.igi-global.com

Editorial Advisory Board

Table of Contents

Detailed Table of Contents

the basic theories in autism and also discusses the technological developments of autism in the present era. With the enrichment in technological developments, researchers and experts focused on the monitoring and improvement of the skills (social, communication, and behavioral) in individuals with autism-related disorders. In conclusion, the work presented in this chapter summarizes that the evolutionary computational interventions have a remarkable possibility for the monitoring and basic skills enhancement in ASD.

The present study aims to find the level of psychological distress in female caregivers of patients with mental illness in the context of Jharkhand and its relations with the socio-demographic variable. The sample was drawn from five blocks of Hazaribagh districts of Jharkhand and the respondents were 200 relatives of the patients with mental illness. A socio-demographic data sheet used for recording the socio-demographic characteristics and Kessler Psychological Distress Scale version 10 (K10) used for assessing their psychological distress. The result shows that female gender is having more psychological distress than male and may lead to common mental disorder under persistent condition. The mean score of female was higher than male (i.e., 26.36 [SD= 9.44] and 22.23 [SD= 8.86], respectively). The difference between both the genders found to be significant at less than 0.001 p values in Man Whitney U test.

The chapter interrogates the explicit and implicit perception of health and well-being among the Jats of Western Uttar Pradesh by using anthropological life cycle approach. The research combined village ethnography and empirical field work to discuss their behavioural choices that they make to maintain good spiritual, mental and physical well-being. For the purpose of the study, both primary and secondary data have been used. Taking a village as a unit is a generally accepted way of the doing research in the social anthropology, and the author has used this approach to gain the overview of health, well-being, wellness, and belief pattern as perceived by the villagers.

Foreword

How much ever wealth one possesses, if good health is not there, will be of no use. If one possesses excellent mental, social, and emotional health that will lead to good character. World Health Organization defines Mental Health is a "state of complete physical, mental, and social well-being and not merely the absence of disease or infirmity". This definition throws much light on mental health. Body and mind are not separate entities. A physical discomfort may lead to less cognitive function. To have good mental health, one has to be better in three domains, such as physical, psychological and social. Another implication from the definition is that the absence of mental illness does not mean that one has got good mental health.

The highest wealth in this world is to have a happy living. Possession of good mental health unleashes one's potential to have better self-awareness, have better communication, have better intra and interpersonal relationship, have problem-solving skill, cope with emotion, and deal with stress.

Our faculty Srinivasan Padmanaban and Chittranjan Subudhi had jointly brought out an edited book on *Psychosocial Perspectives on Mental Health and Well-Being* under IGI Global, an international publisher. Thus, this book exhibits international outlook in psychosocial care.

Aligning to the soul is better than aligning with the material world. This alignment will enrich the self, and this is spirituality. Spirituality is a critical issue which plays a significant role in promoting mental health. That is why three out of fifteen chapters highlight this issue.

The book portrays different connotations on the definition of wellbeing that is perceived from western and eastern countries. Eastern countries view mental health as positive psychology, whereas western countries see it as subjective wellbeing. Emotional intelligence could be a moderator for mental health.

A. P. Dash
Central University of Tamil Nadu, India

Preface

Health is wealth. How much ever one possesses wealth, without sound physical and mental health, that acquired wealth will become unutilized. Hence one has to be physically and mentally fit. People need to cognize about the knowledge, attitude, and process of keeping physically and mentally fit. This book is an attempt to provide that.

Well-being is a complex phenomenon. There is no single factor that brings prosperity. Many psychological and sociological factors are responsible. This book tries to explore the psychosocial ways which are liable to keep a person physically and mentally fit.

Generally, a book serves for a particular professional. For example, a book on technology will be helpful for technicians, and a book on pedagogy will be beneficial for educationists. But there are few books which serve every humanity. This book is one of those.

The following are the brief abstracts of all chapters in this book.

Rajeev Kumar and Ranjit Kumar Dehury from India discussed spirituality as an inevitable component of psycho-social care. The quality of life concerned with the soul is much better than the quality of being concerned with the material world. Psychology is not just science of studying behavior alone; it goes beyond that and analyzes how spirituality has any impact on human. Being spiritual improves health. The authors prescribed few spiritual activities to improve mental health and also free from chronic diseases.

USA's Lynne Orr, Kathrine Pigeon, Linda Weekley, and Brianna Reyes contributed to defining and promoting student well-being. This chapter discusses how wellbeing is defined and described in America and few other countries such as Australia, Lebanon, Turkey, Asia, Europe, India, and Canada. Eastern institutions use positive psychology, psychological wellbeing whereas subjective wellbeing is used by western institutions to determine wellbeing. Few assessment scales on wellbeing and improvement programs on wellbeing were also added.

Gitanjali T Roy and Prapti Suriya of India interpreted the application of the 'Four Paths of Yoga' for positive well-being. This article exposes the influence of Vedic practice on mental health and wellbeing. It discourses on the theory and practice of four yogas such as karma, jnana, bhakti, and raja. The chapter ends with modern trends of the four yoga.

Six authors from Jamaica, West Indies, collaborated and written an article on quality of life and well being of breast cancer patients. The authors are Melisa Anderson, Dwayne Tucker, Fabian Miller, Kurt Vaz, Lennox Anderson-Jackson, and Donovan McGrowder. Two million women get breast cancer every year: breast cancer, the leading case of mortality among women. The authors study the Quality of Life of these patients and provide many conventional and online interventional programs to improve the quality of life of cancer patients.

Vikas Khullar, Harjit Pal Singh, and Manju Bala from India attempted a systematic review of autism spectrum disorders, from the perspective of computer assisted developments. Autism is a mental disorder with less social interaction and communication. According to the Rehabilitation Council of India 1 in 500 Indians are with Autism, and people have low awareness of Autism Disorder. This article spreads awareness by giving a detailed description of the computer-based technological devices that could help people tremendously with autism.

Abhijit Pathak and Chittaranjan Subudhi of India surveyed psychological distress among female caregivers of the patients with mental illness. Distress means a feeling of extreme worry. The sample was drawn from five blocks of Jharkhand state. The results emphasize that women have more pain than men.

Dhananjay Kumar wrote health and well-being among the Jat's of Western Uttar Pradesh of India. The author undertook the medical anthropology of Jat's in a village, and he goes through their lifestyle from pregnancy, birth, infancy, childhood, adolescence, Adulthood, old age, and to till death. All these stages were discussed under the umbrella of health and wellbeing.

Michael Schwartz and Paul Oppold from the USA critically analyzed the role of assistive technology in enhancing the quality of life. Disability can be physical or mental or both. Disabled persons have less than average quality of life. Technologies can be innovated, produced, and provided to those disabled persons to enhance their quality of life. By adopting or utilizing technology, disabled persons may lead to a better experience.

Elavarasi Dhanakotti and Poornima Rajendran, from India, have written a chapter on emotional intelligence as a moderator in reducing academic stress in school students. Various stressors operate among school students to overcome their curricular and co-curricular output. Managing the stress improves the students' overall performance. Hence the authors suggest that management of stress can be better done through the application of emotional intelligence.

Suresh, Manimozhi, and Elango from India trace technological issues in emotional and mental health. Technology is a boon and bane, as well. Technology perturbs society. Hence, there is a disturbance in emotional and mental health by technology. The authors' displays how people are getting distracted through technology and thereby decreasing their emotional and mental health. They also prescribe a few methods to get rid of technology addiction.

Ahu Ergen and Aybike Elif Bolcan, of Turkey, speaks on who lives healthier in a university. Leading a healthier life is inevitable for satisfaction in life. This study explores the level of healthiness among Students, Faculty and Administrative staff of Istanbul University. The dimensions of healthiness are environments, economic, socio-cultural, genetic factor, lifestyle and access to health services. Based on the findings, the author has given some ways and means to achieve a healthy lifestyle.

Italy's Alberta Mazzola compared the interventions given in a mental health center, a school, and in an office. World Health Organization states that Health is a state of complete physical, mental and social well-being and not merely the absence of disease or infirmity. From the definition above, it implies that just because mental illness is absent, the presence of perfect mental health is not assured. The authors compared three different interventions given in three different contexts, the common thread being metal health.

Sanja Tatalović Vorkapić and Renata Čepić from University of Rijeka, Croatia have written on personal and professional well-being among early childhood teachers. This study attempts to find the personal and professional well-being of Croatian early childhood teachers. Teachers from the Kindergarten "Rijeka" have participated in this research as samples. Results showed that early education teachers were moderately satisfied with their work.

Rajeev Kumar and Ranjit Kumar Dehury of India has written on the role of AYUSH on mental health. AYUSH is the acronym of traditional medicinal practices. Ayurveda, Yoga, and Siddha from India, Unani from Greek and Homeopathy from Germany. Allopathy is modern medicine. This article portrays AYUSH in promoting physical and mental health.

Bhanu Prasad Behera from India explains the quote 'sama dana bheda dandopaya,' from Hindu epic. It gives the glimpses about Freud's Id, Ego, and Superego. The author discusses SWOT (Strength, Weakness, Opportunities, and Threat) analyses and suggests various ways to improve mental health.

There are 15 chapters in this book. Each one promotes physical and mental well-being in its way. Thus, this book helps in spreading the practices of keeping good health. A sound mind in a sound body is essential for every human being, and this ensures that they are free from physical and mental discomfort. Hence this book serves a ready reckoner to keep one in good health. By reading the book, one can get knowledge, attitude and practices about maintaining good health. Readers can have good health through a spiritualistic path or by applying emotional intelligence or by stress reduction techniques or by practicing yoga, etc.

Acknowledgment

We thank IGI Global for allowing us to publish in their esteemed publishing house. This opportunity may be a small help offered by them, but it is a big leap to us and put us in the world's academic map. IGI Global has a beautiful management system called eEditoral Discovery. This system helped us in calling of chapters, submission of manuscripts, review management, proofing, and templates for the foreword, preface, and acknowledgment. Thank you, IGI Global.

We express our gratitude to the honorable Vice Chancellor, Prof. A. P. Dash, Central University of Tamil Nadu who has given a foreword for this book, is an internationally reputed zoologist. Prof. Dash is a motivating force behind us, in all our academic endeavors. He is an institution builder and easily approachable, friend, and guide. Thank you, sir.

We thank every author for writing a chapter. They are from different countries possessing expertise in the related social discipline. In spite of the busy schedule, they have given their contribution. Authors have written each chapters meticulously. Without the author's input, this book would not have been possible. Many trees join to form a forest; likewise, many chapters join to create a book. Through this opportunity, we have developed friendship amongst us. Throughout the review process, we can say that authors exhibited their tolerance and carried over the correction. Thank you, authors.

We are indebted to every reviewer. They have put decades of experience and are experts in their respective domains. They have given their precious time in evaluating the chapters. It is because of them, this piece of work has come as a beautiful work, free from errors. Thank you, reviewers, for your honorary work.

Srinivasan Padmanaban

Chittaranjan Subudhi

Chapter 1
Spirituality:
An Inevitable Component of Psycho-Social Care

Rajeev Kumar
Indian Institute of Technology, Kharagpur, India

Ranjit Kumar Dehury
https://orcid.org/0000-0002-3926-9459
School of Management Studies, University of Hyderabad, India

Poulomee Shaw
Mind's, Kolkata, India

ABSTRACT

The World Health Organization (WHO), in its definition of health, considers spirituality as an inseparable segment of health. Spiritualism exists in every human being—it is individualized. Spirituality attracted the attention of mental health professionals despite the advancement in science, technology, quality of life, medical care. Healthcare research conducted in developed countries demonstrated the efficacy of spirituality in medical and psychosocial care and promoting quality of life. There is a significance of integrating spirituality with psychosocial care. Various empirical studies are suggestive of the positive impact of spirituality in the holistic management of various disorders: depression, anxiety disorder, substance abuse, cancer, and AIDS. In the backdrop of the above, the chapter addresses the spirituality of the client and the role of religion in the implementation of psychosocial care plans. This chapter also sheds some light upon the integration of spirituality in nursing care, rehabilitation, and the management of trauma-related disorders.

DOI: 10.4018/978-1-7998-1185-5.ch001

INTRODUCTION

Spirituality and religiosity maintained its space even in the modernized world despite advancements in science, technology, education medical technology, and industrialization, and especially in health and mental health care, and it holds prime importance (Chattopadhyay, 2005). With the advancement of time, the importance of religiosity and spirituality in health care is increasing but in distinct ways. A robust body of literature has documented the relationship between health and spirituality (VanderWeele, Balboni, & Koh, 2017). Globalization, cultural pluralism, social and cultural development, and institutionalization of spirituality have contributed significantly to the resurgence of spirituality (Vanderveer, 2009).

Religiosity and Mental Health

Historically, it has been observed that extreme form of religious practices in irrational ways causes superstitions, and those are harmful to physical and psychological health. While religious beliefs emphasize positive emotions such as peace, forgiveness, and caring for each other. These positive aspects of religions promote quality and quality of life. This positive aspect of religiosity can be seen around the world. In such a way, religiosity enhances positive emotion, generosity, gratitude, kindness, compassion, and hope. And these positive emotions attached to religions are closely associated with positive outcomes of mental health (Falb & Pargament, 2014). This good outcome of mental health is achieved through the social aspect of religiosity. Because religions enhance social network, social support, and connectivity of people in community, which further lead to reciprocation of emotional and instrumental help. This emotional reciprocation is based on win-win approach, giver, and receiver; both are benefitted. The emotional exchange causes emotional fulfillment and instills a sense of personal worth, feeling loved and valued by God or a Higher Power. When a person thinks that he/she is loved and God is taking care of him/her, the person develops the emotional comfort, this psychological comfort help in elevating the coping during the time of distress and diseases (Miller & Thoresen, 2003).

What is Spirituality?

Spirituality is an evitable component of human existence; it relates to something higher power. Human being offered the diverse nomenclature to this higher power. Despite the variety of classification, our relationship with divine power instill the power of life, sense of stability, power, purpose, and a direction (Bullis, 1996; Schuster & Ashburn, 1992). According to the doctrine of various religions, the yardstick of spiritual development is different, and different time levels are decided to achieve spiritual goals; it may be one lifetime or several lives. Spiritual development is connected with normal development milestones of a human being, according to human development theorists (Erikson, 1988; Fowler, 1981). Spiritual growth is correlated with the biological, psychological, and social developmental stages of a human being (Goldman, 1968).

Differences and Similarities Between Religiosity and Spirituality

Spirituality has emerged from the term spirit, and it is related to something pure and sacred in life. Spirituality offers answers to several pertinent questions of life. Those questions are the meaning and purpose of life, hope, transcendence, compassion, and welfare of others. Aldridge (1993) offered 13 definitions of spirituality, the essence of those definitions are related to healing the mind and body, rise above material life, the realization of God of some higher power, exploring the meaning, purpose, and directions in life, and faith healing.

In other definitions, spirituality is closely related to organized religions. For example, in the traditions of Christianity and Judaism, spirituality encompasses personal beliefs and institutional factors (Koenig, George, Meador, Blazer, & Dyck, 1994). Thus according to those definitions, spirituality does not exist without religiosity (Larson, Swyers, & McCullough, 1998). Spirituality carries multidimensional concepts, those mostly subjective and challenging to observe directly. This multifaceted concept includes agreement and disagreement of many societies and community beliefs. Spirituality is the common purpose of all religions of the world (Smith, 1994). Holiness and sacredness are the characteristic properties of all religions (W. R. Miller & Thoresen, 2003; Thoresen, 1998). Besides, a realization of self beyond material world and union with supreme power is the primary component of religiosity; a sum of all the concept of spirituality is broader than religiosity (Astrow, Puchalski, & Sulmasy, 2001).

Spirituality is a subjective experience of our relationship with universal power. Religions are the formal institutionalized system of beliefs and dogmas, creeds, denominational identity, and rituals (Bullis, 1996; Zastro & Kirst-Ashman, 1990). All the religions pave the path for spirituality and emphasize on spiritual development (Swinburne, 1986).

In most cases, the purpose of spirituality is achieved through religious practices. However, some people define their spirituality in pursuing their passions, such as nature, music, commitment to friends, and family, a set of philosophical beliefs (Bisht, 1985). In this way religions can be defined as community effort to realize the transcendental meaning in life, all the faiths encourage spirituality through compassion, forgiveness, and harmony, which are essential components of spirituality;

religions foster the spirituality; beliefs are the process and spirituality is the outcome; however religions are extrinsic, and spirituality is intrinsic in nature (Bisht, 1985).

Why Spirituality is Needed to Integrate with Clinical Practice?

Including India—which has an ancient spiritual tradition—in several other developed countries, there are numerous justifiable reasons to include spirituality in clinical practice. Several reasons appear plausible within the American culture and possibly in different highly industrialized cultures, but these reasons are more relevant to Indian culture, where spirituality has its root. These include the following:

- Old aged people are more inclined to spirituality (Erickson, Erickson, & Kivnick, 1986).
- Disharmonious personal lives, social, and community alienation pushes people toward the spirituality community (Bellah, Madisen, Sullivan, Swidler, & Tipton, 1985; House, Landis, & Umberson, 1988).
- Several pieces of evidence show that spirituality enhances the coping in chronic diseases (Brady, Peterman, Fitchett, Mo, & Cella, 1999; Ehman, Ott, Short, Ciampa, & Hansen-Flaschen, 1999)
- The concept of holistic health lies deeply beyond the disease-free body. Existence, meaning, the purpose of life, quality of interpersonal relations, social, and cultural factors are strong determinants of good health (Ornish, 1999; Ryff & Singer, 1998).
- According to the bio-psychosocial-spiritual model (Sulmasy, 2002), health is not only the outcome of the relationship inside the body (Among various organs of the human body, the biochemical process, the relationship between mind and body). Health is also related to the external environment and transcendence.
- Considering the transcendental perspective, health and diseases appear above than physiological phenomenon, and because of this reason, health-related researches are taking account of spiritual and religious factors (Koenig, 2015).

Spiritual Healing in Different Disorders

In mental health care, religiosity and spirituality hold an essential place in the psychotherapeutic process and therapeutic-relations (Larson, Larson, & Koenig, 2001). Avoidance of spiritual issues weakens the therapeutic relation and therapeutic response (Gockel, 2011). The concept of mind-body relations and its influence on health and diseases are well accepted (Bambling, 2006). Because through cognitive processes, information is passed to physiological functions such as the immune system, central and autonomic systems (Ottaviani et al., 2016).

Pieces of evidence suggested that higher involvement in religious activities alleviates problems related to hypertension, cardiac diseases, strokes, and increase life span. Religious commitment helps in recovery from illness and substantial preventive factors (Park et al., 2017). Considering the psychological component, higher involvement in religious activities promotes well-being and satisfaction in life (Roh et al., 2015). Furthermore, increased religiosity is associated with a lower rate of depression, anxiety, and suicide attempts (AbdAleati, Mohd Zaharim, & Mydin, 2016). And because of this reason, the inclusion of religious beliefs in psychotherapy catalyzes the recovery compared to traditional methods involving traditional methods (Koenig, 2015). The spiritual involvement in health care reduces the economic burden of health care — research evidence estimated the cost-benefit aspect of religiosity and spiritual concern; people having religious and spiritual participation have shorter post-surgery stay in hospital compared to their counterparts (Koenig, 1998). In rehabilitation counseling, spirituality revitalizes the outcome of therapeutic rehabilitation (Waldron-Perrine et al., 2011).

In the treatment and rehabilitation of people suffering from substance use, spirituality plays a pivotal role; because spiritual conflicts deteriorate the recovery of substance use and give the feeling of insecurity, aggressiveness, and poor self-esteem (Coleman, Kaplan, & Downing, 1986). Thus spiritual support among people having a problem with substance use enhances social comfort, resilience, and optimism (Miller, Forcehimes, O'Leary, & LaNoue, 2008). Besides, religious and spiritual involvement reduces the indulgence in substance use (Behere, Muralidharan, & Benegal, 2009).

In the similar connection; a Canadian study conducted by Baetz, Larson, Marcoux, Bowen, & Griffin, (2002) in a mental health care institute reported that people having higher attendance in religious places are less likely to develop depression and alcohol consumption, their satisfaction if life is more elevated than people having less participation in religious places. Studies also recommended that religious and spiritual components can reduce suicidal tendencies (Colucci & Martin, 2008). There is a potent effect of yoga in the prevention and treatment of alcohol and drug dependence problems (Sarkar & Varshney, 2017). Moreover, yogic interventions successfully treat and prevent psychosomatic disorders, geriatric issues, and anxiety disorders (Da Silva, Ravindran, & Ravindran, 2009).

Spiritual Intervention in Coping With Traumatic Events

After the disaster, even the survivors carry traumatic memories; in the inner world of survivors, the theological meanings of meaningfulness, love, care, and peace adopts the negative connotation. The survivors began to question the relationship between the creator and humankind. The belief of caring and loving nature of creator decline to sustain after witnessing the disaster and this is the apparent reaction of any person in the phase of traumatic victimization (Falsetti, Resick, & Davis, 2003). However, a study by (Tran, Kuhn, Walser, & Drescher, 2012) reported the religiously committed persons are less likely to suffer PTSD symptoms compared to non-religious persons.

Spiritual Activities in Clinical Practice

To add spirituality in clinical and group activities, Drescher & Foy (1995) recommended guidelines for group activities. These guidelines are based on two premises: voluntary participation and mutual respect for diverse views. These spiritual activities include a spiritual autobiography, discussion of vital existential issues, silent prayer and meditation, guided imagery, practice in religious ritual, use of selected readings, and attending religious services.

Spiritual Autobiography

Participants are asked to write their life in chronological order. They are asked to highlight their milestones in the development of religious beliefs. The purpose of this exercise is to enable participants to objectify their beliefs in the context of life events, and especially to compare them with concurrent religious beliefs so that they can determine their further direction to pursue.

Discussion of Critical Issues

In this process, group participants are suggested to identify the significant theological and existential matters for debate. Each member shares their experience regarding that. In this process, each member has the opportunity to explore new issues they often face. In a mutual group discussion, many of their doubts are clarified.

Spiritual Exercises

There are exercises to explore self within such as guided meditation, guided imagery, and silent prayer. In addition to inner-exploration, these exercises help in stress alleviation.

Selective Readings and Religious Ritual

Group members collect stories and spiritual teachings of all religions. And each story or teaching is given a particular theme. These themes are associated with relevant perceptions and experiences of participants, and these selective readings are assigned to group members as part of their homework. As well as they are asked to maintain a diary to note down important points so that in subsequent sessions, those experiences can be shared.

Religious Participation Outside Group

The members of the group are suggested to participate in the religious service of their faith. The purpose of this exercise to develop and facilitate the social-communication and interaction beyond their limited network or to extend their social support network. The second purpose of this exercise to instill hope and realistic ideas of the world – as the construction and destruction both are natural, and they are the two aspects of one world, and it should be accepted without having a conflict with it. The third purpose of this exercise is to re-establish the connection with the faith in which they are born and brought up. The fourth purpose of this exercise is to explore a new dimension of their religious expression, which can further provide them comfort.

Spirituality in Nursing Care

Nurses are the closest health care provider for indoor-patients. Nurses can implement a spiritual component in health care. In this view, Amenta & Bohnet (1986) prescribed four spiritual tools in health care. These spiritual techniques are the following:

1. An active and empathetic listening skill
2. A manifestation of physical and emotional presence
3. Acceptance of patience, and their experience
4. Judicious self-disclosure, whenever it is required.

Psycho-Synthesis: A Discipline of Personal and Spiritual Development

Assagioli (1965) propounded the concept of Psycho-synthesis; it is a blend of psychology and mysticism. Earlier psychology was viewed in a very dispassionate manner, as it is based on the hard facts and rationality, and the excess of rationality took away its charm. It was felt that adding the component of soul and meaning of life, make the psychology more interesting, psycho-synthesis is the blend of mysticism and core scientific nature of psychology (Assagioli, 1974).

Psycho-synthesis was more evolved to cater to the need for growth and healing. Since his time, the various premises of psycho-synthesis were: development of different faculties of mind and maintain balance among them, emphasis the personal and spiritual growth as well, and the development of the unique creative potential of each individual. Psycho-synthesis recognizes that each need to realize his/her relation with the universe in a unique way (Hardy, 2016).

Shreds of evidence proved augmentation of the spiritual component and spiritual identity in the psychotherapeutic process boost the quality and outcome of psychotherapy, especially while dealing with spiritual crisis and drug dependence; techniques of psycho-synthesis handled these issues successfully (Firman & Gila, 2012).

Challenges of Inclusion of Spirituality in Psychotherapy

There are several challenges to include the spiritual component in psychotherapy.

There is an overlapping of boundaries between psychotherapies and spirituality. There may be subjective differences in religiosity between therapists and patients; these individual differences are because of the non-acceptance of religious and spiritual beliefs (Vaughan, 1991).

Even within the same religious or spiritual paths, there are several schools and denominations, where the set of beliefs varies. And to challenge these belief systems are complicated because they are very deep-rooted. In fact, within academic boundaries, there is diversity of norms and expectations related to psychotherapeutic schools, and somewhere these academic dogma makes challenging to accept the models outside the boundaries of their schools (Gonsiorek, Richards, Pargament, & McMinn, 2009). The border of comfort zone is infringed considering spiritual issues; because of this reason, therapists avoid the discussions of spiritual problems (Schultz-Ross & Gutheil, 1997).

Spiritual issues arise in dealing with families with rigid religious beliefs. The pathological family pattern is associated with strict religious beliefs. Because these families are often involved in abusive parenting (Bowman, 1989). Consequently, these children develop a negative image of supreme power, which is defined as one type of spiritual crisis (Josephson, 1993).

The Indian Scenario in Clinical and Spiritual Practice

Spiritual practice is the backbone of the Indian lifestyle. According to (Wig, 1990), Indian spiritual and religious scriptures have given the importance to search for the supreme power, spiritual meaning, and detachment to material life. The mystic-metaphysical tradition of Indian spiritual life greatly influenced the practice of psychotherapy in Indian mental health care set up; psychotherapy in India has been widely influenced by Mystico-metaphysical cultures (Neki, 1984). There is a difference in evolution of western and Indian psychotherapeutic practices. The socio-ethnic-dynamics of Judaism and Christianity greatly influenced psychotherapy traditions. Since India has variety of cultural beliefs, therefore development of psychotherapy was fewer patients centric.

The professionalism between patient and therapist is not in the tradition in the Indian therapeutic scenario. Because from the centuries, the relationship between a guru (teacher) and chela (disciple) was of the nature to receive and impart knowledge, such ties were meant to resolve the personal, interpersonal, and worldly issues; as it is mentioned in the Upanishads (Indian Spiritual scriptures). So the patients or clients see an image of Guru in the therapist, who can resolve his/her issues and change his/her life, unlike the professional therapeutic relationship (Neki, 1974).

CONCLUSION AND FUTURE RECOMMENDATION

From the above discussion, it is evident that the advancement of science and technology could not hinder the importance of spirituality. In India, healing practice for various mental and physical disorders has emerged from religiosity and spirituality. Under the British colonial rule, it was merged with the western method of healing. After independence under the influence of rapid advancement, the component of spirituality was seemed to ignore. But now from a decade, it is coming back to its roots after synthesis with western psychotherapy and in its modified form. The above mentioned various empirical research has proved the efficacy of spirituality in psychotherapy in holistic management of the different disorders. But further, the integration of spirituality in psychotherapy needs caution to take care the diversity of Indian culture.

REFERENCES

AbdAleati, N. S., Mohd Zaharim, N., & Mydin, Y. O. (2016, December 1). Religiousness and Mental Health: Systematic Review Study. *Journal of Religion and Health*. doi:10.100710943-014-9896-1

Aldridge, D. (1993). Is there evidence for spiritual healing? *Advances*, *9*(4), 4–21.

Amenta, M., & Bohnet, N. (1986). *Nursing Care of the Terminally ill*. Boston, MA: Little, Brown, and Company.

Assagioli, R. (1965). *Psychosynthesis: A manual of principles and techniques*. Oxford, UK: Hobbs, Dorman & Co., Inc.

Assagioli, R. (1974). Jung and psychosynthesis. *Journal of Humanistic Psychology*, *14*(1), 35–55. doi:10.1177/002216787401400104

Astrow, A. B., Puchalski, C. M., & Sulmasy, D. P. (2001). *Religion, spirituality, and health care: Social ethical and practical consideration*. Academic Press.

Baetz, M., Larson, D. B., Marcoux, G., Bowen, R., & Griffin, R. (2002). Canadian psychiatric inpatient religious commitment: An association with mental health. *Canadian Journal of Psychiatry*, *47*(2), 159–166. doi:10.1177/070674370204700206 PMID:11926078

Bambling, M. (2006). Mind, body and heart: Psychotherapy and the relationship between mental and physical health. *Psychotherapy in Australia*, *12*(2), 52–59.

Behere, R. V., Muralidharan, K., & Benegal, V. (2009). Complementary and alternative medicine in the treatment of substance use disorders-A review of the evidence. *Drug and Alcohol Review*, *28*(3), 292–300. doi:10.1111/j.1465-3362.2009.00028.x PMID:21462415

Bellah, R. N., Madisen, R., Sullivan, W., Swidler, A., & Tipton, S. (1985). *Habits of the heart: Individualism and commitment in American life*. Berkeley, CA: University of California Press.

Bisht, D. B. (1985). *Spiritual Dimension of Health*. New Delhi: Directorate General of Health Services.

Bowman, E. S. (1989). Understanding and responding to religious material in the therapy of multiple personality disorder. *Dissociation: Progress in the Dissociative Disorders*, *2*(4), 231–238.

Brady, M. J., Peterman, A. H., Fitchett, G., Mo, M., & Cella, D. (1999). A case for including spirituality in quality of life measurement in oncology. *Psycho-Oncology*, *8*(5), 417–428. doi:10.1002/(SICI)1099-1611(199909/10)8:5<417::AID-PON398>3.0.CO;2-4 PMID:10559801

Bullis, R. (1996). *Spirituality in social work practice*. Washington, DC: Taylor & Francis.

Chattopadhyay, S. (2005). Spiritual and religious themes in psychiatric management: A proposed biopsychosocial model. *The Internet Journal of World Health and Societal Politics, 2*(1).

Coleman, S. B., Kaplan, J. D., & Downing, R. W. (1986). Life Cycle and Loss— The Spiritual Vacuum of Heroin Addiction. *Family Process*, *25*(1), 5–23. doi:10.1111/j.1545-5300.1986.00005.x PMID:3956709

Colucci, E., & Martin, G. (2008). Religion and Spirituality Along the Suicidal Path. *Suicide & Life-Threatening Behavior*, *38*(2), 229–244. doi:10.1521uli.2008.38.2.229 PMID:18444780

Da Silva, T. L., Ravindran, L. N., & Ravindran, A. V. (2009). Yoga in the treatment of mood and anxiety disorders: A review. *Asian Journal of Psychiatry*, *2*(1), 6–16. doi:10.1016/j.ajp.2008.12.002 PMID:23051013

Drescher, K. D., & Foy, D. W. (1995). *Spirituality and Trauma Treatment: Suggestions for Including Spirituality as a Coping Resource - the National Center for Post Traumatic Stress Disorder Napa County, California*. Retrieved November 5, 2019, from http://napa.networkofcare.org/veterans/library/article.aspx?id=384&cat=473

Ehman, J. W., Ott, B. B., Short, T. H., Ciampa, R. C., & Hansen-Flaschen, J. (1999). Do patients want physicians to inquire about their spiritual or religious beliefs if they become gravely ill? *Archives of Internal Medicine*, *159*(15), 1803–1806. doi:10.1001/archinte.159.15.1803 PMID:10448785

Erickson, E. H., Erickson, J. M., & Kivnick, H. W. (1986). *Vital involvement in old age*. New York: Norton.

Erikson, J. M. (1988). *Wisdom and the senses*. New York: W.W. Norton.

Falb, M. D., & Pargament, K. I. (2014). Religion, Spirituality, and Positive Psychology: Strengthening Well-Being. In Perspectives on the Intersection of Multiculturalism and Positive Psychology. Cross-Cultural Advancements in Positive Psychology (7th ed.). Dordrecht: Springer.

Falsetti, S. A., Resick, P. A., & Davis, J. L. (2003). Changes in religious beliefs following trauma. *Journal of Traumatic Stress*, *16*(4), 391–398. doi:10.1023/A:1024422220163 PMID:12895022

Firman, J., & Gila, A. (2012). *Psychotherapy of Love, A: Psychosynthesis in Practice*. Albany, NY: State University of New York Press.

Fowler, J. W. (1981). *Stages of faith: The psychology of human development and the quest for meaning*. San Francisco: Harper and Row.

Gockel, A. (2011). Client perspectives on spirituality in the therapeutic relationship. *The Humanistic Psychologist*, *39*(2), 154–168. doi:10.1080/08873267.2011.564959

Goldman, R. (1968). *Religious thinking from childhood to adolescence*. New York: Seabury.

Gonsiorek, J. C., Richards, P. S., Pargament, K. I., & McMinn, M. R. (2009). Ethical challenges and opportunities at the edge: Incorporating spirituality and religion into psychotherapy. *Professional Psychology, Research and Practice*, *40*(4), 385–395. doi:10.1037/a0016488

Harding, R., Powell, R. A., Kiyange, F., Downing, J., & Mwangi-Powell, F. (2010). Provision of Pain- and Symptom-Relieving Drugs for HIV/AIDS in Sub-Saharan Africa. *Journal of Pain and Symptom Management*, *40*(3), 405–415. doi:10.1016/j.jpainsymman.2009.12.025 PMID:20685071

Hardy, J. (2016). *A psychology with a soul: Psychosynthesis in evolutionary context*. Routledge. doi:10.4324/9781315562124

House, J. S., Landis, K. R., & Umberson, D. (1988). Social relationships and health. *Science*, *241*(4865), 540–545. doi:10.1126cience.3399889 PMID:3399889

Josephson, A. M. (1993). The Interactional problems of Christian families and their relationship to developmental psychopathology: Implications for treatment. *Journal of Psychology and Christianity*, *12*(4), 312–328.

Koenig, H. G. (1998). Religious attitudes and practices of hospitalized medically ill older adults. *International Journal of Geriatric Psychiatry*, *13*(4), 213–224. doi:10.1002/(SICI)1099-1166(199804)13:4<213::AID-GPS755>3.0.CO;2-5 PMID:9646148

Koenig, H. G. (2015). Religion, spirituality, and health: A review and update. *Advances in Mind-Body Medicine*, *29*(3), 19–26. PMID:26026153

Koenig, H. G., George, L. K., Meador, K. G., Blazer, D. G., & Dyck, P. B. (1994). Religious affiliation and psychiatric disorder among protestant baby boomers. *Hospital & Community Psychiatry*, *45*(6), 586–596. doi:10.1176/ps.45.6.586 PMID:8088740

Larson, D. B., Larson, S. S., & Koenig, H. G. (2001). The patient's spiritual/religious dimension: A forgotten factor in mental health. *Directions in Psychiatry*, *21*(4), 10–15.

Larson, D. B., Swyers, J. P., & McCullough, M. E. (1998). *Scientific research on spirituality and health: A consensus report*. Rockville, MD: National Institute for Healthcare Research.

Miller, W. R., Forcehimes, A., O'Leary, M. J., & LaNoue, M. D. (2008). Spiritual direction in addiction treatment: Two clinical trials. *Journal of Substance Abuse Treatment, 35*(4), 434–442. doi:10.1016/j.jsat.2008.02.004 PMID:18657945

Miller, W. R., & Thoresen, C. E. (2003). Spirituality, religion, and health: An emerging research field. *The American Psychologist, 58*(1), 24–35. doi:10.1037/0003-066X.58.1.24 PMID:12674816

Neki, J. S. (1974). A reappraisal of the guru-chela relationship as a therapeutic paradigm. *International Mental Health Research Newsletter, 16*(2), 2–7.

Neki, J. S. (1984). Psychotherapy in India traditions and trends. In A. De Souza & M. D. A. De Souse (Eds.), *Psychiatry in India* (pp. 339–342). Bhalani Book Depot.

Ornish, D. (1999). *Love and survival: 8 pathways to intimacy and health.* New York: Harper Collins.

Ottaviani, C., Thayer, J. F., Verkuil, B., Lonigro, A., Medea, B., Couyoumdjian, A., & Brosschot, J. F. (2016). Physiological concomitants of perseverative cognition: A systematic review and meta-analysis. *Psychological Bulletin, 142*(3), 231–259. doi:10.1037/bul0000036 PMID:26689087

Park, C. L., Masters, K. S., Salsman, J. M., Wachholtz, A., Clements, A. D., Salmoirago-Blotcher, E., ... Wischenka, D. M. (2017). Advancing our understanding of religion and spirituality in the context of behavioral medicine. *Journal of Behavioral Medicine, 40*(1), 39–51. doi:10.100710865-016-9755-5 PMID:27342616

Roh, S., Kim, Y., Lee, K. H., Lee, Y. S., Burnette, C. E., & Lawler, M. J. (2015). Religion, Social Support, and Life Satisfaction Among American Indian Older Adults. *Journal of Religion & Spirituality in Social Work, 34*(4), 414–434. doi:10.1080/15426432.2015.1097094

Ryff, C. D., & Singer, B. (1998). The Contours of Positive Human Health. *Psychological Inquiry, 9*(1), 1–28. doi:10.120715327965pli0901_1

Sarkar, S., & Varshney, M. (2017). Yoga and substance use disorders: A narrative review. *Asian Journal of Psychiatry, 25*, 191–196. doi:10.1016/j.ajp.2016.10.021 PMID:28262148

Schultz-Ross, R. A., & Gutheil, T. G. (1997). Difficulties in integrating spirituality into psychotherapy. *The Journal of Psychotherapy Practice and Research, 6*(2), 130–138. PMID:9071663

Schuster, C. S., & Ashburn, S. S. (1992). *The process of human development: A holistic lifespan approach* (3rd ed.). New York: Lippincott.

Smith, H. (1994). *The world's religions: A guide to our windows traditions.* San Francisco: Harper Collines.

Sulmasy, D. P. (2002). A Biopsychosocial-Spiritual Model for the Care of Patients at the End of Life. *The Gerontologist, 42*(3suppl_3), 24–33. doi:10.1093/geront/42.suppl_3.24 PMID:12415130

Swinburne, R. (1986). *The evolution of the soul.* Oxford, UK: Oxford University Press.

Thoresen, C. E. (1998). Spiritual health and science, the coming revival? In S Roth Roemer, S Korpivas Robinson, & C. C. (Eds.), The emerging role of counseling psychology in health care. New York: Norton.

Tran, C. T., Kuhn, E., Walser, R. D., & Drescher, K. D. (2012). The Relationship between religiosity, PTSD, and depressive symptoms in veterans in PTSD residential treatment. *Journal of Psychology and Theology, 40*(4), 313–322. doi:10.1177/009164711204000406

Vanderveer, P. (2009). Spirituality in Modern Society. *Social Research, 76*(4), 1097–1120.

VanderWeele, T. J., Balboni, T. A., & Koh, H. K. (2017, August 8). Health and spirituality. *JAMA - Journal of the American Medical Association.* doi:10.1001/jama.2017.8136

Vaughan, F. (1991). Spiritual issues in psychotherapy. *Journal of Transpersonal Psychology, 23*(2), 105–119.

Waldron-Perrine, B., Rapport, L. J., Hanks, R. A., Lumley, M., Meachen, S. J., & Hubbarth, P. (2011). Religion and Spirituality in Rehabilitation Outcomes Among Individuals With Traumatic Brain Injury. *Rehabilitation Psychology, 56*(2), 107–116. doi:10.1037/a0023552 PMID:21574729

Wig, N. N. (1990). Indian concepts of mental health and their impact on the care of the mentally ill. *International Journal of Mental Health, 18*(3), 71–80. doi:10.1080/00207411.1989.11449136

Zastro, C., & Kirst-Ashman, K. (1990). *Understanding human behavior and the social environment.* Chicago: Nelson-Hall.

Chapter 2
Defining and Promoting Student Well-Being:
American and International Colleges

Lynne Orr
Walden University, USA

Kathrine Pigeon
Walden University, USA

Brianna Reyes
William Paterson University, USA

Linda Weekley
Walden University, USA

ABSTRACT

The chapter includes a summary of how American and international colleges define students' wellbeing. American colleges began using wellbeing within the practice of positive psychology. Now, colleges in the United States use the term health and wellness, which encompasses a multidimensional meaning including psychological, social, physical, and spiritual wellbeing. The international colleges primarily define wellbeing as subjective wellbeing, dependent upon the students' perceptions, culture, and social support. A few wellness assessments will be introduced. The remainder of the chapter discusses varying wellness programs conducted on today's American college campuses.

DOI: 10.4018/978-1-7998-1185-5.ch002

INTRODUCTION

Well-being is a term that is most commonly applied to persons but is never intersected with their circumstances—more specifically, with college students. In this chapter, the authors will use a global discussion of how well-being is defined, in conjunction with how it is discussed and normalized, to compare the American standard. The authors will also compare the assessments American college campuses are utilizing to the ones used by their global counterparts. Applying well-being to college students would add more to the conversation regarding their academic success, retention rates, and likelihood to graduate. Colleges have become increasingly concerned about their students' health and well-being.

DEFINING STUDENT WELL-BEING ON AMERICAN COLLEGE CAMPUS

Seligman, Ernst, Gillham, Reivich, and Linkins (2009) mention three factors on why colleges should be concerned with students' well-being. First, the prevalence of depression and anxiety among adolescents has increased. Second, Americans are less satisfied with life and happiness, in comparison to 50 years ago. Third, improved well-being leads to better learning. According to Seligman et al., "more well-being is synergistic with better learning" (p. 294). Seligman et al. (2009) believe well-being can be taught in school "as a vehicle for increasing life satisfaction, and as an aid to better learning and more creative thinking" (p. 294).

Subjective Well-Being

Overall, four models of well-being on American college campuses are currently available. One of these models is subjective well-being (SWB). SWB comes from a psychological perspective which influences a person's level of anxiety and depression. There seems to be some overlap of subjective well-being with positive psychology, yet there is a greater emphasis on measuring neurosis and creating implementation strategies for improving neurosis. Ratelle, Simard, and Guay's (2013) study mentions the importance of SWB among college students, because "SWB has also been associated with important outcomes, such as educational aspirations, academic engagement, class attendance, educational track/choice of field of study, and academic achievement, and dropout" (p. 894). The study's purpose was to examine students perceived social support. Kim and Kim (2017) studied the impact social networking has on SWB. Munzel, Meyer-Waarden, and Galan (2018) also investigated the influence of social networking upon students' SWB. Overall, many of the studies on college students' SWB have been primarily conducted in other countries. Thus, the use of SWB among American colleges has been less popular, in comparison to Asian, European, and Canadian colleges. Hartman, Evans, and Anderson (2017) implemented a credit-based leisure education course to promote adaptive coping skills and SWB.

Positive Psychology

Seligman et al. (2009) are considered as leaders in positive psychology. Positive psychology grew from the psychological clinical field, which, instead of focusing on psychopathologies and comorbidities, put emphasis on happiness, life satisfaction, and well-being (Marshall, 2016). Seligman et al. (2009) explained three realms of Positive Psychology exist. The first is positive emotions, such as pleasure, contentment, joy, and love. The second component revolves around an "engaged life", "flow," and being fully present (p. 296). The third realm includes a "meaningful life," relating to people's connections to others, as well as knowing their highest strengths (Seligman, 2002).

Many different studies have been conducted on elements of positive psychology. One of these studies (Marshall, 2016) investigated college students' grit, life satisfaction, positive affect, and optimism in predicting executive functioning. Other scholars focused on the concept of hope as a component of positive psychology (Ingram, Warlick, Ternes, & Krieshok, 2018; Selvaraj & Bhat, 2018; Vela, Smith, Whittenberg, Guardiola, & Savage, 2018).

The following studies all included hope as a component of positive psychology. Ingram et al.'s study (2018) integrated the concept of hope among college students. Hope was conceived as a concept where individuals would demonstrate "decreasing negative affective states, while also promoting well-being and stress management" (para. 2). Vela et al.'s (2018) study on American colleges investigated hope and mindfulness as predictors of psychological grit. They defined psychological grit as the "presence of meaning in life, search for meaning in life, hope, life satisfaction, and mindfulness" (p. 2). Finally, Selvaraj and Bhat's (2018) research investigated how the strengthening of positive psychology, such as hope, resilience, efficacy, and optimism, would advance college students' positive mental health. McDermott et al. (2017) also investigated hope as a function of positive psychology, in relation to help-seeking behavior.

Hope is defined as a positive aspect of one's thinking and belief, which impact on suicidal actions. Given the increase in suicides among college students, some studies have been conducted on the prevention of suicide. The stress college students experience could potentially increase the risk of suicide, therefore Matel-Anderson,

Bekhet, and Garnier-Villarreal's (2019) scholarship reviewed the influence of social support and positive thinking on suicide efficacy.

Implementing Positive Psychology Practices

A wide variety of studies have investigated the implementation of the principles of positive psychology. Shushok and Hulme (2006) investigated the impact of students finding and using their personal strengths upon their well-being. Another study implemented a two-week nature-based well-being intervention (Passmore & Holder, 2017). Feldman and Dreher (2012) research included a goal-setting session, to evaluate if students became more hopeful. Nagata, Conoley, Arnadottir, White, and Shishim's (2011) study implemented three positive psychology interventions with first year college students: "Three Good Things," "Using Signature Strengths," and the "Gratitude Visit" (Nagata et al., 2011, para. 2). A final positive psychology study investigated an online stress management intervention (Meredith et al., 2014). Wilson (2016) studied gratitude as another area of positive psychology. Wilson discussed the impact of gratitude practices on college students' resilience to learning. Renshaw and Rock (2018), instead, studied gratitude as a thinking intervention.

Psychosocial Wellness and Wellness Models on College Campuses

The American College Health Association represents over 1,100 institutions of higher education, helping students with their health and wellness needs. On most college campuses, health centers have combined departments with counseling to serve students' health and wellness. The rise of mental illness among college students has become a major concern for universities (Cressy, 2011). Cressy (2011) clearly stated that "to help manage stress and promote overall well-being, students need to develop wellness strategies and make active healthy living a habit" (para. 3). Thus, a health and wellness model includes various dimensions of a student, such as physical, emotional, social, financial, educational, and spiritual wellness. Similar studies applied the term psychosocial wellness (Beauchemin, Gibbs, & Granello, 2018; Reymann, Fialkowski, & Stewart-Sicking, 2015).

American colleges are also concerned with retaining and graduating students. Tinto's (1975, 1987) departure theory suggested the students' level of engagement impacts whether the student completes a degree or withdraws. Thus, Tinto's theory recommends that a student engages with the university. Others mention the importance of belonging to the university (Cressy, 2011).

College recreation centers often include programing for fitness and well-being and offer a place for students to feel as if they belong. There is a need for collaboration among the recreation center staff and the health staff to further help foster the students' sense of well-being. Cressy (2011) recommended the following:

Fitness and health professionals can work together with student leaders to support broad-based active healthy living initiatives across campus. Such collaborative initiatives need to employ innovative, coordinated strategies that increase awareness among both students and staff of the relationship between physical activity, healthy eating, mental health, social integration and student success (para. 56).

Vasold, Deere, and Pivarnik (2018) investigated the influence of recreation sports on psychosocial and physical health. The study measured the overall well-being, sense of belonging, and overall health of college students participating in recreational sports. Robino and Foster (2018) investigated the psychosocial predictors of wellness among college students. Conley, Travers, and Bryant (2013) measured stress management and promotion of psychosocial adjustment, as well as the benefits of engagement in a psychosocial wellness seminar. Cressy (2011) discussed the *Learning Reconsidered* document, while Cressy stated about the document:

The recommendation is to replace our traditionally distinct categories of student learning and academic learning with a fused, integrated, and comprehensive vision of transformative learning that is centered on and responsive to the whole student. Approaching health and wellness as a vital part of student development is an example of valuing the whole student including their mind, body, emotions, and spirit. Applying the learning reconsidered principles to campus recreation, including broad-based wellness programs, calls for staff and faculty to take a holistic perspective of student's well-being. Collaborative partnerships must be developed across interconnected divisions, with leaders valuing learning as a transformative process that occurs beyond the classroom (para. 3).

Application of Psychosocial Wellness and Wellness Programs in Colleges

In addition to the collaboration of faculty and staff to fully implement students' wellness, there are other programs on college campuses. Gieck and Olsen (2007) discussed holistic wellness as a means for developing healthy behavior of college students. The study implemented an 11-week program to determine the impact on their holistic wellness (Gieck & Olsen, 2007). Other colleges have implemented a mobile application (Booc, San Diego, Tee, & Caro, 2016), mindfulness training (Dvořáková et al., 2017), as well as a wellness course (Beauchemin et al., 2018). Schweitzer, Ross, Klein, Lei, and Mackey (2016) implemented an electronic wellness program to improve college students' diet and exercise. One of the chapter's author helped develop a well-being course as part of the universities' general education requirement. Further, both chapter's authors observed and taught freshman seminar courses which incorporated aspects of wellness for college students.

Assessing College Students' Well-Being

The Academic Emotions Questionnaire

The academic emotions questionnaire (AEQ) can be used to measure student enjoyment, ego, relief, fury, shame, uneasiness, sorrow, and boredom, along with a cognitive-motivational model of achievement effects of emotions and control value theory to study students (Pekrun, Goetz, Frenzel, Barchfeld, & Perry, 2011). The AEQ assesses students' achievement emotions as domain-general and trait-like constructs, such as test anxiety. Recent research has revealed that students' emotions are organized in a domain-specific way, to a certain extent (Pekrun et al., 2011).

Respondek, Seufert, Stupnisky, and Nett (2017) applied the AEQ and discovered most of the bivariate Pearson correlations were consistent with earlier research. While Pekrun, Lichtenfeld, Marsh, Murayama, and Goetz (2017) conducted a longitudinal study applying the AEQ while measuring attitudes related to Mathematical academics. Pekrun et al. (2017) noticed positive effect influenced positive achievement.

The Satisfaction with Life Scale

Life satisfaction can be described as a comprehensive and universal assessment of the quality of life, which is dependent on items and criteria the individual considers important (Pettay, 2008). Positive and negative affect and life satisfaction make up SWB (SWB) or happiness. Diener, Emmons, Larsen, and Griffin developed the Satisfaction with Life Scale (SWLS) to measure the life satisfaction variable of SWB (Pettay, 2008). The SWLS is an inventory containing five items and a 7-point scale; the five items include: (1) In most ways my life is close to ideal; (2) the conditions of my life are excellent; (3) I am satisfied with my life; (4) so far, I have gotten the important things I want in life; (5) if I could live my life over, I would change almost nothing. Studies have shown the SWLS has strong internal reliability and medium validity, which highlights the long-term consistency of life satisfaction over time (Pettay, 2008). Ilies, Yao, Curseu, and Liang (2019) applied the SWLS scale to the variable of education, job fit, and life satisfaction, and discovered, "financial, job and health satisfactions were specified as predictors of general life satisfaction" (p. 165).

Personal Well-Being Index for Adults

Personal well-being is positive psychological development, which emphasizes the whole person and influences intrinsic motivation (Sayler, Boazman, Natesan, & Periathiruvadi, 2015). The Personal Well-being Index for adults (PWI) is used to measure satisfaction with life and contains an 8-item questionnaire. The PWI measures subjective cognitive dimensions of quality of life. The PWI includes items pertaining to different domains related to life, such as success, the standard of living, community connectedness, meeting goals, relationships, future security, and health (Weinberg, Seton, & Cameron, 2018).

The International Well-Being Group has developed numerous PWI instruments to assess well-being across diverse groups and ages of people. A few factors contribute to the variance in well-being: Having close relationships, being optimistic and showing gratitude, spirituality, having greater education, intelligence, and/or income (Sayler et al., 2015). The PWI can assist counselors to improve wellness by using a holistic approach in working with students to improve satisfaction (Ranney, Kleinpeter, & Potts, 2018). In comparison to other SWB assessments which only measure general life satisfaction, the items which make up the PWI were chosen because each contributes significant original variance in a multiple regression analysis, which predicts general life satisfaction (Weinberg et al., 2018). Chopik, Newton, Ryan, Kashdan, and Jarden (2019) found there was near zero effect of age on gratitude and well-being.

College Student Subjective Well-Being Questionnaire

The college student subjective well-being questionnaire (CSSWQ) is a 15-item self-report rating scale which is used to measure four classes of college-specific well-being behavior. These classes of behavior are academic efficacy, academic satisfaction, school connectedness, and college gratitude (Renshaw, 2018). Current revised versions of the CSSWQ standardizes the response options for all items to a unified 7-point Likert-type scale, 1 equaling strongly disagree to 7 equaling strongly agree. Renshaw (2018) revealed the convergent validity and structural validity of the CSSWQ was favorable, the contextual perspective was limited.

Recommended Practices for Student Well-Being Services in American Colleges

First-Year Experience Programs

First-Year Experience (FYE) programs consist of first-year seminars for students and student success courses which universities use to better integrate students on an academic, social, and emotional level to improve the transition to college and promote resiliency. These courses and seminars form the students' experience from their first day to the end of the semester and is a high-impact practice which can improve student engagement and outcomes (Rockey & Congleton, 2016). In these programs, peer grouping is used. Common goals of these courses and seminars are to assist in student adjustment to college life, to promote peer connections, and to support general wellness information. Eighty percent of colleges offer FYE courses and seminars, but only 20% require student participation (Rockey & Congleton, 2016). FYE programs have the potential to meet students' needs that contribute to their success: Building social relationships, building commitment and focusing on aspirations, making college life attainable, and developing college readiness skills (Rockey & Congleton, 2016). Institutions need to implement FYE programs in a way which promotes student success.

Well-Being Courses

Research shows that, upon completing a well-being course, students can achieve a heightened sense of psychological well-being. Courses emphasizing well-being can facilitate the exploration of emotional states which support processes involving self-actualization, which improves overall college student well-being (Crowley & Munk, 2017). Integrating practices which enhance attention to awareness of current experiences and reality supports well-being and improves students' overall functioning and life satisfaction. Gaining insights and skills developed during well-being courses can lead college students to a sense of mastery and acceptance of present life circumstances (Crowley & Munk, 2017). By learning to focus on the present, attention should shift from focusing on the unknown future or an outcome, and anxiety can be lowered. Concentrating on the present decreases negative effects and increases the sense of well-being, which contributes to a more overall positive outlook on life. Well-being courses aim at facilitating a deeper understanding, internal acceptance, and an acceptance of current life experiences.

Mindfulness

One way to promote a healthy transition to college is by mindfulness training. In a Learning to Breath program (L2B), a universal mindfulness program is adapted to match the developmental tasks of college transition. Mindfulness can be described as a practice of accepting present thoughts and feelings with a non-judgmental attitude, which determines the groundwork for intrapersonal and interpersonal awareness (Dvořáková et al., 2017). Raising awareness and attention, while adopting sensitive attitudes towards physical body sensations, thoughts, and emotions, is needed for students to learn necessary stress management skills and emotion regulation skills. Mastering mindfulness assists students in making healthy choices, developing positive relationships, and promotes resilience during challenges (Dvořáková et al., 2017). A pilot study at a large public university in Pennsylvania aimed to evaluate the effectiveness of the mindfulness program to promote students' health and well-being. The results showed the program was associated with a significant increase in students' life satisfaction and a significant decrease in depression and anxiety (Dvořáková et al., 2017). Mindfulness-based programs are shown to be an effective strategy to promote healthy transitions to college. To address current issues in colleges, education needs to broaden its reach and facilitate the development of the whole person (Dvořáková et al., 2017).

Positive Psychology

Positive institutions are a component within positive personal psychology. Individual character strengths should be emphasized in the development of happiness since this enables positive experiences and enjoyment. Multiple factors account for well-being and happiness. Practicing positive psychology by addressing life's experiences can improve student satisfaction and condition while supporting well-being and flourishment (Lambert, Passmore, & Holder, 2015). Positive experiences, traits, and institutions are the three pillars of positive psychology and, in the authors' experience, faculty and educators have access to the students, which can have a significant influence on student evaluation of experiences.

INTERNATIONAL PERSPECTIVE: COLLEGE STUDENTS' WELL-BEING

The authors conducted a peer-reviewed article search on studies from 2000-2019, applying the term well-being in its different spellings "well-being," "well being," and "wellbeing." The researchers found a wide variety of studies was conducted with college students attending their countries' universities. In these articles, their authors used additional key terms: Positive psychology, positive education, subjective well-being, college counseling, psychological well-being, life satisfaction, and school well-being. The studies which were conducted in Australia, Lebanon, Asia, and India applied both subjective well-being and positive psychology. On the other hand, Turkish studies viewed subjective well-being as a concept to measure comorbidity. Also, the European studies began studying psychological well-being in relation to psychological disorders; at the same time, they investigated stress and the transition to college. Overall, the analysis was limited to recent studies and the use of well-being as a keyword of the search criteria. The following sections detail the above-mentioned articles.

Australian College Students

The Australian studies primarily viewed subjective well-being following positive psychology and the framework of Seligman's model of well-being (Kern, Waters, Adler, & White (2015). Several studies investigated international students attending an Australian college (Fisher, 2009; Lu, Dear, Johnston, Wootton, & Titov, 2014; Rosenthal, Russell, & Thomson, 2008), while the final study investigated spiritual well-being (Fisher & Wong, 2013). Kern et al. (2015) suggested well-being is a multidimensional concept including "cross-sectional associations with life satisfaction, hope, gratitude, school engagement, growth mindset, spirituality, physical vitality, physical activity, somatic symptoms, and stressful life events" (p. 262).

Kern et al. (2015) applied Seligman's model and hypothesized that defining subjective well-being would allow schools to better understand, measure, and promote well-being as a whole (Kern et al., 2015). Seligman et al. (2009) conducted studies with grammar school age children in Australia. Overall, they supported the need for positive education as a classroom intervention as a component of positive psychology (Seligman et al., 2009). Most of the studies which were conducted in Australia were with grade school students, on developing character education (Seligman et al., 2009), or high school students (Kern et al., 2015). The reports about college students either discussed international students attending an Australian university (Fisher, 2009; Lu et al., 2014; Rosenthal et al., 2008) or the results of studies on spiritual well-being (Fisher & Wong, 2013).

Lebanese University Students

Most psychological studies which were conducted in Lebanon focused upon violence and the civil war, and their effects on psychological pathology (Moghnie & Kazarian, 2012). The newer studies centered around subjective well-being and the focus on positive psychology, which provided a new perspective for studying Lebanese college students. The studies in Lebanon investigated well-being, as it connects to a cultural concept of happiness (Moghnie & Kazarian, 2012).

Nauffal, Ammar, and Sbeity (2013) conducted a study researching the role of perceived social support in foretelling subjective well-being among Lebanese college students. This study applied subjective well-being as a term meaning and a construct describing emotions and life satisfaction. Nauffal et al. (2013) discovered Lebanese students experienced a high level of perceived social support through their family, friends, and significant others, which positively correlated with a students' well-being and life satisfaction. Ayyash-Abdo and Sánchez-Ruiz (2012) researched Lebanese university students' subjective well-being in relation to students' multilingualism. Self-esteem was higher among multilingual students (Ayyash-Abdo & Sánchez-Ruiz, 2012). Moghnie and Kazarian's (2012) research investigated Lebanese college students' subjective happiness. Moghnie and Kazarian (2012) defined college students' subjective well-being as "realizing their potentials, pursuing their interests, and maintaining their mental health" (p. 204). The study aimed to investigate happiness as a cultural concept (Moghnie & Kazarian, 2012).

Sabbah, Sabbah, Khamis, Sabbah, and Droubi, (2013) explored the health-related quality of life of Lebanese college students. Sabbah et al. (2013) defined health as follows: "A state of complete physical, mental, and social well-being, and not merely the absence of disease and infirmity, is an important factor for academic achievement at school and in higher education" (p. 2). Offering the context of universities helps promote health and well-being as a means for fostering learning.

Turkish College Students

Evidence shows more studies from Turkey, in comparison to Lebanon, focused upon college-level students and their well-being. Three articles centered upon varying implications, such as college counseling (Sivis-Cetinkaya, 2013), medical students and stressful life events (Aktekin et al., 2001), and the effectiveness of an online strengths-based intervention (Koydemir & Sun-Selışık, 2016). Sivis-Cetinkaya (2013) investigated subjective well-being regarding psychological strengths. Aktekin et al. (2001) specifically investigated medical students in Turkey from a more psychological comorbidity perspective. The study measured anxiety, depression, and stressful life events. Koydemir and Sun-Selışık (2016) applied Seligman's well-being theory. Koydemir and Sun-Selışık (2016) summarized Seligman's (2011) definition of well-being as follows: "Positive emotions, engagement, relationships, meaning, and accomplishment are components of flourishing life, and...they should be part of positive interventions" (p. 435). Tümkaya's (2011) study investigated humor styles and demographic variables as predictors of subjective well-being. Thus, additional studies investigating the well-being of Turkish college students exist; yet, the use of well-being remains a mixed perspective of the term.

Asian College Students

College students in China consisted of 37 million in 2015. This is considered the greatest number in the world and accounts for approximately one-fifth of the total world. Given the extensive number of traditional college-age students and the likelihood of high risk for developing mental disorders (Zhang, Shang, Zhang, Shang, & Fang, 2018), the studies among college Chinese students also applied research terms of social support, as well as introduced the term resilience (Peng et al., 2012; Zheng, Xie, & Ding, 2018).

Zheng et al.'s (2018) study focused on college students' psychological stress in terms of psychological distress. Psychological distress was described as a milder form of mental health. More specifically, they investigated how resilience and social support influenced mental health. Further, the study determined the relationship between resilience and social support. Also, Peng et al.'s (2012) study applied the terms of social support and resilience to measure Chinese medical students' mental health. Chen (2016) investigated the influence of resilience and coping skills on subjective well-being. Other studies on Chinese college students continued with the use of subjective well-being and added an oriental cultural context to the studies investigation (Liu, Peng, Zeng, Zhao, & Zhang, 2019).

Continued studies on Chinese college students investigated well-being and social support and added the concept of gratitude (Sun, Jiang, Chu, & Qian, 2014). Tackett, Wright, Lubin, Li, and Pan (2017) added empathy as a personal construct influencing subjective well-being. Four additional studies investigated various additional components of subjective well-being. Hou et al. (2018) examined religion and subjective well-being, while Norvilitis and Mao (2013) investigated attitudes towards credit and finance as an influential factor of Chinese college students' well-being. Two other studies researched social media and Internet behavior: Zheng et al. (2018) considered the relationship between Internet altruistic behavior and subjective well-being, Wang, Jackson, Gaskin, and Wang (2014) researched the impact of social networking on subjective well-being.

Several studies were conducted with Thai college students. All of them applied the term psychological well-being to excessive smartphone usage (Tangmunkongvorakul et al., 2019), and Internet addictions (Varma, Cheaskul, & Poonpol, 2018). A Korean study measured the influence of taking a Pilates class on college students psychological well-being (Roh, 2018). Lastly, a study in China investigated the effect of taking a Baduanjin exercise class on physical and psychological well-being (Zheng et al., 2013).

European College Students

The studies which were conducted in Northern Ireland with college students applied the well-being term "mental health". McLafferty et al. (2017) researched student well-being as co-morbidity rates, thus as a more psychological disorder. O'Reilly, Ryan, and Hickey (2010) investigated psychological well-being and sociocultural adaptation. Another study among Irish college students sought to discover the help-seeking behavior for mental well-being (Goodwin, Behan, Kelly, McCarthy, & Horgan, 2016). Denovan and Macaskill (2017) commented that previously there was limited research on UK college students, yet, over the last few years, the students seem to have experienced more stress. This UK study discussed stress and subjective well-being. Also, Bewick, Koutsopoulou, Miles, Slaa, and Barkham's (2010) analysis discovered UK college students experienced heightened distress during college, which impacted students' psychological well-being, and recommended a need to offer services to strengthen college students' psychological well-being to better handle stress throughout the college years (Bewick et al., 2010; Denovan & Macaskill, 2017).

El Ansari et al. (2011) considered the health behaviors and lifestyle characteristics of over 3,000 European college students and recommended colleges include health promotion programs. Collings, Swanson, and Watkins (2014) investigated the impact of a peer mentoring program on student well-being and retention of the university. Topham and Moller (2011) researched subjective well-being and the impact of academic performance; their focus was on psychological distress and students transition to college. Galante et al. (2016) expressed the increase of mental health problems, with the largest trigger being academic pressure. The study investigated the impact of a mindfulness intervention to support well-being and resilience to stress (Galante et al., 2016).

College Students from India

Two articles were published on college students in India, and both applied the term "psychological well-being." Krishnamurthy and Chetlapalli (2015) investigated Internet addiction from a psychological disorder perspective. Lolla (2018) conducted a study on the impact of mantras on college students' psychological well-being and as a help to relieve depression and pressure. Another study on medical students in India analyzed the effect of Mind Sound Technology on college students' psychological well-being (Dayalan, Subramanian, & Elango, 2010). Kumar et al., (2009) researched with dental university students and discussed how students' stress can impact their psychological well-being.

Canadian Research with College Students

Mongrain and Anselmo-Matthews (2012) repeated Seligman et al.'s (2005) study to determine if positive psychology interventions would strengthen happiness. Marcotte and Levesque (2018) investigated the role identity plays on the impact of anxiety and well-being. Van Slingerland, Durand-Bush, and Rathwell (2018) specifically looked at student athletes' mental health functioning. Finally, Bilodeau and Meissner (2018) measured the effects of a combined academic and personal counseling initiative upon the retention of students from a Canadian university.

FUTURE RESEARCH

Overall, the colleges need to implement best practices which promote students' well-being. Future research could promote well-being programs and assess their effectiveness. Recommendations are to employ one leader over FYE (First-Year Experience) programs and build an interdepartmental team and faculty across disciplines to support the design and implementation of FYE programs (Rockey & Congleton, 2016). FYE programs benefit from the use of institutional research professionals who develop ways to measures program effectiveness. Universities are institutions where FYE programs can use positive psychology to promote student resilience and well-being. Based on the authors' experience, raising student awareness and teaching them to view themselves positively can shape their life experience and determine their desire to continue academically. Interest in using mindfulness programs such as L2B to support college students' personal growth and well-being by teaching awareness and insight is rising.

CONCLUSION

Subjective well-being seems to be which has been the most studied term among Western colleges. On the other hand, positive psychology, psychological well-being, and health and wellness are the most used terms among Eastern colleges. All the countries' colleges are concerned about the well-being of their students. They have discovered college students are under stress and need to further develop their resiliency and coping skills to be successful in college. They have also discovered current traditional students are beginning college with depression and anxiety issues. American colleges are also concerned with the retention and attrition rates of their institutions. Given the multiple studies on effective strategies for developing students' well-being, it is time to continue implementing these strategies and assess their effectiveness.

REFERENCES

Aktekin, M., Karaman, T., Senol, Y. Y., Erdem, S., Erengin, H., & Akaydin, M. (2001). Anxiety, depression and stressful life events among medical students: A prospective study in Antalya, Turkey. *Medical Education, 35*(1), 12–17. doi:10.1046/j.1365-2923.2001.00726.x PMID:11123589

Ayyash-Abdo, H., & Sánchez-Ruiz, M. J. (2012). Subjective well-being and its relationship with academic achievement and multilinguality among Lebanese university students. *International Journal of Psychology, 47*(3), 192–202. doi:10.1080/00207594.2011.614616 PMID:22047001

Beauchemin, J., Gibbs, T., & Granello, P. (2018). Wellness promotion courses in university settings: A review of the outcome research. *Building Healthy Academic Communities Journal, 2*(1), 36–49. doi:10.18061/bhac.v2i1.6344

Bewick, B., Koutsopoulou, G., Miles, J., Slaa, E., & Barkham, M. (2010). Changes in undergraduate students' psychological well-being as they progress through university. *Studies in Higher Education, 35*(6), 633–645. doi:10.1080/03075070903216643

Bilodeau, C., & Meissner, J. (2018). The effects of a combined academic and personal counselling initiative for post-secondary student retention. *Canadian Journal of School Psychology, 33*(1), 8–25. doi:10.1177/0829573516644554

Booc, C. E. R., San Diego, C. M. D., Tee, M. L., & Caro, J. D. (2016). A mobile application for campus-based psychosocial wellness program. In *Proceedings of the 2016 7th International Conference on Information, Intelligence, Systems & Applications (IISA)* (pp. 1-4). IEEE. 10.1109/IISA.2016.7785426

Chen, C. (2016). The role of resilience and coping styles in subjective well-being among Chinese university students. *The Asia-Pacific Education Researcher, 25*(3), 377–387. doi:10.100740299-016-0274-5

Chopik, W. J., Newton, N. J., Ryan, L. H., Kashdan, T. B., & Jarden, A. J. (2019). Gratitude across the life span: Age differences and links to subjective well-being. *The Journal of Positive Psychology, 14*(3), 292–302. doi:10.1080/17439760.2017.1414296 PMID:31105762

Collings, R., Swanson, V., & Watkins, R. (2014). The impact of peer mentoring on levels of student wellbeing, integration and retention: A controlled comparative evaluation of residential students in UK higher education. *Higher Education*, *68*(6), 927–942. doi:10.100710734-014-9752-y

Conley, C. S., Travers, L. V., & Bryant, F. B. (2013). Promoting psychosocial adjustment and stress management in first-year college students: The benefits of engagement in a psychosocial wellness seminar. *Journal of American College Health*, *61*(2), 75–86. doi:10.1080/07448481.2012.754757 PMID:23409857

Cressy, J. (2011). The roles of physical activity and health in enhancing student engagement: Implications for leadership in post-secondary education. *The College Quarterly*, *14*(4), n4. Retrieved from https://search-ebscohost-com.ezp.waldenulibrary.org/login.aspx?direct=true&db=eric&AN=EJ967640&site=eds-live&scope=site

Crowley, C., & Munk, D. (2017). An examination of the impact of a college level meditation course on college student well-being. *College Student Journal*, *91*(1). Retrieved from https://search-ebscohost-com.ezp.waldenulibrary.org/login.aspx?direct=true&db=edsgea&AN=edsgcl.487602756&site=eds-live&scope=site

Dayalan, H., Subramanian, S., & Elango, T. (2010). Psychological well-being in medical students during exam stress: Influence of short-term practice of mind sound technology. *Indian Journal of Medical Sciences*, *64*(11), 501. doi:10.4103/0019-5359.102122 PMID:23051942

Denovan, A., & Macaskill, A. (2017). Stress and subjective well-being among first year UK undergraduate students. *Journal of Happiness Studies*, *18*(2), 505–525. doi:10.100710902-016-9736-y

Diener, E., Wirtz, D., Tov, W., Kim-Prieto, C., Choi, D. W., Oishi, S., & Biswas-Diener, R. (2010). New well-being measures: Short scales to assess flourishing and positive and negative feelings. *Social Indicators Research, 97*(2), 143–156. doi:10.100711205-009-9493-y

Dvořáková, K., Kishida, M., Li, J., Elavsky, S., Broderick, P. C., Agrusti, M. R., & Greenberg, M. T. (2017). Promoting healthy transition to college through mindfulness training with first-year college students: Pilot randomized controlled trial. *Journal of American College Health*, *65*(4), 259–267. doi:10.1080/07448481.2017.1278605 PMID:28076182

El Ansari, W., Stock, C., John, J., Deeny, P., Phillips, C., Snelgrove, S., ... Mabhala, A. (2011). Health promoting behaviours and lifestyle characteristics of students at seven universities in the UK. *Central European Journal of Public Health, 19*(4), 197–204. doi:10.21101/cejph.a3684 PMID:22432394

Feldman, D. B., & Dreher, D. E. (2012). Can hope be changed in 90 minutes? Testing the efficacy of a single-session goal-pursuit intervention for college students. *Journal of Happiness Studies, 13*(4), 745–759. doi:10.100710902-011-9292-4

Fisher, J. W. (2009). Investigating Australian education students' views about spiritual well-being, as compared with teachers in schools. *International Journal of Children's Spirituality, 14*(2), 151–167. doi:10.1080/13644360902830358

Fisher, J. W., & Wong, P. H. (2013). Comparing levels of spiritual well-being and support among pre-service teachers in Hong Kong and Australia. *Religious Education Journal of Australia, 29*(1), 34.

Galante, J., Dufour, G., Benton, A., Howarth, E., Vainre, M., Croudace, T. J., ... Jones, P. B. (2016). Protocol for the Mindful Student Study: A randomised controlled trial of the provision of a mindfulness intervention to support university students' well-being and resilience to stress. *BMJ (Clinical Research Ed.), 6*(11), 1–8. doi:10.1136/bmjopen-2016-012300 PMID:28186934

Gieck, D. J., & Olsen, S. (2007). Holistic wellness as a means to developing a lifestyle approach to health behavior among college students. *Journal of American College Health, 56*(1), 29–36. doi:10.3200/JACH.56.1.29-36 PMID:17711823

Goodwin, J., Behan, L., Kelly, P., McCarthy, K., & Horgan, A. (2016). Help-seeking behaviors and mental well-being of first year undergraduate university students. *Psychiatry Research, 246*, 129–135. doi:10.1016/j.psychres.2016.09.015 PMID:27693865

Hartman, C. L., Evans, K. E., & Anderson, D. M. (2017). Promoting adaptive coping skills and subjective well-being through credit-based leisure education courses. *Journal of Student Affairs Research and Practice, 54*(3), 303–315. doi:10.1080/19496591.2017.1331852

Hou, Y., Feng, X., Yang, X., Yang, Z., Zhang, X., & Koenig, H. G. (2018). Religion and subjective well-being in Chinese college students: Does meaningfulness matter? *Archiv Für Religionspsychologie. Archiv für Religionspsychologie, 40*(1), 60–79. doi:10.1163/15736121-12341351

Ilies, R., Yao, J., Curseu, P. L., & Liang, A. X. (2019). Educated and Happy: A Four-Year Study Explaining the Links Between Education, Job Fit, and Life Satisfaction. *Applied Psychology*, *68*(1), 150–176. doi:10.1111/apps.12158

Ingram, P. B., Warlick, C. A., Ternes, M. S., & Krieshok, T. S. (2018). Examining the feasibility of the integrated hope scale in American college students. *Counselling Psychology Quarterly*, *31*(3), 336–352. doi:10.1080/09515070.2017.1318111

Kern, M. L., Waters, L. E., Adler, A., & White, M. A. (2015). A multidimensional approach to measuring well-being in students: Application of the PERMA framework. *The Journal of Positive Psychology*, *10*(3), 262–271. doi:10.1080/17439760.2014.936962 PMID:25745508

Kim, B., & Kim, Y. (2017). College students' social media use and communication network heterogeneity: Implications for social capital and subjective well-being. *Computers in Human Behavior*, *73*, 620–628. doi:10.1016/j.chb.2017.03.033

Koydemir, S., & Sun-Selışık, Z. E. (2016). Well-being on campus: Testing the effectiveness of an online strengths-based intervention for first year college students. *British Journal of Guidance & Counselling*, *44*(4), 434–446. doi:10.1080/03069885.2015.1110562

Krishnamurthy, S., & Chetlapalli, S. K. (2015). Internet addiction: Prevalence and risk factors: A cross-sectional study among college students in Bengaluru, the Silicon Valley of India. *Indian Journal of Public Health*, *59*(2), 115. doi:10.4103/0019-557X.157531 PMID:26021648

Kumar, S., Dagli, R. J., Mathur, A., Jain, M., Prabu, D., & Kulkarni, S. (2009). Perceived sources of stress amongst Indian dental students. *European Journal of Dental Education*, *13*(1), 39–45. doi:10.1111/j.1600-0579.2008.00535.x PMID:19196292

Lambert, L., Passmore, H. A., & Holder, M. D. (2015). Foundational frameworks of positive psychology: Mapping well-being orientations. *Canadian Psychology*, *56*(3), 311–321. doi:10.1037/cap0000033

Liu, H., Peng, F., Zeng, X., Zhao, J., & Zhang, X. (2019). Authoritarian personality and subjective well-being in Chinese college students: The moderation effect of the organizational culture context. *Personality and Individual Differences*, *138*, 79–83. doi:10.1016/j.paid.2018.09.030

Lolla, A. (2018). Mantras help the general psychological well-being of college students: A pilot study. *Journal of Religion and Health*, *57*(1), 110–119. doi:10.100710943-017-0371-7 PMID:28271341

Lu, S. H., Dear, B. F., Johnston, L., Wootton, B. M., & Titov, N. (2014). An Internet survey of emotional health, treatment seeking, and barriers to accessing mental health treatment among Chinese-speaking international students in Australia. *Counselling Psychology Quarterly*, *27*(1), 96–108. doi:10.1080/09515070.2013.824408

Marcotte, J., & Lévesque, G. (2018). Anxiety and well-being among students in a psychoeducation program: The mediating role of identity. *Journal of College Student Development*, *59*(1), 90–104. doi:10.1353/csd.2018.0006

Marshall, S. (2016). Predicting college students' positive psychology associated traits with executive functioning dimensions. *College Student Journal*, *50*(2), 179–190. Retrieved from https://search-ebscohost-com.ezp.waldenulibrary.org/login.aspx?direct=true&db=a9h&AN=116190967&site=eds-live&scope=site

Matel-Anderson, D. M., Bekhet, A. K., & Garnier-Villarreal, M. (2019). Mediating effects of positive thinking and social support on suicide resilience. *Western Journal of Nursing Research*, *41*(1), 25–41. doi:10.1177/0193945918757988 PMID:29460692

McDermott, R. C., Cheng, H.-L., Wong, J., Booth, N., Jones, Z., & Sevig, T. (2017). Hope for help-seeking: A positive psychology perspective of psychological help-seeking intentions. *The Counseling Psychologist*, *45*(2), 237–265. doi:10.1177/0011000017693398

McLafferty, M., Lapsley, C. R., Ennis, E., Armour, C., Murphy, S., Bunting, B. P., ... O'Neill, S. M. (2017). Mental health, behavioural problems, and treatment seeking among students commencing university in Northern Ireland. *PLoS One*, *12*(12), e0188785. doi:10.1371/journal.pone.0188785 PMID:29236727

Meredith, L. N., Frazier, P. A., Paulsen, J. A., Greer, C. S., Howard, K. G., Belgrade, A., & Kim, S. (2014). *Assessing the efficacy of an online stress management intervention for community college students*. doi:10.1037/e555772014-001

Moghnie, L., & Kazarian, S. S. (2012). Subjective happiness of Lebanese college youth in Lebanon: Factorial structure and invariance of the Arabic Subjective Happiness Scale. *Social Indicators Research*, *109*(2), 203–210. doi:10.100711205-011-9895-5

Mongrain, M., & Anselmo-Matthews, T. (2012). Do positive psychology exercises work? A replication of Seligman et al. (2005). *Journal of Clinical Psychology*, *382*(4). doi:10.1002/jclp.21839 PMID:24469930

Munzel, A., Meyer-Waarden, L., & Galan, J.-P. (2018). The social side of sustainability: Well-being as a driver and an outcome of social relationships and interactions on social networking sites. *Technological Forecasting and Social Change*, *130*, 14–27. doi:10.1016/j.techfore.2017.06.031

Nagata, C. M., Conoley, C., Arnadottir, V., White, S., & Shishim, M. (2011). *Using positive psychology interventions in a college prevention context*. doi:10.1037/e708082011-001

Nauffal, D., Ammar, D., & Sbeity, R. (2013). The role of perceived social support in predicting subjective well-being in Lebanese college students. *Happiness & Well-Being, 116*. Retrieved from: https://laur.lau.edu.lb:8443/xmlui/handle/10725/4075?show=full

Norvilitis, J. M., & Mao, Y. (2013). Attitudes towards credit and finances among college students in China and the United States. *International Journal of Psychology*, *48*(3), 389–398. doi:10.1080/00207594.2011.645486 PMID:22397472

O'Reilly, A., Ryan, D., & Hickey, T. (2010). The psychological well-being and sociocultural adaptation of short-term international students in Ireland. *Journal of College Student Development*, *51*(5), 584–598. doi:10.1353/csd.2010.0011

Passmore, H. A., & Holder, M. D. (2017). Noticing nature: Individual and social benefits of a two-week intervention. *The Journal of Positive Psychology*, *12*(6), 537–546. doi:10.1080/17439760.2016.1221126

Pekrun, R., Goetz, T., Frenzel, A. C., Barchfeld, P., & Perry, R. P. (2011). Measuring emotions in students' learning and performance: The Achievement Emotions Questionnaire (AEQ). *Contemporary Educational Psychology*, *36*(1), 36–48. doi:10.1016/j.cedpsych.2010.10.002

Pekrun, R., Lichtenfeld, S., Marsh, H. W., Murayama, K., & Goetz, T. (2017). Achievement emotions and academic performance: Longitudinal models of reciprocal effects. *Child Development*, *88*(5), 1653–1670. doi:10.1111/cdev.12704 PMID:28176309

Peng, L., Zhang, J., Li, M., Li, P., Zhang, Y., Zuo, X., ... Xu, Y. (2012). Negative life events and mental health of Chinese medical students: The effect of resilience, personality, and social support. *Psychiatry Research*, *196*(1), 138–141. doi:10.1016/j.psychres.2011.12.006 PMID:22405636

Pettay, R. F. (2008). *Health behaviors and life satisfaction in college students* (Doctoral dissertation). Kansas State University.

Ranney, M., Kleinpeter, C. B., & Potts, M. (2018). Personal well-being, depression, and alcohol use among community college students receiving services from a student health center. *The International Journal of Health, Wellness & Society*, *8*(2), 9–16. doi:10.18848/2156-8960/CGP/v08i02/9-16

Ratelle, C. F., Simard, K., & Guay, F. (2013). University students' subjective well-being: The role of autonomy support from parents, friend, and the romantic partner. *Journal of Happiness Studies*, *14*(3), 803–910. doi:10.100710902-012-9360-4

Renshaw, T. L. (2018). Psychometrics of the revised college student subjective well-being questionnaire. *Canadian Journal of School Psychology*, *33*(2), 136–149. doi:10.1177/0829573516678704

Renshaw, T. L., & Rock, D. K. (2018). Effects of a brief grateful thinking intervention on college students' mental health. *Mental Health and Prevention*, *9*, 19–24. doi:10.1016/j.mhp.2017.11.003

Respondek, L., Seufert, T., Stupnisky, R., & Nett, U. E. (2017). Perceived academic control and academic emotions predict undergraduate university student success: Examining effects on dropout intention and achievement. *Frontiers in Psychology*, *8*, 243. doi:10.3389/fpsyg.2017.00243 PMID:28326043

Reymann, L. S., Fialkowski, G. M., & Stewart-Sicking, J. A. (2015). Exploratory study of spirituality and psychosocial growth in college students. *Journal of College Counseling*, *18*(2), 103–115. doi:10.1002/jocc.12008

Robino, A., & Foster, T. (2018). Psychosocial predictors of wellness in college students. *Adultspan Journal*, *17*(1), 3–13. doi:10.1002/adsp.12049

Rockey, M., & Congleton, R. (2016). *Exploring the role of first-year experiences in enhancing equity & outcomes. Insights on Equity and Outcomes, 14*. Office of Community College Research and Leadership.

Roh, S. Y. (2018). The influence of physical self-perception of female college students participating in Pilates classes on perceived health state and psychological well-being. *Journal of Exercise Rehabilitation*, *14*(2), 192–198. doi:10.12965/jer.1836088.044 PMID:29740551

Rosenthal, D. A., Russell, J., & Thomson, G. (2008). The health and well-being of international students at an Australian university. *Higher Education*, *55*(1), 51–67. doi:10.100710734-006-9037-1

Sabbah, I., Sabbah, H., Khamis, R., Sabbah, S., & Droubi, N. (2013). Health related quality of life of university students in Lebanon: Lifestyles behaviors and socio-demographic predictors. *Health*, *5*(7), 1–12. doi:10.4236/health.2013.57A4001

Sayler, M. F., Boazman, J., Natesan, P., & Periathiruvadi, S. (2015). Subjective well-being of gifted American college students: An examination of psychometric properties of the PWI-A. *Gifted Child Quarterly*, *59*(4), 236–248. doi:10.1177/0016986215597748

Schweitzer, A. L., Ross, J. T., Klein, C. J., Lei, K. Y., & Mackey, E. R. (2016). An electronic wellness program to improve diet and exercise in college students: A pilot study. *JMIR Research Protocols*, *5*(1), e29. doi:10.2196/resprot.4855 PMID:26929118

Seligman, M. (2011). *Flourish: A visionary new understanding of happiness and well-being*. New York, NY: Simon & Schuster.

Seligman, M. E. P. (2002). *Authentic happiness: Using the new positive psychology to realize your potential for lasting fulfillment*. New York, NY: Free Press.

Seligman, M. E. P., Ernst, R. M., Gillham, J., Reivich, K., & Linkins, M. (2009). Positive education: Positive psychology and classroom interventions. *Oxford Review of Education*, *35*(3), 293–311. doi:10.1080/03054980902934563

Seligman, M. E. P., Steen, T. A., Park, N., & Peterson, C. (2005). Positive psychology progress: Empirical validation of interventions. *The American Psychologist*, *60*(5), 410–421. doi:10.1037/0003-066X.60.5.410 PMID:16045394

Selvaraj, P. R., & Bhat, C. S. (2018). Predicting the mental health of college students with psychological capital. *Journal of Mental Health (Abingdon, England)*, *27*(3), 279–287. doi:10.1080/09638237.2018.1469738 PMID:29733236

Shushok, J. F. Jr, & Hulme, E. (2006). What's right with you: Helping students find and use their personal strengths. *About Campus: Enriching the Student Learning Experience*, *11*(4), 2–8. doi:10.1002/abc.173

Sivis-Cetinkaya, R. (2013). Turkish college students' subjective wellbeing in regard to psychological strengths and demographic variables: Implications for college counseling. *International Journal for the Advancement of Counseling*, *35*(4), 317–330. doi:10.100710447-013-9185-9

Sun, P., Jiang, H., Chu, M., & Qian, F. (2014). Gratitude and school well-being among Chinese university students: Interpersonal relationships and social support as mediators. *Social Behavior and Personality*, *42*(10), 1689–1698. doi:10.2224bp.2014.42.10.1689

Tackett, S., Wright, S., Lubin, R., Li, J., & Pan, H. (2017). International study of medical school learning environments and their relationship with student well-being and empathy. *Medical Education, 51*(3), 280–289. doi:10.1111/medu.13120 PMID:27896846

Tangmunkongvorakul, A., Musumari, P. M., Thongpibul, K., Srithanaviboonchai, K., Techasrivichien, T., Suguimoto, S. P., ... Kihara, M. (2019). Association of excessive smartphone use with psychological well-being among university students in Chiang Mai, Thailand. *PLoS One, 14*(1), e0210294. doi:10.1371/journal.pone.0210294 PMID:30615675

Tinto, V. (1975). Dropout from higher education: A theoretical synthesis of recent research. *Review of Educational Research, 45*(1), 89–125. doi:10.3102/00346543045001089

Tinto, V. (1987). *Leaving college: Rethinking the causes and cures of student attrition* (2nd ed.). Chicago, IL: University of Chicago Press.

Topham, P., & Moller, N. (2011). New students' psychological well-being and its relation to first year academic performance in a UK university. *Counselling & Psychotherapy Research, 11*(3), 196–203. doi:10.1080/14733145.2010.519043

Tümkaya, S. (2011). Humor styles and socio-demographic variables as predictors of subjective well-being of turkish university students. *Egitim ve Bilim, 36*(160), 158-170. Retrieved from http://search.ebscohost.com/login.aspx?direct=true&db=edselc&AN=edselc.2-52.0-84885637295&site=eds-live&scope=site

Van Slingerland, K. J., Durand-Bush, N., & Rathwell, S. (2018). Levels and prevalence of mental health functioning in Canadian university student-athletes. *Canadian Journal of Higher Education, 48*(2), 149–168. doi:10.7202/1057108ar

Varma, P., Cheaskul, U., & Poonpol, P. (2018). The influence of parenting styles on academic adjustment and psychological well-being among Thai university students mediated by Internet addiction and self-regulation: A path model. *Journal for Leadership and Instruction, 17*(2), 13–24. Retrieved from https://ezp.waldenulibrary.org/login?url=https://search.ebscohost.com/login.aspx?direct=true&db=eric&AN=EJ1199679&site=eds-live&scope=site

Vasold, K. L., Deere, S. J., & Pivarnik, J. M. (2018). Self-reported wellness benefits of recreational sports use in college freshmen: 1328 Board# 136 May 31 9. *Medicine and Science in Sports and Exercise, 50*(5S), 316. doi:10.1249/01.mss.0000536122.63367.fc

Vela, J. C., Smith, W. D., Whittenberg, J. F., Guardiola, R., & Savage, M. (2018). Positive psychology factors as predictors of Latina/o college students' psychological grit. *Journal of Multicultural Counseling and Development*, *46*(1), 2–19. doi:10.1002/jmcd.12089

Wang, J.-L., Jackson, L. A., Gaskin, J., & Wang, H.-Z. (2014). The effects of social networking site (SNS) use on college students' friendship and well-being. *Computers in Human Behavior*, *37*, 229–236. doi:10.1016/j.chb.2014.04.051

Weinberg, M. K., Seton, C., & Cameron, N. (2018). The measurement of subjective well-being: Item-order effects in the Personal Well-being Index—Adult. *Journal of Happiness Studies*, *19*(1), 315–332. doi:10.100710902-016-9822-1

Wilson, J. T. (2016). Brightening the mind: The impact of practicing gratitude on focus and resilience in learning. *The Journal of Scholarship of Teaching and Learning*, *16*(4), 1–13. doi:10.14434/josotl.v16i4.19998

Zheng, G., Li, M., Lan, X., Yan, X., Lin, Q., Chen, L., ... Fang, Q. (2013). The effect of Baduanjin exercise for physical and psychological wellbeing of college students: Study protocol for a randomized controlled trial. *Trials*, *14*(1), 422. doi:10.1186/1745-6215-14-422 PMID:24308310

Zheng, X., Xie, F., & Ding, L. (2018). Mediating role of self-concordance on the relationship between Internet altruistic behaviour and subjective well-being. *Journal of Pacific Rim Psychology*, *12*, e1. doi:10.1017/prp.2017.14

ADDITIONAL READING

Baldwin, D. R., Towler, K., Oliver, M. D. II, & Datta, S. (2017). An examination of college student wellness: A research and liberal arts perspective. *Health Psychology Open*, *4*(2). doi:10.1177/2055102917719563 PMID:29379611

Balon, R., Beresin, E. V., Coverdale, J. H., Louie, A. K., & Roberts, L. W. (2015). College mental health: A vulnerable population in an environment with systemic deficiencies. *Academic Psychiatry*, *39*(5), 495–497. doi:10.100740596-015-0390-1 PMID:26327172

Bhochhibhoya, A., Dong, Y., & Branscum, P. (2017). Sources of social support among international college students in the United States. *Journal of International Students*, *7*(3), 671–686.

Center for the Advancement of Well-Being. (2018). Retrieved from https://wellbeing.gmu.edu

Downs, N. S., Alderman, T., Schneiber, K., & Swerdlow, N. R. (2016). Treat and teach our students well: College mental health and collaborative campus communities. *Psychiatric Services (Washington, D.C.)*, *67*(9), 957–963. doi:10.1176/appi.ps.201500465 PMID:27181737

Eisenberg, D., & Ketchen Lipson, S. (2017). *The healthy minds study*. Retrieved from http://healthymindsnetwork.org/system/resources/W1siZiIsIjIwMTcvMDkvMTIvMTNfMjZfMDRfMTgzX0hNU19uYXRpb25hbC5wZGYiXV0/HMS_national.pdf

Häfner, A., Stock, A., & Oberst, V. (2015). Decreasing students' stress through time management training: An intervention study. *European Journal of Psychology of Education*, *30*(1), 81–94. doi:10.100710212-014-0229-2

Kilgo, C. A., Mollet, A. L., & Pascarella, E. T. (2016). The estimated effects of college student involvement on psychological well-being. *Journal of College Student Development*, *57*(8), 1043–1049. doi:10.1353/csd.2016.0098

Mofidi, T., El-Alayli, A., & Brown, A. A. (2014). Trait gratitude and grateful coping as they relate to college student persistence, success, and integration in school. *Journal of College Student Retention*, *16*(3), 325–349. doi:10.2190/CS.16.3.b

Pawelski, J. O. (2016). Bringing together the humanites and the science of well-being to advance human flourishing. In D. W. Harward (Ed.), *Well-being and higher education: A strategy for change and the realization of education's greater purposes* (pp. 207–216). Washington, DC.

Schiffrin, H. H., & Liss, M. (2017). The effects of helicopter parenting on academic motivation. *Journal of Child and Family Studies*, *26*(5), 1472–1480. doi:10.100710826-017-0658-z

Seldon, A., & Martin, A. (2017, September 21). *The positive and mindful university*. Retrieved from http://www.hepi.ac.uk/2017/09/21/positive-mindful-university/

Shatkin, J. P., Diamond, U., Zhao, Y., DiMeglio, J., Chodaczek, M., & Bruzzese, J. M. (2016). Effects of a risk and resilience course on stress, coping skills, and cognitive strategies in college students. *Teaching of Psychology*, *43*(3), 204–210. doi:10.1177/0098628316649457

Shimer, D. (2018, January 26). Yale's most popular class ever: Happiness. *The New York Times*. Retrieved from https://www.nytimes.com/2018/01/26/nyregion/at-yale-class-on-happinessdraws-huge-crowd-laurie-santos.html

Sliney, C. (2018, April 3). Penn's second 'Campus Conversation,' designed to highlight students, saw low student turnout. *The Daily Pennsylvanian*. Retrieved from https:// http://www.thedp.com/article/2018/04/second-campus-conversation-lack-of-turnout-ivyleague-upenn-mental-wellness-health

Strom, R. E., & Savage, M. W. (2014). Assessing the relationships between perceived support from close others, goal commitment, and persistence decisions at the college level. *Journal of College Student Development*, *55*(6), 531–547. doi:10.1353/csd.2014.0064

Suh, H., Gnilka, P. B., & Rice, K. G. (2017). Perfectionism and well-being: A positive psychology framework. *Personality and Individual Differences*, *111*, 25–30. doi:10.1016/j.paid.2017.01.041

VIA Institute on Character. (2018). Bring out the best in others. Retrieved from http://www.viacharacter.org/www/Professionals

Yeager, D. S., & Dweck, C. S. (2012). Mindsets that promote resilience: When students believe that personal characteristics can be developed. *Educational Psychologist*, *47*(4), 302–314. doi:10.1080/00461520.2012.722805

Yeager, D. S., Walton, G. M., Brady, S. T., Akcinar, E. N., Paunesku, D., & Keane, L. … Dweck, C. S. (2016). Teaching a lay theory before college narrows achievement gaps at scale. *Proceedings of the National Academy of Sciences, 113*(24), E3341–E3348. 10.1073/pnas.1524360113

KEY TERMS AND DEFINITIONS

Health and Wellness: Higher education institutions apply this term to students' health and wellbeing.

Positive Psychology: A term applied in higher education as the study of the life satisfaction and happiness of a person.

Psychosocial Wellbeing: Refers to both the psychological and social wellbeing of a person.

Subjective Wellbeing: Refers to the individual perceptions on their own wellbeing.

Wellbeing: Interchangeable with wellness, a state of wellness.

Wellness: Interchangeable with wellbeing, a state of wellness.

Chapter 3
An Interpretation and Application of the 'Four Paths of Yoga' for a Positive Well-Being

Gitanjali Tamal Roy
The Maharaja Sayjirao University of Baroda, India

Prapti Suriya
The Maharaja Sayajirao University of Baroda, India

ABSTRACT

The objective of this chapter is to introduce a conceptual framework and application of the four paths of yoga in modern times to strip the human mind of all its impurities and see the stream of consciousness is clear as crystal and capable of reflecting whole reality. The conceptual framework is formulated from the ancient Indian scriptures and literature. Karmayoga, jnanayoga, bhaktiyoga, and rajayoga are the four yoga or spiritual paths significant for improving individual and society wellbeing. The chapter includes trends of each yoga with respect to modern times.

INTRODUCTION

Every individual aspires for a positive wellbeing and its absence brings a sense of burden in living. Both Western and Indian perspective of psychology emphasises on positive wellbeing (PW) from different perspectives. Commonly, a good state of body and mind are considered for positive well-being. Various scholars of both

DOI: 10.4018/978-1-7998-1185-5.ch003

the perspectives have different ways to define positive wellbeing. To begin with, the Oxford English and Cambridge dictionaries define wellbeing as the state of being comfortable, healthy, or happy. Seligman (2002) said it's "life satisfaction", whereas Pollard and Lee (2003) stated a sense-of well-being as "happiness". Tehrani, Humpage, Willmott, and Haslam (2011) epitomises an encompassing bio-psycho-social construct (of well-being) that comprises of physical, psychological, and social well-being, subsequently being more inclusive that mere avoidance of physical illness or sickness. VandenBos (2015) characterised well-being as a state of contentment, satisfaction, happiness, low levels of distress and illness, good physical and mental health, a positive outlook, or good quality of life. Wellbeing comprises objective descriptors and subjective evaluations of physical, material, social and emotional wellbeing, together with the extent of personal development and purposeful activity, all weighted by a set of values' (Felce & Perry, 1995). These definitions point to positive psychological, physical and social states as important ingredients of wellbeing. For a deeper understanding, one has to dig in philosophy and Indian philosophy provides a holistic structure of explanation.

The Indian Knowledge Tradition

In the Indian knowledge tradition, the concept of wellbeing collates with happiness. Happiness and wellbeing are paved as fundamental elements of human life goal specifically in Vedas, Upanishads, and other ancient scriptures. They have comminute 'wellbeing' and 'happiness' into qualities such as being non-materialistic, desire less, faith, religion, spiritual, consciousness, caring about social relations, being aware about self, human potentials and personality. Indian knowledge system propounds two perspectives of wellbeing, the materialistic and transcendental. When the sole criterion of wellbeing is pleasure fulfilment specifically sensory desires, like Lord Brahaspati and Charvaka's views, it is the materialistic view. Charvaka's philosophy denies the Vedic concepts such as metaphysical existence of a Consciousness (*Atman*), existence of God, values (*dharma*), theory of rebirth (law of *karma*) etc. Charvaka considered consciousness and mind (*manas*) as a characteristic that lasts with the bodily wellbeing and mind helps in knowing the world through the senses (Raju, 1992). Charvaka's philosophy stated that our lives belong and ends in this material world, so one should try to make the best of it by doing anything possible to enhance pleasure and avoid pain. This system of philosophy is similar to the hedonic perspective and did not gain importance in ancient India. The transcendent perspective, similar to eudemonic, advocates happiness and wellbeing as subjective, something that do not depend on any objective conditions of reality, including one's state of body-mind. It has a universal vision that aspires for the wellbeing of everyone in the universe. The basis or foundation of the transcendental view was born out of experience of pure consciousness or *shuddhachaitanya* of yogis and is essence of Vedic tradition. When we try to categorise people in either of the above two perspectives, most of them would be a misfit because they would manifest qualities of both materialistic or hedonic and transcendent or eudemonic. They represent a collective or mixed perspective. On this basis, ancient sages established a social structure with ground rules for good life to ensure the wellbeing of all and documented as scriptures like *Bhagavad Gita, Darshansastras, Manusmriti* and *Yogasutras.* They contain the knowledge that leads to a holistic way of living i.e. balancing inner harmony and wellbeing of physical, social, mental and spiritual spheres. In times like today, one feels robbed of inner peace due to dynamic changes in society and technology dependency. With our hands full, our mind still wants more to feel alive and healthy. A thorough understanding and following of these scriptures will restore inner peace.

Positive Wellbeing in Ancient Indian Scriptures

According to Seligman and Ciskszentmihalyi (2000) in stable, prosperous and peaceful cultures, questions related to thriving of human existence are positive wellbeing. Indian philosophy is focused on good action, good character and their role in making life most worthwhile. Vedas, upanisads and other scriptures chart wellbeing in different traditions.

The Vedas outline the principles of life to attain eternal freedom but as time went by, these principles propounded as Manusmriti, the foundation scripture of Vedic laws. Manusmriti contains the outlines of *dharma*, an elaboration of do's and don'ts; and for a healthy and prosperous living, laid four principle *dharma* or duties for all classes- nonviolence, truthful, non-stealing and control over desires. It focused more on the positive wellbeing for every individual, irrespective of class, caste and creed, or gender. The Vedic and Upanishadic scholars and sages emphasized on understanding the *nitya* (eternal) and *satya* (true) knowledge and not pursue *mithya* (not true), *kshara (*negative*)*and *kshanika* (temporary). The ultimate goal of human kind was set to fulfil the quest for fundamental and ultimate truth for liberation, *moksha*. Ancient sages walked this path to unfold answers of physiological, psychological, social, ethical and moral nature. Hence, one needs to worship and follow this path like words in a gospel. They meditated for *Brahman*, the permanent and ultimate reality and cause the existence of individual's consciousness as transcendental self or *Atman*; and realized *atman* through *satya* and *nitya,* the single way to escape suffering and experience bliss or *ananda*.

Taittiriya Upanishad states happiness or *ananda* as an original condition of every human being, covered by five *koshas* or sheaths namely, *annamaya, pranamaya, manomaya, vijnanamaya,* and *anandamaya kosha*. Each *kosha* represents a unique dimension of awareness- food or physical body, prana or vital force, cognitive functions, instinctive faculty and blissfulness respectively. Each *kosha* ascertain the self on different levels and unfolding of each *kosha* or dimension alters the sense of self-identity progressively to bliss (*anandmaya kosha*). Any obstruction in *koshas* via blockage in mental abilities, inertia, depression etc. causes sufferings by inhibiting wellbeing and happiness.

Sankhya Darshan recognizes bliss as a state of *gunateet*, where the self is evolved beyond the effects of three *gunas* to experience closeness with the ultimate reality. Kapil muni, propounder of Sankhya Darshan, emphasized on increasing *Sattva* over *rajas* and *tamas guna* because it brings illumination of mind and then grows out of the three *gunas* to experience bliss, freedom from *bhautika, adhunika* and *adhyatmika* sufferings and pains. The three *gunas* constitute *prakriti*, which evolves under the influence of *purusha*, leading to evolution. The evolutes have varied effects of the three *gunas* and thus determining uniqueness in human personality. Hegemony traits of each *guna* (Roy, 2018) are helpful in personality profiling. Roy (2018) suggested eleven traits of *triguna* to profile individual personality for a descriptive psychological and physiological understanding. Subjugation of *sattvic* traits leads to physiological and psychological difficulties. So, one must increase and maintain *sattva* in personality to experience positive wellbeing. Lord Krishna explained *Triguna* descriptively in Bhagavad Gita for common man.

Teachings from Bhagavad Gita focus on character building and values indoctrination for positive wellbeing. Being indifferent to pain and pleasure, success and failure (B.G.2.68), prevents attachment that results into physiological and psychological ailments. People should fulfil their duties towards society, humanity and God and not be preoccupied by the results of those actions (B.G. 3.3); since results are not in our control, hovering over it gives anxiety, fear and cowardice. Detachment from materialistic world and relations bring a man close to his self and he finds peace (B.G. 5.21). According to Dilip et al. (2014), Bhagavad Gita has certain components of wisdom that should be taught and learned in developing psychotherapeutic interventions that could be more holistic than present therapies and aim at improving well–being over psychiatric symptoms. Dabas and Abha (2018) found teaching from Bhagavad Gita as intervention resulted in significant increase in optimism, hope and resilience compared to intervention based on western positive psychology; and for character building and positive constructs, culture and faith reposed in certain cultural creations like scriptures can be considered as an important practice.

Yoga Darshan gives importance to physical-mental-spiritual wellbeing. Patanjali's yogasutra (1.13) suggests that one should be a proactive observer of thoughts that keep mind pre-occupied; because proactive observation of thoughts, actions and emotions bring discipline, commitment and renunciation. Sri Aurobindo recognised that yoga means union with the Divine- a union either transcendental (above the Universe) or cosmic (Universal) or individual or, all three together. It means getting into a state of consciousness where one is no longer bounded by the personal ego, personal vital and body but it is in union with the Supreme self, the Universal consciousness so that one is aware of his soul, inner being and of the truth of existence.

Tapering the above definitions and meaning in few points define wellbeing- a state of being happy and healthy with culture, values, relationships and social structure, physical and mental health as significant influencing factors. The knowledge and principles of life outlined by Vedas, Upanishads and other scriptures are amended in form of cultural rituals and customs, for common man to follow and experience positive physical, psychological and spiritual growth. Following sections elaborate four spiritual paths or paths of yoga and their significance with positive wellbeing.

FOUR PATHS OF YOGA AND POSITIVE WELLBEING

In Indian knowledge system, external happiness and internal state of blissfulness is wellbeing. The chapter intentionally focus on Bhagavad Gita teaching an integration of values with lifestyle, relationships, education and spirituality to avoid physical and psychological ailments, achieve Positive Wellbeing for attaining the final goal of human life i.e. self-realization through the four paths of yoga.

In the battle of Kurukshetra, Arjuna was prepared to fight until he took a closer look at enemies. Arjun was facing a conflict of fighting against his kith and kin. He felt mental agonies and bodily weaknesses because he feared of generations of misfortunes on killing his family. At the moment of Arjuna's physiological and psychological infirmity, Lord Krishna recited four yogas to Arjuna and resolved his infirmities. The teachings of *Bhagavad Gita* characterises the qualities of yogi who follow these four paths. Swami Vivekananda advocated that everyone identifies with mind, intellect, heart and body, and hence he must practice techniques from each path. Further, he emphasised on choosing a suitable yoga according to temperament, since spiritual paths improve wellbeing of individual and society; and all the paths lead to union with God or Supreme Power or Brahman.

Karma Yoga

On listening to Lord Krishna, Arjuna became aware of his duties as a *Kshatriya*, one of the four *varnas*, who pledge to fight and protect for sanity of the society. They establish goodness in society by defeating and bring evil to justice. Under stress and conflict, one tends to misstep duties according to social roles, agitated and tranquillity and end up making wrong decisions. As darkness brings in the need to search for the light, the fear and misery of the soul creates a need to find an anchor to hold and *nitya* knowledge with *nishkama karma* (self-less action) is the best choice. Lord Krishna guided Arjuna to acquire mental balance and peaceful consciousness, and experience body consciousness for maximum wellbeing, followed by a greater discovery of Higher Presence of Supreme Power. Lord Krishna promoted philosophical analysis of situation according to the duties of individual, true knowledge and surrendered to the almighty. Krishna's directions bring change in senses, body and soul. The *nitya* knowledge from Lord re-oriented Arjuna on the path of a dutiful warrior, i.e. standing against wrongful people who indeed are kith and kin required courage. Any person would feel timid in the beginning but with proper guidance and counselling as done by Lord, gives strength to stand for the righteousness. If the soul is symbolized as Arjuna, Hasthinapur as destination of soul and *Kauravas* as hindrances of progressing towards the destination, then in order to reach to the destination *Gita jnana* by Lord shall help in fighting in the battlefield of Kurukshetra like fighting the desires, greed and temptation for throne and conducting for the rightful reasons. Any path of progress requires struggle and might bring suffering due to resistance to desires. With the progressive conversations between Lord Krishna and Arjuna, the dramatic elements of the battlefield disappears (Radhakrishnan, 1923). As one focuses his mind on *karma, jnana, bhakti* everything in the background diminishes and our mind becomes more focused.

The Gita *jnana* is like the milking the cow of knowledge. The more one milks the more enlightened we make. In the chapter three of Bhagavad-Gita, Lord Krishna conveys about Karma Yoga.

लोकेऽस्मन्दि्वविधािलोकेऽस्मन्निष्ठिापुराप्रोक्तामयानघ।ज्ञानयोगेनसाङ्ख्यानांकर्मयो
गेनयोगनिाम्॥ ३-३॥

Lord Krishna explains two paths for the man to follow– the path of wisdom of the empirical philosophers and the path of action that must be performed. In face of conflict situation we make a tough decision either by choosing the path of wisdom suggested by wise men or we follow the path of righteous action.

Lord Krishna further stated:

यस्त्वन्दि्रयिाणमिनसानयिम्यारभतेऽर्जुन।कर्मेन्द्रयिैःकर्मयोगमसक्तःसवशिष्यि
ते॥ ३-७॥

A person who gains control over his senses and mind, and engages them on the path of selfless actions is a karma yogi, superior of other human beings. When one makes a decision without engaging in sensory desires, not for immediate gratification but for the welfare of people of society, one is said to be wise and superior human being. *Nishkama karma* or selfless actions of a yogi, drives him on the path of karma yoga for salvation or liberation.

Trends of Karma Yoga

In our lives, most of our actions are motivated by selfish desires revolving around words like "my benefit, my earnings, it is about me and my reputation …" etc. This gradually leads us on the path of 'I-centric actions' and everything we perceive becomes about 'me'. It's is anything but *nishkama karma.* 'I' is a very powerful word, it denotes ego and self-awareness but once magnified it represents *ahankara* or egotistical attitude. An 'I-centric' attitude gives rise to similar society i.e. selfish, motivated by desires and self-fulfilling prophecy kind. One can only imagine a society with doctors, engineers, lawyers, teachers, police, mother, father, brothers and sisters, so selfish and dominated by the egotistical need satisfaction functioning smoothly. Such a self-centric society will not be a society to live for; it will only be a society of corruption, mistrust and mental ill-health. *Karma*, not sanctioned by scriptures, if performed brings an illusion of satisfaction and happiness but corrodes the sanctity of *atman*. Karma yoga disapproves any action that is performed for the benefit or welfare of one personal intention on the cost of social detriment. All it can cause is moral chaos and spiritual deterioration. For the true benefit of the society one must adhere to the *nitya* knowledge of Karma yoga not because it will raise you above others, but it is the right thing. If one continues to follow *mithya* knowledge, s/he will find limitation of psychological and spiritual growth and a pathological attachment (*aasakti*) with impermanent worldly labels, designations or possessions.

In 21st century, with technological awareness, fast speed internet and various facilities to make lifestyle easy, we are moving ahead on worldly or physical dimension but completely neglecting the true spiritual dimension where we are gradually deteriorating without any notice. This deterioration is latent but manifests strong various physical and psychological ailments. We see a lot of people working long hours, compromising their family life, neglecting physical health and most important they announce to be in love with their jobs and positions. They get so attached to their role, designation, reputation, success and failures that their 'self 'and 'ego' starts identifying with it. They drift away from spirituality to growth in worldly matters; they search for happiness outside themselves whereas it lies within. Hence, a sudden change in life makes them tremble and scared because they do not have anything to hold on to. They lose their calm and patience, get emotionally disturbed, psychologically imbalanced, and experience ego conflict with people around them. They have difficulty in letting go of any wrongful experiences with people around them. So they carry the weight of these emotional baggages with them for a very long time, resulting into stress related conditions, psychological disorientations, forgetful, careless, and absenteeism. The hard earned money is then spent in curing physical conditions. The sense of positive wellbeing is crushed under the load of egoism, expectations and emotional turmoil. One cannot find it in their environment because it truly reaps from within.

How Karma Yoga can bring positive wellbeing in our lives? Karma yoga teaches us to stay focused on the actions. Observe the Sun rising every day from east and setting in west, animals leaving their younger ones to fall, fly or walk, Mother Nature taking its turns on seasons. Did you ever witness them changing their course of routine activities? It is like mundane and predictive actions. We need to learn from them to live our lives and engage in activities like it is our duty. Imagine if the Sun, the moon and the Mother Nature refuse to perform their task, say Sun refuses to set in the west or the Mother Nature refuses rain after summer. Being an emotional person is helpful in understanding people and analysing situations but emotional attachment gives rise to expectations, a sense of pride, a desire to control or dominate and finally dissatisfaction of none of them are achieved. Attachments bind us to materialistic pleasures, impermanent relationships and perishable body. It blinds us from the truth of non-attachment which brings freedom from desires, whims and anxieties. As you start performing actions without emotional attachments then the locus of our mental and physical energy is the work.

The 'intention' of performing any task is very important because they are the source of attachments. For a student, studying is a duty appropriate for his role but if his intentions are to gain parental or societal approval then he is not sincere in performing the role appropriate duty. With this intension, he would be worried and be anxious about the result and outcome of the study and not gain any knowledge. For a teacher, providing the disciples with proper knowledge is a role appropriate duty. If a teacher becomes greedy or too attached with the disciple then he tends to be bias in his duties. The disciple will go without proper knowledge, learn to be greedy and emotionally attached results and tasks. So every individual needs to learn, understand and practice the philosophy of non-attachment and working with right intentions. When you decide and practice karma yoga, you start working without attachments, like a philanthropist, to reaches the higher spiritual path and without attachments with the results. To attain spiritual evolution and excellence of lifestyle through actions, man should practice Karma Yoga.

Bhakti Yoga

Like a young boy, Arjuna, with folded hands and innocence asked Lord- Whom do you consider a *Bhakta*. The one who constantly glorify Lord or the one who believes in Lord's qualities those are impersonal and imperishable. Lord Krishna answered him in following verses of the 12th chapter of Bhagavad-Gita-

मय्यावेश्यमनोयेमांनत्ियुक्ताउपासते।श्रद्धयापरयोपेताःतेमेयुक्ततमामताः॥ १२-२॥

Of those who fix their minds upon almighty, constantly glorify him and possess great faith – is considered as a *Bhakta* (B.G.12.2).

येत्वक्षरमनर्दिेश्यमव्यक्तंपर्युपासते।सर्वत्रगमचनि्त्यञ्चकूटस्थमचलन्ध्रुवम्॥१२-३॥

Those who control their senses, remain mentally composed in all situations, remain dedicated to help all living beings and worship almighty profoundly is also accepted as a *Bhakta* (B.G.12.3).

सन्नयिम्येन्द्रयिग्रामंसर्वत्रसमबुद्धयः।तेप्राप्नुवन्तमिामेवसर्वभूतहतिरताः॥१२-४॥

A *Bhakta* accepts almighty as impersonal, inconceivable, unchanging, with all-pervading qualities (B.G.12.4).

येतुसर्वाणकिर्माणमियसिंन्यस्यमत्पराः।अनन्येनैवयोगेनमांध्यायन्तउपासते॥१२-६॥

तेषामहंसमुद्धर्तामृत्युसंसारसागरात्।मृत्युसंसारसागरात्भवामनिचरित्पार्थमय्यावेशति
चेतसाम्॥१२-७॥

A *Bhakta* is the one who surrenders his actions to the almighty and accepts to remain under his shelter, he is immersed meditating for the communion with almighty; such a *Bhakta* attains the ultimate goal of human existence i.e. *moksha* (salvation) (B.G.12.6 & 7).

मय्येवमनआधत्स्वमयबुिद्धनिविशय।नविसष्यिसमियि्येवअतऊर्ध्वंनसंशयः॥१२-८॥

For *Bhakti yoga*, the yogi needs to fixate his *manas* (mind) and *buddhi* (intellect) on almighty and extent to him (B.G.12.8).

अथचति्तंसमाधातुंनशक्नोषमियसि्थरिम्।स्थरिम्अभ्यासयोगेनततोमामचि्छाप्तुंधनञ्
जय॥१२-९॥

If a yogi makes regular attempts to try to make almighty a pivotal of his *manas*, practice *bhakti yoga*, he can reach almighty (B.G.12.9).

Bhakti yoga is the path of devotion to the almighty. A *bhakta* finds peace being devotee, is emotionally attached to God, and considers everyone equal and forgives easily. A *Bhakta* remains completely absorbed in the devoutness of almighty, shows his love for almighty by chanting *mantras* (holy couplets), singing *bhajan* (devotional songs) and meditating to feel his presence. In *gauna bhakti*, the *bhakta* presents offerings to the idol and in *para bhakti*, the *bhakta* worships *nirguna-nirakar-saguna-*

sakaraishwara (the one who has all the qualities and forms and still is quality less and formless). The latter is considered to be more superior compared to former, but the intention lays the same for both i.e. surrendering self and ego to almighty. The worship is for *bhakta's* peace of mind and not a pretentious act for satisfying social needs. They surrender success and failures to God and. *Bhakti yogi* are not fanatics or delusional, but pure and innocent believer. Ramakrishna Paramhansa and Meera are few *bhakti yogis* who renounce themselves to the almighty.

Trends in Bhakti Yoga

In India, spirituality, religion and *bhakti* are interchanged and misunderstood and hence the purpose of bhakti can be misguiding. With the diversity in culture, the forms of almighty and offering customs vary. If we look around in our society, people who visit temples or any other worship place have no uniform intention. Few visit these places with an intention to achieve societal approval; few have an intention to please the almighty for some gains such as monetary, health, etc., whereas very few have the qualities of a *Bhakta* with the sole intention to surrender themselves to almighty. Why this variation does exist? A very strong reason is lack of scripture knowledge among the people makes them not a *Bhakta* but puppets in the hands of so called spiritual guides. Knowledge is powerful and shall be used to rescue one from the darkness of ignorance. The spiritual teachers must adhere to spread the true meaning of spirituality and *bhakti*. These teachers must try to bring in emotional changes in followers to become unanimous without any boundaries. We often see people manipulate and quarrel over the meanings of scriptures in order to establish the superiority of one spiritual belief over another. Whereas all the spiritual scriptures describe similar qualities of a *Bhakta* and *bhakti*, with the sole purpose of attaining emotional stability by surrendering oneself to the almighty, holding on to him in adversity and find peace of mind in this process. A *Bhakta* has a forgiving nature, sees everyone as a part of Divine soul, treats everyone equally, believes in almighty for any happenings in his life, and offers his prayers without any expectations. Such qualities if acquired can help an individual to become ego-less, proud-less, desire-less. Such a person would love and respect everyone, see himself as a medium to fulfil almighty wishes, free from effects of negative emotions and most importantly, he will be happy and have a positive wellbeing. A *Bhakta* or follower of *Bhakti yoga* not necessarily spends all the time of the day in front of an idol, but believes in the supremacy of almighty and entrusts him to be the source of existence and happenings. If a person who has faith in almighty like a *Bhakta* gets delayed for office because of light traffic or vehicle problem, his perception and reaction will not be frustration and anger, but he would surrender these happening to almighty and believe that there must have been some reason, he won't mind being apologetic to people expecting him and his patience and positive nature would resist others to be angry. Whereas if we use prayers and idols to win over any dispute or discriminate, it does not bring peace within or outside. It becomes a war of egoism where no one can really win because everyone has an inflated ego and absence of true knowledge.

In conversation with the spiritual teachers (female) of Islam, Christianity, Sikhism and Hinduism, about their spiritual beliefs, religious practices, customs and their intentions, the authors learned various similarities in intentions and the difference in customs and practices prevailed due to their ecology. *Bhakti* brings people close to each other on spiritual and emotional dimension of life. It manifests harmony in diversity, congruence of self, and releases egoism from our mind to bring in happiness. It is not hallucination, fanaticism or hooliganism of my idol or my almighty over yours, it is about believing, surrendering and being emotionally stable, for being a part of divinity one must experience happiness that originates from within and lasts forever. It is not about making people follow a custom or culture by installing fear, punishments, but creating a world of conditional love and acceptance. This happiness takes the *Bhakta* on the path of salvation and Samadhi to grow out of worldly attachments, needs and emotions, to connect with the divine.

In face of adversity, emotional turmoil or difficulty, people hold on to alcohol, smoking, drugs, and lately internet and social media. If only they could develop some belief in almighty and surrender their pleasure and pain to him, there is no better anchor than faith in him to hold on to. In this world we find ourselves in a juxtaposition of attachments and insecurities, to let-go or obsess over our possessions. If we let go, it bring social shame and labels whereas obsessing over desires leads to nothing but time wastage and social acceptance. It is a shame when we cannot feel strong within and look for appreciation and affiliations outside. It is a shame when we cannot value time and emotions over materialistic possessions.

Mothers and fathers are overly attached with their achievements, aspirations and ambitions and later try to compensate for their quality time with child by spending lavish over toys, holidays and gadgets. They work hard to build a career and save a lot of money for their child, but the most important function of parenting they skip on is character building which requires only their quality time. As the parents grow older they develop insecurities and tend to bury their children with it. If only they practice surrender and believe in almighty, they can lead a healthier life than spending loads of money to buy happiness. Surrender of ego and self is both a necessary component and subsequent consequence of *Bhakti yoga* as it tends to develop an inner strength to hold on separation or non-attachment. Thus, practice of Bhakti *yoga* is the way to the liberation in modern times.

Jnana Yoga

In the fourth chapter of Bhagavad-Gita, Lord Krishna tells Arjuna that of the four yogas, *Jnana Yoga* is one of the most difficult for a yogi to pick as a path of spirituality because it requires acquiring scripture knowledge (*nitya*) for salvation or liberation. A *Jnana Yogi* longs for *nitya* knowledge specifically from scriptures and thus seeking it as the sole purpose of life. Education till the age of fourteen is mandatory and efficient for basic survival of an individual in India. It is known as formal education which qualifies one for senior school education and further higher educational programs like graduation, post-graduation, doctorate etc. We see people around us getting qualified with various higher education but few of them qualify as *Jnana Yogi*. This might sound contradictory statement because one, who acquires high educational degrees, can be known as a knowledge longing person. Be contradictory but if you ask around the reason for such an aspiration, you might come across answers like- 'I got a degree for the sake of job, or under parental influence or just to find an eligible suitor', but none of these reasons collate with the real intentions to acquire knowledge. What are the qualities of a *Jnana Yogi*?

Lord Krishna states that one who has selfless desires to learn, acts to gain *nitya* knowledge and aspires to devote all his actions for the sake of knowing is a wise person (B.G.4.9).

यस्यसर्वेसमारम्भाःकामसङ्कल्पवर्जिताः।ज्ञानाग्निदग्धकर्माणंतमाहुःपण्डितंबु
धाः॥४-१९॥

Jnana Yogi is the one who has freed himself from the attachments like social, work-place, relational etc. and is focused on spiritual knowledge to become aware about himself, his soul and the almighty. The freedom of self makes him patient and mentally balanced. They do not react with respect to the situation, although they experience every emotion and feelings but remain unattached to their long lasting effects (B.G.4.23). When you have a good day or a bad at work and return home, you tend to carry those good and bad feelings. Your behaviour and thoughts are manifested significantly by emotions, say if it was a bad day or you had a bad experience with your boss or colleague, you might displace the anger or frustration on family members or friends although they were not the original source of the bad feelings and emotions. This displacement tends to begin a vicious cycle of emotions in form of anger bouts or frustration, which perturbs relationships. You start hurting people with your words and cause an irreparable emotional damage. But if you practice detachment like a *jnana yogi* the cycle of bad emotions would not begin. A *jnana yogi* understands the impermanent nature of everything and everyone around him. He understands the permanence of atman and almighty. Their intentions for every action is surrendered to almighty because they are enlighten with the *nitya* knowledge. Hence, their *karma* is performed by being detached and liberated, and by sacrificing their selves (not dying) for the almighty and thus they attain *moksha* i.e. freedom from karma chakra (karmic cycle).

What is sacrifice? Why *jnana yogi* has to make a sacrifice for higher spiritual knowledge? Lord Krishna answered this with verse 4.23 in Bhagavad Gita.

गतसङ्गस्यमुक्तस्यज्ञानावस्थितिचेतसः।यज्ञायाचरतःकर्मसमग्रंप्रविलीयते॥४-२३॥

On the occasion of festivals and marriages, *hawan* or small fire place is prepared to pour various pious things such as ghee, wood etc. Fire has an importance in Vedic tradition as it is considered to be impeccable, pure, unbiased and capable of changing the forms (by burning them) of everything in this nature. Hence anything offered to holy fire becomes pure to be offered to almighty, and any vows made in its presence is sanctioned by almighty and Vedas (such as marriages). *Yagna* or a ritual sacrifice made to the holy fire is prepared by a person (mostly Brahmin, one who belongs to highest of the four *varnas*) who has the knowledge of Vedas and mantras. To put offerings in the holy fire, with an intention to surrender is sacrifice. These actions are accompanied by physical offering of few belongings and psychological offerings ego, emotions, thoughts, self, etc. so anything offered in the *yagna* is a pure sacrifice. The sacrifice involves accepting the reality of almighty as the highest and *nitya*, and giving away themselves in his grace. Hence, every material possession is considered menial compared to almighty. *Jnana yoga* teaches that every action culminates in knowledge (B.G.4.33). Our offerings in *yagna* are considered a pious action, similarly offering our self to knowledge-*yagna* is pious for *Jnana Yoga*.

श्रेयान्द्रव्यमयाद्यज्ञाज्ज्ञानयज्ञःपरन्तप।सर्वंकर्माखलिंपार्थज्ञानेपरसिमाप्य
ते॥४-३३॥

Surrendering to knowledge with an intention of enlightenment is difficult because it requires discipline of body and mind, control over needs and desires and faith in scriptures. Once the yogi finding himself on this path, he can see a change in his intellect, behaviour, emotions and belief system. On this path of spirituality (alike others) *karma* does not bind a person because he is renounced. Knowledge helps him overcome any doubts and let him realize the true nature of his self (B.G. 4.41).

योगसंन्यस्तकर्माणंज्ञानसञ्छन्निसंशयम्।ज्ञानसञ्छन्निसंशयम्आत्मवन्तंनकर्माणनिि
बध्ननन्तधिनञ्जय॥४-४१॥

A *jnana yogi* analyses and reflects on the knowledge acquired from various sources. They are emotionally calm and physically composed compared to other without any knowledge. Like a swan that separates water and milk, *jnana yogi* requires *viveka* i.e. conscious, deliberate and continuous use of intellect for discriminating real from unreal. They are required to detach from worldly possessions, ego and see things as a third person like a *vairagi*. Being indifferent does not mean to be unconcern or unaware about the surrounding, *vairagya* is about keeping our-self unaffected and free from emotional and physical attachments. It leads to *mumukshutva* i.e. a sense of liberation from the worldly sufferings and be committed to the path of self-realization by acquiring knowledge. To stabilize our mind and emotions, we need to see beyond the physical world. How? Is there some specialised tool or method? Yes, *Shad-sampati*trains our mind and emotions to perceive reality beyond this world. The word *shadsampati* means six methods to be followed religiously to stay calm and focused to stay on the path of Jnana Yoga- *shama, dama, uparati, titiksha, shraddha* and *samadhana*. Here, *shama* is to keep our mind at peace byregulating its reaction to external stimuli. *Dama* is strengthening and controlling our mind and senses, and use them only as instruments to perceive our environment (not to satisfy desires). *Uparati* is abandonment of *adharma*. The *dharma* or dutiful actions those sanctioned by scriptures to have a simple lifestyle. *Titiksha* is to tolerate non-conducive situations that commonly produce excitement or suffering such as success and failure, pleasure and pain etc. *Shraddha* is to trust and believe in guru (teacher), scriptures and the yogic path for liberation or salvation. *Samadhana* is to be focused and remain single minded for any task. *Viveka, Vairagya, Shat-Sampati* and *Mumukshutva* are the four pillars of *Jnana Yoga*. They hold the utmost importance in practice of *Jnana Yoga*.

Trends of Jnana Yoga

In the modern time, just like *Karma Yoga* and *Bhakti Yoga, Jnana Yoga* is also relevant. Real knowledge liberates us from the three impurities of human existence, namely egoism, desire ridden actions and the illusion. Knowledge releases the earnestness that binds us from the worldly matters. Thus a *jnana yogi* detaches from effects of social, personal, professional etc. spheres of life to become aware about self, experience mental and emotional stability, and focus on spiritual development and almighty.

The social power and fame, achievements and pride are like moral vices that makes one feel superior to others. People get addicted them like smoking, alcohol etc for social approval and false boost to self-esteem. The media promotes notifications or warnings against the vices and their harmful effects to physical, mental and social health (Hellman, 2017) people throw away their lives for these vices. This faulty self-perception makes one believe that achievements are owned by individual and not by the mercy of almighty. One forms attachments with these vices and starts identifying with them. With time, as achievements and fame start fading away, people experience emotional and psychological pain as if they were real and permanent. Like the piece of chocolate gives pleasure only till it's on palate and not after consumption. The faulty self-perception is undergirding of ignorance, due to absence of true knowledge. Tanesini (2016) explain this ignorance generated by intellectual arrogance by fostering intellectual vices of timidity and servility towards others and self-delusion. Once ignorance is removed and perception is cleared, the emotional stability and detachment from world makes the *jnana yogi* non-reactive and non-submissive to anything but spiritual knowledge.

A *jnana yogi* finds his path of liberation via seeking spiritual knowledge and acknowledges the almighty by surrendering to him; he frees himself from the impurities and experiences stability, calmness, focus and determination to acquire knowledge for the sake of spiritual development. The ethics and virtues cultivate goods in person such as wisdom, understanding, reasoning, self-reflection and truth. Baird and Calvard (2018) outline business ethics and recognize management and implications of vices as illegitimate practices. Indian managers and leaders should outline their work ethics and follow them for the benefit of organization and country. As leaders, they set role models for future generation and as an inheritance they can nurture the future generation with ethical and spiritual knowledge to become a better person instead of being rich, proud and greedy professional. Vices give rise to incapability that hinders the professionalism in every field. Similar ideas can be found in the writings of Bruin (2015) that brings into light incompetence and greed as responsible factors for global financial crisis. The former is personal quality resultant of the latter, a vice. In principle, vice charging is possible but difficult in practice (Kidd, 2016). Hence, Bhagavad Gita and writings of Swami Vivekananda urge every individual to strengthen themselves morally and spiritually, to stand strong in the face of obstacles while on the path of virtues and righteousness.

Raja Yoga

Raja Yoga determines union of *atman* with almighty by building physical strength, control of breath, stabilising our mind and then become conscious of the communion with almighty. *Raja yoga* or *ashtang yoga* can be better known as lifestyle.

ब्रह्मण्याधायकर्माणसिङ्गंत्यक्त्वाकरोतयिः।लप्ियतेनसपापेनपद्मपत्रमविाम्भ
सा॥५-१०॥

Lord Krishna explains Arjuna that for a yogi, fixating his mind on almighty by disposing his desires and possessions and living in isolation to control his body and mind is necessary (B.G.5.10). This is *Raja Yoga* intending to strengthen body to contain healthy mind, and a healthy mind is well prepared for a communion with almighty.

कायेनमनसाबुद्ध्याकेवलैरन्द्रियैरपि।योगनिःकर्मकुर्वन्तसिङ्गंत्यक्त्वात्मशुद्ध
ये॥५-११॥

युक्तःकर्मफलंत्यक्त्वाशान्तमिाप्नोतनैष्ठकीम्।नैष्ठकीम्अयुक्तःकामकारेणफलेसक्तो
नबिध्यते॥५-१२॥

How can one attain a healthy body and a healthy mind? Most of the medical practitioners would suggest balanced diet, ample amount of water and regular exercise. Here, *Raja yoga* suggests different set of practices for a healthy body and mind. A yogi must find a clean sitting environment that is not too high or low, covered with soft grass, a deerskin (not necessarily) or a clean cloth. In this clean place, he must be single-mindedly focused on a point, controlling all the activities of the mind and senses, and practice yoga for purification of body and mind (B.G. 5.11 &5.12).

सर्वकर्माणमिनसासंन्यस्यास्तेसुखंवशी।नवद्वारेपुरेदेहीनैवकुर्वन्नकारयन्॥५-१३॥

After a proper sitting, yogi must hold his body; head and neck straight, remain still and steady, fix his gaze at the tip of the nose (B.G. 5.13). This is yoga position, indicating the beginning of yoga. By holding body still, one experiences steadiness in mind and feel an inflow of positive energies. This stillness shall not be confused with catatonic condition. A steady body helps in proper functioning of various systems like improved respiration, digestion, circulation etc. A straight posture is promoted by physicians and if body is strong, posture is straight and body systems function properly, positive wellbeing is attained.

नकर्तृत्वंनकर्माणलोिकस्यसृजतप्रिभुः।नकर्मफलसंयोगंस्वभावस्तुप्रवर्तते॥५-१४॥

After attaining yoga position, yogi experiences no disturbance outside and inside him, no fear and vows celibacy. Celibacy here means abstinent of sexual desires and needs, as it causes more interference than any other desire or need. Then he controls his mind by thinking of almighty, focuses his mental energies to unite his *atman* with the supreme power (B.G. 6.14). With all this, our mind is now ready to receive *nitya* knowledge.

नादत्तेकस्यचत्पिापंनचैवसुकृतंवभिुः।अज्ञानेनावृतंज्ञानंतेनमुह्यन्तजिन्तवः॥५-१५॥

Regular practice makes one experience inner peace and spiritual growth. So, in this way yogi controls his mind and withdraws from materialistic desires to experience calmness, peace and liberation from worldly attachments (B.G. 5.15).

इहैवतैर्जतिःसर्गोयेषांसाम्येस्थतिंमनः।नर्दिोषंहसिमंब्रह्मतस्माद्ब्रह्मणतिस्थ
ताः॥५-१९॥

When the steady mind is fixed exclusively upon the self, then one becomes free from all material desires – such a person is said to be situated in yoga (B.G. 5.18).

वद्यिावनियसम्पन्नेब्राह्मणेगवहि्स्तनि।शुनचैवश्वपाकेचपण्डताःसमदर्शनिः॥५-१८॥

Just as a flame does not flicker in a windless place, the mind of a yogi never wavers in its concentration on the self (B.G. 5.19). Meditation is found to reduce activations in a brain network area, responsible for self-related thoughts and mind wandering (Garrison, Zeffiro, Scheinost, Constable and Brewer, 2015).

Such a focused mind and high concentration was of Swami Vivekananda who could read and remember each word from a book that he would just scroll. If we practice and increase the focus of mind and concentration, there would be no reason for conditions such as exam stress, forgetfulness, absenteeism, difficulty in remembering and recalling, etc. Each school must inculcate these practices in their curriculum for mental growth of their students and teachers.

ज्ञानेनतुतदज्ञानंयेषांनाशतिमात्मनः।तेषामादत्यिवज्ज्ञानंप्रकाशयततित्परम्॥५-१६॥

Intake of food is limited for raja yogi because over or under eating causes ill-health like indigestion, gastric problems etc. Similar rule stands valid for sleep because excess of sleep results into lethargy and shortage of sleep reduces physical energy. Hence neither over nor under sleep and food is favourable for yogi (B.G.5.16).

तद्बुद्धयस्तदात्मानस्तन्नष्ठिास्तत्परायणाः।गच्छन्त्यपुनरावृत्तज्ञिाननर्धि्‌ूतकल्म
षाः॥५-१७॥

A proper schedule or routine of sleep and food can resolve a lot many problems such as stress; obesity, etc. Yoga prevents the physical and mental sufferings with a moderate food intake and gets proper sleep for physical relaxation, and performs all activities timely (B.G. 5.17).

नप्रहृष्येत्प्रयिंप्राप्यनोद्वजित्प्राप्यचाप्रयिम्।चाप्रयिम्स्थरिबुद्धरिसम्मूढोब्रह्मविद्ब्रह्मणस्थितिः॥५-२०॥

बाह्यस्पर्शेष्वसक्तात्मावन्दित्यात्मनयित्सुखम्।यत्सुखम्सब्रह्मयोगयुक्तात्मासुखमक्षयमश्नुते॥५-२१॥

येहसिंस्पर्शजाभोगादुःखयोनयएवते।आद्यन्तवन्तःकौन्तेयनतेषुरमतेबुधः॥५-२२॥

शक्नोतीहैवयःसोढुंप्राक्शरीरवमिोक्षणात्।प्राक्शरीरवमिोक्षणात्कामक्रोधोद्भवंवेगंसयुक्तःससुखीनरः॥५-२३॥

When our mind is restrained and detached from material desires it experiences inner strength and peace by the practice of Raja Yoga. Thus we can unite our self with almighty and attain happiness. This bliss, happiness and positive wellbeing is beyond the experience of the mundane situations like festivals, and being in this spiritual requires an intellect that can discriminate reality from a non-existent world. Growing out of emotions and maturing on spiritual dimension bring tranquillity to remain undisturbed in the midst of any greatest calamities (B.G. 5.20-5.23).

Maharshi Patanjali propounded the knowledge of *Raja yoga* into eight steps also known as *Ashtang*-Yoga. *Asht* means eight and *ang* means limbs, thus the eight limbs are – *Yama,Niyama, Aasan, Pranayam, Pratyahar, Dharana, Dhyana* and *Samadhi*. The first two limbs contain conducts and practices common to all spiritual paths and religions.

Yama refer to the moral conducts for individual to practice in order for soothe the functioning of the society. It includes *ahimsa, satya, asteya, aparigraha,* and *brahmacharya. Ahimsa* means refraining from injuring any living creature in thoughts, words or deeds. *Satya* means not lying under any circumstance. Truthfulness and straightforwardness is the way to happiness. *Asteya* refers to non-stealing, *Aparigraha, is a*bstention from greed. *Brahmacharya* means moderation in all sensual pleasures: *Brahmacharya* implies disciplining of the senses and moderation in diet and other sensual activities, i.e. celibacy.

Niyama are personal conducts for an individual to follow for cleaning of body and mind. They are *Saucha, Santosh, Tapas, Swadhyaya* and *Ishwarpranidhana*. *Saucha* is physical and mental cleaning by regular shower, oral hygiene etc. The practice of *Saucha* develops order and discipline of the body and mind. *Santosha, means* contentment *and it* helps to develop tolerance, appreciation and awareness. *Tapa* is austerity or self-discipline that requires regular practice of *yama* and previous *niyam*. *Swaadhyaaya* of self-education requires study of the Scriptures. Taking some time out daily to study scripture and meditate to bring change in our thought processes and perspectives on life. *Ishwarapranidhaana* is about surrendering the worldly achievements, failures, happiness and sorrows, pains and pleasures to God. We should work hard and give the best shot at the job, and then we need to surrender our actions and its results to the Almighty. It involves you in activities that are uplifting and beneficial for the spiritual growth.

The third limb, *Asana* is the ability to sit comfortably in a steady, erect posture. In order to meditate, one has to reach a stage where the body is no longer in pain or displeasure. *Asana* make one's body strong and flexible. For beginners, the *asanas* differ from intermediate and advanced *raja yogi*. The asana begins with small muscles of body from head to toe, exercising and stretching for releasing the tension. Further asana for internal and external parts of the body are prescribed by yoga expert for regular use. Cowen and Adams (2005) pointed at physical benefits of asana such as regulation of blood pressure, increased upper body and trunk muscles, body endurance and flexibly. Once the body is in align with mind, the breath is regularized by the yogi.

The fourth limb, *Pranayama* aims at controlling *prana* or breath. *Prana* or breath is the source of life for every living organism on this earth. In human beings, breathing is the sign of life. One of its constituent, oxygen is important for various physiological and cognitive processes. Vaksh, Pandey and Kumar (2016) reported improvement in academic performance of school students after six months of *pranayam*. Indian mythologies and cultural stories about sages are common among the Indian community, where the sages have an undergird control over breath and could survive under water, earth, also in adverse conditions. The control of *prana* through breathing exercises leads to control of the mind which leads to control over vital organs and senses. Such a control magnifies the capabilities of an individual to perform various physical and psychological processes energetically. Kuppuswamy, Kamaldeen, Pitani, Amaldas and Shanmugam (2017) reported benefitial effects of *bhramari pranayam* such as decrease in heart rate and blood pressure, improvement in cognitive functioning, significant reduction in irritability, depression and anxiety associated with tinnitus, and reduction in stress level. Thus, one can conclude that *pranayam* is extremely beneficial and effective for physical and mental health.

The fifth limb, *Pratyahara* is the withdrawal of the senses from objects or the withdrawal of the mind from the senses. One gets mental purity through *yama* and *niyama*, when the body becomes steady through asana practice and the *prana* also comes under control through *pranayama*.

The sixth limb, *Dharana* means concentration i.e. as the mind is withdrawn and remains focused on its object of concentration for an extended period of time, without any distraction and has mastered concentration. *Dharana* emphasises on adapting a lifestyle of yogi by adhering to the above mentioned steps. This stage is achieved only after the yogi aligns his body and mind with breath. He grows out of emotional, social and worldly bonds and associates himself with the almighty.

The seventh limb, *Dhyana* means meditation which is a state of mind which is one-pointed and steady. *Dhyana* or meditation is practice of sitting and thinking with quiet inner and outer environment about self. Meditation brings out a sense of relaxation and peace of mind, thus improving cognitive processes. Since ancient times, the effects of meditation are experienced by sages and scholars and they have documented these experiences as a step closer to blissfulness and Almighty. Modern science and their scientist are making efforts to understand the neurological effects of meditation in human body. Such studies vary from healthy to unhealthy individuals. Shapiro (2017) provided clinical and psychological comparisons and benefits of meditation over self-control strategies-hypnosis, biofeedback and progressive muscular relaxation techniques. Meditation has shown effective results in post-traumatic stress disorder and depressive symptoms (Hilton, Maher, Colaiaco, Apaydin, Sorbero, Booth, Shanman & Hempel, 2017).

Finally, the eighth limb, *Samadhi* or the Transcendental State, is called as *Turiya*, the fourth state of consciousness (the other three states are- waking, dreaming and dreamless sleep). Swami Vivekananda is proclaimed *raja yogi* who achieved the state of *Samadhi* and successfully popularised practice of all the above seven stages for spiritual, moral, physical and psychological development. Anand, Chhina and Singh (2017) wrote a chapter titled 'Some aspects of Electroencephalographic studies in yogis' to bring together various experimentally validating the claims made by *raja yoga* i.e. in the state of *Samadhi*, one is unaware to external and internal environment but the higher nervous activities remain in the state of ecstasy. Their efforts concluded with few experimental observations on yogis i.e. in the state of *Samadhi* the ECG read a persistent, well modulated and unblocked alpha activity.

The practice of eight limbs of *raja yoga* employs yogic methods from muscular relaxation, memory enhancement to voluntary control over visceral muscles (autonomic functions) (Wenger & Bagchi, 1961; Yamashiro, 2015; Rao, 2017) and attention enhancement (Singh & Srinivasan, 2019).

Trends of Raja Yoga

Raja Yoga affects cognition, behaviour, personality, mood, emotions and physiology of individual. *Raja Yoga* increases the flexibility of the spine, improves body's physical condition and heightened awareness to the importance of relaxation in both healthy and unhealthy people.

To practice yoga (*raja yoga, asanas, kundalini yoga, hath yoga* and mindful yoga etc.), age, gender, physical and mental condition is not a limitation. Over the years, various studies have shown children, adults, old age population, people with physical and mental illnesses benefitting from yoga. An exploratory study by Butzer, Over, Taylor and Khalsa (2015) suggest that yoga has a protective effect on academic performance. Razza, Dessa and Raymon (2015) studied the significant effects of mindful yoga intervention on increasing attention, delay of gratification and inhibitory control among the pre-schoolers. Authors have seen in clinical practice that children with ADHD can learn to relax and gain self control by breathing exercises and *asanas*. Eyre, Siddarth, Acevedo and Dyk (2017) found significant improvement in executive functioning, depressive symptoms and resilience in older participants (≥55 years of age) as a result of effect of *kundalini yoga* as compared to memory enhancement training. Yoga is a beneficial exercise for cognitive processes in relapsing and remitting multiple sclerosis (Sandroff, Hillman, Benadict & Molt, 2015). Bernstein, Bar, Ehrman, Golubic and Roizen (2014) found *yoga asana* benefits in behavioural change, weight reduction and its management; they emphasizes on practicing yoga slowly, coordinating body movement with the breath, pausing motionless in each position and always with full concentration. Hath yoga can effectively reduce the cognitive complaints of breast cancer survivors' (Derry, Jaremka, Bennett, Peng, Andridge, Shapiro, Malarkey, Emery, Layman, Mrozek, Glaser, Keicol-Glaser, 2014).

We regularly get referrals of patients/clients who are incapable of handling lifestyle stress and anxiety (non-clinical). As an intervention, they are prescribed practice of yogic methods. Their qualitative and experiential feedback reports soothing and calming effect all over body by paying attention to breath and breathing mechanism. Similar qualitative and experiential feedbacks are received for conditions like insomnia, fatigue and forgetfulness. Yoga is effective in treating variety of autoimmune diseases (Guthrie, 2010; Bartlett, Moonaz, Mill, Bernatsky, & Bingham, 2013; Roger & MacDonald, 2015) because it can reduce the symptoms these diseases often cause, such as stiffness, melancholy, fatigue, and weakness. Thus, regular practice of *Raja Yoga* strengthens body and mind, to prepare for the path of spirituality, and meditate daily to reach the ultimate goal i.e. liberation.

CONCLUSION

In modern times, one tends to side-track teaching from scriptures, and adds technological advancements and mental agonies to our lives. This brings in the lowest condition of the mental and physical wellbeing. The root cause of our sufferings and sorrows is incongruence with true self, i.e. atman, due to ignorance to reality, over indulgence in desires, and lack of spiritual growth. The four spiritual paths of yoga teach different ways to attain knowledge of self and union with the almighty for salvation or liberation. *Karma yoga* is the path of performing self-less actions to eradicate the egotistical attitude and let go attachments. *Bhakti yoga* is the path of surrender and unconditional devotion to the Almighty. It is the process of inner purification and teaches us to surrender our ego and self to the Almighty through prayers, worship, and reading scriptures. *Jnana yoga* is the path of attaining true knowledge with a sense of discrimination of real from unreal. Removal of ignorance and attachments gives an opportunity to mind to imbibe knowledge that enlightens our self. *Raja yoga* is the path of meditation by strengthening and aligning body, breath and mind. It teaches to develop a strong body in order to contain a strong mind, so that the impurities of mind can be removed by regular physical and mental exercises. Yoga must be practices vigorously and fearlessly (Nikhilananda, 1996). Each individual needs to decide which yoga best corresponds to their self.

A common question or dilemma crossing every mind is - How anyone becomes more aware about choosing a particular yoga path? A person who likes being active and believes that working is like praying, must choose *karma yoga*. People who are emotional and devotional shall choose *bhakti yoga*. People with strong will power, zeal to keep physical strength and mental strength aligned must choose *raja yoga*. *Jnana yoga* is for one with logical, rational, and philosophical and has longing for true knowledge from scriptures. Traditionally, an enlightened teacher or a guru provides the yogi a path to follow based on their personality and temperament. Although, the four paths seem to be different, but their goal is freedom from attachments and realization of true self closer to the Almighty for liberation.

REFERENCES

Anand, B. K., Chhina, G. S., & Singh, B. (2017). Some aspects of Electroencephelographic studies in yogis. In D. Shapiro (Ed.), *Meditation: Classic and Contemporary Perspectives* (pp. 475–476). New York: Routledge. doi:10.4324/9780203785843-50

Baird, C. & Calvard, T.S. (2018). Epistemic Vices in Organizations: Knowledge, Truth and Unethical Conduct. *Journal of Buisness Ethics*. doi:10.100710551-018-3897-z

Bartlett, S. J., Moonaz, S. H., Mill, C., Bernatsky, S., & Bingham, C. O. III. (2013). Yoga in rheumatic diseases. *Current Rheumatology Reports*, *15*(12), 387. doi:10.100711926-013-0387-2 PMID:24173693

Bernstein, A., Bar, J., Ehrman, J. P., Golubic, M., & Roizen, M. (2013). Yoga in management of Overweight and Obesity. *Journal of Lifestyle Medicines*, *8*(1), 33–41. doi:10.1177/1559827613492097

Bhagavad Gita. (n.d.). Gita Press.

Bruin, B. (2015). *Ethics and the Global Financial Crisis*. Cambridge University Press. doi:10.1017/CBO9781139237093

Cowen, V., & Adams, T. (2005). Physical and Perceptual Benefits of Yoga Asana Practice: Results of a Pilot Study. *Journal of Bodywork and Movement Therapies*, *9*(3), 211–219. doi:10.1016/j.jbmt.2004.08.001

Dabas, P & Sing, A. (2018). Bhagavad Gita teachings and positive psychology: Efficacy for semi-urban Indian students of NCR. *Cogent Psychology, 5*(1).

Derry, H., Jaremka, L., Bennett, J., Peng, J., Andridge, R., Shapiro, C., ... Keicol-Glaser, J. (2014). (2014). Yoga and self-reported cognitive problems in breast cancer survivors: A randomized controlled trial. *Journal of Psychological. Social and Behavioural Dimensions of Cancer*, *24*(8), 958–966. PMID:25336068

Diener, E., & Suh, M. E. (1998). Subjective Well-Being and Age: An International Analysis. In K. W. Schaie & M. P. Lawton (Eds.), *Annual Review of Gerontology and Geriatrics: Focus on Emotion and Adult Development*. New York, NY: Springer Publishing Company.

Dilip, V., Jeste, M. D., Ipsit, V., & Vahia, M. D. (2014). Comparison of the conceptualization of wisdom in ancient Indian literature with modern views: Focus on the Bhagavad Gita. *Psychiatry*, *71*, 197–209. PMID:18834271

Eyre, H., Siddarth, P., Acevedo, B., & Dyk, K. (2017). A Randomized controlled trial of Kundalini Yoga in mild cognitive impairment. *International Psychogeriatrics*, *29*(4), 557–567. doi:10.1017/S1041610216002155 PMID:28088925

Garrison, K., Zeffiro, T., Scheinost, D., Constable, R., & Brewer, J. (2015). Meditation leads to reduced default mode network activity beyond an active task. *Cognitive, Affective & Behavioral Neuroscience*, *15*(3), 712–720. doi:10.375813415-015-0358-3 PMID:25904238

Guthrie, C. (2010). *Befriending the Body: Find Peace and Relief from Autoimmune Disorders through Yoga*. Retrieved from https://www.yogajournal.com/lifestyle/befriend-the-body

Hellman, M. (2017). *Promoting Vices- An Introduction to Research on the Advertising of Coercive Products*. University of Helsinki.

Hilton, L., Maher, A. R., Colaiaco, B., Apaydin, E., Sorbero, M. E., Booth, M., ... Hempel, S. (2017). Meditation for posttraumatic stress: Systematic review and meta-analysis. *Psychological Trauma: Theory, Research, Practice, and Policy*, *9*(4), 453–460. doi:10.1037/tra0000180 PMID:27537781

Kidd, I. J. (2016). Charging Others with Epistemic Vices. *The Monist*, *99*(2), 181–197. doi:10.1093/monist/onv035

Kuppuswamy, M., Kamaldeen, D., Pitani, R., Amaldas, J., & Shanmugam, P. (2017). Effects of Bhramari Pranayam on Health - A Systematic Review. *Journal of Traditional and Complementary Medicine*, *8*(1), 11–16. doi:10.1016/j.jtcme.2017.02.003 PMID:29321984

Pollard, E. L., & Lee, P. D. (2003). Child Well-being: A Systematic Review of the Literature. *Social Indicators Research*, *61*(1), 59–78. doi:10.1023/A:1021284215801

Radhakrishnan, S. (1923). *Indian Philosophy* (Vol. 1). New Delhi: Oxford University Press.

Raju, P. T. (1992). *The philosophical traditions of India*. New Delhi: Motilal Banarasidass Pub. Ltd.

Rao, K. (2017). Empirical studies of Meditation. In *Foundations of Yoga Psychology* (pp. 137–174). Singapore: Springer. doi:10.1007/978-981-10-5409-9_6

Razza, R., Dessa, B., & Raymond, K. (2015). Enhancing preschoolers' Self-regulation via Mindful yoga. *Journal of Child and Family Studies*, *24*(2), 372–385. doi:10.100710826-013-9847-6

Rogers, K. A., & MacDonald, M. (2015). Therapeutic Yoga: Symptom Management for Multiple Sclerosis. *Journal of Alternative and Complementary Medicine (New York, N.Y.)*, *21*(11), 655–659. doi:10.1089/acm.2015.0015 PMID:26270955

Roy, G. (2018). *To construct and test multi-component trait model of personality in Indian psychology* (Unpublished thesis). The Maharaja Sayajirao University of Baroda, Vadodara.

Sandroff, B., Hillman, C., Benadict, R., & Molt, R. (2015). acute effects of walking, cycling and yoga exercise on cognition in person with relapsing-remitting multiple sclerosis without impaired cognitive processing speed. *Neuropsychology*, *37*(2), 209–219. PMID:25658772

Seligman, M. E. P. (2002). *Authentic happiness: Using the new positive psychology to realize your potential for lasting fulfillment*. New York, NY: Free Press.

Seligman, M. E. P., & Csikszentmihalyi, M. (2000). Positive psychology: An Introduction. *The American Psychologist*, *55*(1), 5–14. doi:10.1037/0003-066X.55.1.5 PMID:11392865

Shapiro, D. (2017). *Meditation: Classic and Contemporary perspectives*. New York: Routledge. doi:10.4324/9780203785843

Singh, A., & Srinivasan, N. (2019). Concentrative (Sahaj Samadhi) meditation expands subjective time. *PsyCh Journal*, *8*(1), 28–35. doi:10.1002/pchj.265 PMID:30788909

Swami Nikhilananda. (1996). *Vivekanana: Yogas and other works*. Chennai Mission Publication.

Tanesini, A. (2016). 'Calm Down, Dear': Intellectual Arrogance, Silencing and Ignorance. *Aristotellian Society Supplementary*, *90*(1), 71–92. doi:10.1093/arisup/akw011

Tehrani, N., Humpage, S., Willmott, B., & Haslam, I. (2011). *What's happening with well-being at work?* London, UK: Chartered Institute of Personnel and Development.

Vaksh, S., Pandey, M., & Kumar, R. (2016). Study the Effect of Pranayam on Academic Performance of School Students of IX and XI Standards. *Scholars Journal of Applied Medical Sciences*, *4*(5D), 1703–1705.

VandenBos, G. R. (Ed.). (2015). *APA Dictionary of Psychology* (2nd ed.). Washington, DC: American Psychological Association; doi:10.1037/14646-000

Wenger, M. A., & Bagchi, B. K. (1961). Studies of autonomic functions in practitioners of yoga in India. *Behavioral Science*, *6*(4), 312–323. doi:10.1002/bs.3830060407 PMID:14006122

Yamashiro, J. (2015). Brain basis of Samadhi: The Neuroscience of Meditative Absorption. *The New School Psychology Bulletin*, *13*(1), 1–10.

Yoga Sutra. (n.d.). New Delhi: Vijay Goyal Publisher.

ADDITIONAL READING

Foresight Mental Capital and Wellbeing Project. (2008). *Final Project report*. London, UK: The Government Office for Science. Retrieved from https://www.gov.uk/government/uploads/system/uploads/attachment_data/file/292450/mental-capital-wellbeing-report.pdf

King, M., Renó, V., & Novo, E. (2014). The Concept, Dimensions and Methods of Assessment of Human Well-Being within a Socio-ecological Context: A Literature Review. *Social Indicators Research*, *116*(3), 681–698. doi:10.100711205-013-0320-0

Safaya, R. (1976). *Indian Psychology*. New Delhi: Munshiram Manoharlal Publishers Pvt. Ltd.

Shah, H., & Marks, N. (2004). *A well-being manifesto for a flourishing society*. London, UK: NEF (The New Economics Foundation). Retrieved from http://b.3cdn.net/nefoundation/813660812dc0c82af5_vkm6vve98.pdf

Yadav, S. K. (2015). *Importance of yoga in daily life*. doi:10.13140/RG.2.1.4538.3842

Chapter 4
Quality of Life and Well-Being of Breast Cancer Patients

Melisa Anderson
College of Health Sciences, University of Technology, Jamaica

Dwayne Tucker
Department of Pathology, Faculty of Medical Sciences, The University of the West Indies, Jamaica

Fabian G. Miller
https://orcid.org/0000-0002-5821-1711
Faculty of Education, The Mico University College, Jamaica

Kurt Vaz
Department of Pathology, Faculty of Medical Sciences, The University of the West Indies, Jamaica

Lennox Anderson-Jackson
Department of Pathology, Faculty of Medical Sciences, The University of the West Indies, Jamaica

Donovan McGrowder
Department of Pathology, Faculty of Medical Sciences, The University of the West Indies, Jamaica

ABSTRACT

Breast cancer is a disease in which there is increased proliferation of malignant breast cells. This disease is more likely to begin in the ducts or lobules rather than the connective tissue. Globally, breast cancer is the most regularly diagnosed cancer. It is also a leading cause of cancer-related mortality in females. While cancer of the breast affects the physical aspect of patients, it can also negatively impact the quality of life (QoL) of survivors. There is a dearth of information, especially in the last decade, on the negative impact of breast cancer and treatment modalities on the QoL of patients. This review of the literature will examine the QoL and well-being of breast cancer patients to present a current perspective on the topic. Major findings of past and present articles that have contributed to improving the care of breast cancer patients will be summarized and included.

DOI: 10.4018/978-1-7998-1185-5.ch004

INTRODUCTION

Over the last decade, there have been advances in treatment strategies and early detection of breast cancer in developed countries, including the United States, the United Kingdom, and other European countries. This has resulted in an increased prevalence of breast cancer survivors (Brady et al., 2018). However, breast cancer survivors usually have health concerns related to treatment and an increased risk of developing other conditions like cardiovascular disease, metabolic syndrome, and recurrence of the disease (Dieli-Conwright et al., 2014). Over the last several years, a variety of measures have been employed to assess the QoL in breast cancer survivors. In evaluating the short- and long-term effects of breast cancer on the QoL of patients, a number of valid cancer-specific health-related QoL (HRQL) instruments have been established, including (Gordon & Siminoff, 2010):

- European Organization for Research and Treatment of Cancer Care Cancer QoL Questionnaire Core 30 (EORTC QLQ-C30) and its breast cancer specific complementary measure (EORTC QLQ-BR23)
- Life in Adult Cancer Survivor Scale (QLACS)
- Functional Adjustment to Cancer Therapy (FACT)
- Cancer Rehabilitation Evaluation System (CARES)
- Functional Living Index - Cancer (FLIC).

Demographic and socioeconomic factors (i.e., older age, lack of education, low income) have been found to be negatively related to QoL in breast cancer patients. Gender influences the degree of impairment of QoL. The literature suggests that low income is a risk factor of psychological distress. This is more likely among older females with breast cancer who may be on a fixed income compared with their younger counterparts. However, older females may possess a greater degree of psychological adaptation due to prior life experiences, exposure with healthcare systems, and observing other females diagnosed with the disease (Campbell-Enns & Woodgate, 2015).

This article will review information in the literature on the QoL and well-being of breast cancer patients. It will also examine how social support and physical exercise improve the QoL of these patients during and after treatment. The article will also discuss findings from the literature relating to rehabilitation intervention of breast cancer patients and how these improve QoL and well-being.

Method of Article Selection

A literature search was conducted for all English-language literature published prior to April 2019. The search was conducted using electronic databases, including PubMed, Embase, Web of Science, and Cochrane Library. The search strategy included keywords like breast cancer, QoL, well-being, treatment, intervention, social support, physical exercise, and QoL scales. The authors include several interventional and observational studies with reported findings, particularly recently published journal articles.

BACKGROUND

Epidemiology of Breast Cancer

Globally, breast cancer is the most frequently diagnosed malignancy in women and the leading cause of cancer-related deaths (Bray et al., 2018). It is estimated that about 2.1 million women are affected each year (WHO, 2018). Based on GLOBOCAN estimates, breast cancer was predicted to be the second leading cause of cancer after lung cancer in 2018 (Bray et al., 2018). It was estimated that there were 2,088,849 incident cases and a global mortality burden of 626,679 in 2018, which accounted for 11.6% of total cancer cases (Bray et al., 2018). In 2018, breast cancer accounted for about 15% of cancer-related mortality among women (WHO, 2018). Globally, the incidence of breast cancer in females is expected to rise to 3.2 million cases annually by 2050 (Tao et al., 2015). Moreover, the projected lifetime risk is one in eight women (12.5%; Saki, Ebrahim, & Tehranian, 2011). There has been a surge in the incidence of breast cancer in most countries, particularly in those with historically relatively low rates (Bray et al., 2018).

There is compelling evidence that the risk of breast cancer increases with age. The rate of abnormal cell changes increases gradually with time, which may elevate the risk of breast cancer with age. In the U.S., 81% of breast cancer cases occur in women ages > 50 years, with a median age at diagnosis of 62 years (DeSantis, Ma, Goding Sauer, Newman, & Jemal, 2017). Furthermore, 89% of breast cancer mortality was observed in women in this age group (Desantis et al., 2017). The median age at death was 68 years for women diagnosed with breast cancer (Desantis et al., 2017). There are reports supporting that breast cancer is becoming increasingly prevalent among women of younger age. It was recently reported that breast cancer is the most widespread cancer in women aged 15-39 years; many women in this age group die from the disease (Suter & Pagani, 2018).

QoL OF LIFE SCALES USED TO ASSESS BREAST CANCER

Cancer-specific HRQOL instruments have been created to assess the impact of short- and long-term effects of cancer on the QoL of cancer patients (Abu-helalah, Al-hanaqta, Alshraideh, & Hijazeen, 2014). Most reported studies focus on the QoL of long-term survivorship (between 5 and 10 years). Despite being relevant, studies seldom include assessments of the impact of diagnosis and initial intervention measures between years one and four (Tan et al., 2014). One of the most common HRQOL for assessing QoL of breast cancer survivors is the EORTC core questionnaire, more specifically the EORTC QLQ-C30 and EORTC QLQ-BR23 (Abu-helalah, Al-hanaqta, Alshraideh, & Hijazeen, 2014; Montazeri, 2008). The QLQ-C30 is a general QoL instrument; the QLQ-BR23 is specific for breast cancer.

EORTC QLQ-C30 and EORTC QLQ-BR23 Scales

The EORTC QLQ-C30 instrument is used to assess the impact of cancer on the following parameters or scales: physical, role, emotional, cognitive and social functioning, global health status or QOL scales, fatigue, pain, nausea and vomiting, constipation, diarrhoea, dyspnoea, insomnia, appetite loss, and financial difficulties (Tan et al., 2014). These parameters are assessed using a 30-item instrument designed to incorporate both multi-item and single-item parameters. These parameters are inclusive of five functional scales, three symptom scales, a global health status/QoL scale, and six single items (Fayers et al., 2001). A linear score ranging from 0 to 100 is used to represent each scale, as well as single-item parameters. A high score is indicative of a stronger response weight. Thus, a high score for functional scale represents a healthy level of functioning. A high score for global health status/QoL represents high QoL. However, a higher score in relation to a symptom represents a more severe symptom item (Fayers et al., 2001).

The EORTC QLQ-BR23 is a breast cancer module appropriate for patients at different stages of the disease across a spectrum of different therapies, including partial or total mastectomy, radiotherapy, and chemotherapy (with or without hormonal therapy; Abu-helalah, Al-hanaqta, AlshraideFayers, & Hijazeen, 2014). It has 23 questions covering five multi-item parameters, as well as three single-item parameters. Multi-items assess body image, arm symptoms, breast symptoms, side effects of systemic therapy, and sexual functioning. Single items address sexual enjoyment, hair loss, and future perspective. Scoring for the QLQ-BR23 is similar in principle to that of the single-items in the QLQ-C30 (Fayers et al., 2001).

Different versions of the QLQ-EORTC QLQ-C30 and EORTC QLQ-BR23 are utilized globally. The Moroccan Arabic version was used to assess QoL in breast cancer patients undergoing different types of treatment. The QoL was significantly improved one year posttreatment and the instruments were found to be quite useful in identifying early those patients with low scores on the functional scale (Traore et al., 2018). Furthermore, poor QoL was observed across a wide spectrum of health domains in a cross-sectional study of breast cancer patients undergoing radiation treatment (Jafari et al., 2013), and reasonably fair QoL in women with breast cancer after receiving adjuvant treatment post-surgery (Spatuzzi et al., 2016).

Quality of Life in Adult Cancer Survivors (QLACS) Scale

Quality of Life in Adult Cancer Survivors (QLACS) is widely used to evaluate the HRQL of long-term cancer survivors ≥ 5 years in many cancers, including female breast cancer (Sohl et al., 2015). QLACS addresses some of the limitations of generic measures and those associated with scales that focus primarily on treatment following diagnosis and treatment-related effects (Avis et al., 2005). Despite being originally established for long-term cancer survivors, QLACS also captures pertinent information associated with early transition cancer survivors (Sohl et al., 2015).

QLACS comprises a 47-item questionnaire, measuring 12 domains (five are cancer specific and seven are generic; Sohl et al., 2014). The cancer-specific domains capture information associated with having had cancer, including appearance concerns, financial problems, family-related distress, distress about recurrence, and benefits of having cancer (Sohl et al., 2015). Conversely, the generic domains address areas not specifically about cancer but pertinent to cancer survivorship (Sohl et al., 2015). The generic domains address areas like social avoidance, cognitive problems, physical pain, sexual problems, positive or negative feelings, and fatigue (Sohl et al., 2015). Cancer-specific and generic scores are separately generated by addition of the constituent domain scores, eliminating domains associated with cancer benefits (Avis et al., 2005). Domain scores are done in such a way that higher scores characterize poor QoL (Avis et al., 2005).

QLACS was reported to have appropriate convergent and divergent validity and good internal consistency (Sohl et al., 2015). A study of posttreatment breast cancer survivors between 1.5-2.0 years evaluated the psychometric properties of QLACS and supported that QLACS is also a suitable indicator for measuring the QoL for breast cancer patients during early transition survivorship (Sohl et al., 2015). In addition, the QLACS-SF was validated in Spanish breast cancer survivors and the findings demonstrated fairly good reliability and validity. The authors concluded that it can be useful in assessing QoL in short-term survivors (Escobar et al., 2015). Similarly, this instrument was found to be effective in evaluating HRQL among long-term breast cancer survivors and demonstrated an elevated level of responsiveness to life changes (Avis, Ip & Foley, 2006).

Functional Assessment of Cancer Therapy (FACT)

FACT is a 27-item questionnaire that can be altered to a more specific instrument, such as FACT Breast (FACT-B), provided that a module of 10 breast cancer-specific items were added (Cheung, Luo, Ng, & Lee, 2014). FACT-B is one of two instruments that specifically examined the QoL of breast cancer survivors (Nguyen et al., 2015). It is categorized in the general cancer subscale domain and breast cancer-specific subscale domain (Nguyen et al., 2015). FACT-B, a 37-item instrument, measures the following five domains: (1) social/family well-being; (2) physical well-being; (3) functional well-being; (4) emotional well-being; and (5) additional concerns for breast cancer (Cheung et al., 2014). Five-point Likert scales are used to rate the items. The FACT-B total score is determined by summing the scores of social/family, physical, functional, and emotional well-beings (Cheung et al., 2014). Higher scores are associated with better QoL of patients. FACT-B has been reported to be a valid and reliable measurement of the QoL in breast cancer patients (Nguyen et al., 2015).

The FACT-B (Version 4) have also been reported to demonstrate good reliability and validity in assessing QoL in a sample of 280 English-speaking women participating in a clinical trial for breast cancer therapy (Hahn et al., 2015). It is believed to provide useful information for evaluating the overall burden of breast cancer and the efficacy of intervention (Hahn et al., 2015). The Italian version of FACT-B (Version 4) evaluated in a cohort of 55 women who had been treated surgically for breast cancer, showed acceptable reliability results that are similar to Spanish and English versions (Di Bella et al., 2018).

The FACT have used to investigate QoL of breast cancer patient in a number of studies where the level of social support was also investigated. In a study by Zang et al. (2017) breast cancer patients with social support had higher mean scores of resilience and QoL. In an earlier reported study of 1,160 Chinese females with newly diagnosed breast cancer higher QoL scores were associated with adequate social support from family members, neighbors and friends, as well as medical insurance plans and higher household income (Yan et al., 2016). Furthermore, in a more recent study involving the use of FACT-B to assess QoL in 653 breast cancer survivors, low values in each domain was associated with declines in social support and family well-being (Goyal et al., 2018).

TREATMENT OF BREAST CANCER

Localized Treatment: Surgery and Radiotherapy

The literature covering the impact of surgery on the QoL of breast cancer patients invokes the notion that surgery type may be a key indicator of post-surgery QoL for patients (Montazeri, 2008; Paterson et al., 2015). Supporting evidence of this was also found in a 2016 report of a study involving Italian women. The data showed differences in QoL parameters among patients who had the following surgery types: mastectomy, reconstructive surgery post-mastectomy, and breast-conserving surgery (BCS; Spatuzzi et al., 2016).

Body image perception is perhaps one of the strongest impediments to QoL in women who undergo breast cancer surgery (both physical and psychological implications). Paterson et al. (2015) reported that women who undergo some type of reconstructive or BCS generally have better body image than those who received mastectomies (Paterson et al., 2015). The study data provided by Andrzejczak et al. (2013) showed that 31% of that study group felt less attractive after their mastectomy; 30% were perceived as less attractive by their partners (Andrzejczak et al., 2013).

Montazeri (2008) detailed that mastectomies, whether partial or total, had similar impacts on long-term QoL. The short- and long-term distress from each was dependent on the age at diagnosis (Montazeri, 2008). A meta-analysis published in 2016 outlined that greater issues relating to body image, sexuality, and intimacy were reported in younger women who underwent breast cancer surgery. The study data further explained that breasts are more important symbols of sexuality and femininity among that demographic (Paterson et al., 2015).

There are a number of studies that have evaluated the impact of radiotherapy on the QoL of breast cancer patients. Radiotherapy, a progressive and improved method to treat breast cancer, minimizes side effects (Muszalik et al., 2016). Nonetheless, radiotherapy is associated with fatigue, which threatens the QoL of breast cancer patients (Montazeri, 2008; Muszalik et al., 2016). A 2016 report outlined that fatigue and overall QoL in response to radiotherapy is also age dependent. In this study, women over the age of 71 years had better QoL scores than women between 51 and 70 years (Muszalik et al., 2016).

Other studies that have investigated the impact of radiotherapy on the QoL of breast cancer patients reported negative effect posttreatment (Yucel et al., 2014), decreased QoL during treatment (Whelan, Levine, Julian, Kirkbride & Skingley, 2000) and no significantly change in QoL during and up to one year post-radiotherapy (Xiao et al., 2016).

Systemic Therapy: Chemotherapy

Systemic therapies, such as adjuvant chemotherapy, have a considerable impact on the QoL of breast cancer patients. According to a study published in 2013, breast cancer patients treated with chemotherapy presented with diminished physical, emotional, and functional well-being, as well as greater breast cancer-specific anxieties as measured by FACT-B (Hwang, Chang, & Park, 2013). Moreover, a prospective study concluded that adjuvant chemotherapy showed significantly lower QoL in breast cancer patients vs. hormonal or radiotherapy alone (Galalae et al., 2005).

A 2013 cross-sectional study compared the QoL in women who received chemotherapy vs. those who did not receive the treatment. The findings of this study strongly aligned with the general literature and a 2002 follow-up study noting that chemotherapy patients generally receive poorer scores on QoL scales (Ganz, 2002). Depression and unmet sexual needs were found to be key contributors to QoL impairment in women who received chemotherapy. The study further highlighted that the impact of adjuvant chemotherapy was somewhat dependent on survival time post-surgery (Hwang et al., 2013). After examining three groups in relation to time, the study showed significant impairment to QoL (assessed by FACT-BC) among patients with less than one-year post-surgery (group 1) and greater than three-years post-surgery survival (group 3). Group 1 generally had poorer scores than group 3 in relation to depression and unmet sexual needs (Hwang et al., 2013). Chemotherapy is also associated with early onset of amenorrhea and infertility due to oestrogen imbalances. This impacts QoL scores (assessed by QLQ-EORTC QLQ-C30 and EORTC QLQ-BR23) in both the functional and symptom scales, especially in premenopausal women (Ganesh, Lye, & Lau, 2016). The distress of being infertile weighs heavily on the mental and emotional faculties of premenopausal women who are of reproductive years. Consequently, they exhibit poorer QoL (Ganesh et al., 2016; Hopwood, Haviland, Mills, Sumo, & Bliss, 2007). Nonetheless, studies have shown that most breast cancer patients experience an improvement in QoL scores after adjuvant therapy (Grimison & Stockler, 2007). These patients progress without long-term effects except for vasomotor symptoms and sexual dysfunction (Ahmed et al., 2018; Grimison & Stockler, 2007).

Hormonal Therapy

Most breast cancer diagnoses occur at postmenopausal age. They are usually hormone receptor-positive tumors in which adjuvant endocrine therapy is used to improve survival. However, optimal endocrine therapy has a typical five-year treatment course, including aromatase inhibitors like exemestane given up front or sequentially following tamoxifen (van Nes et al., 2012). These treatments have adverse impacts on survivors. As such, there has been a concerted effort to examine the effect of endocrine therapy on the QoL of these survivors. A Dutch clinical trial outlined the impact of exemestane and tamoxifen on postmenopausal early breast cancer patients. The study reported that both treatment options result in the development of various menopausal symptoms, including insomnia and sexual problems due to reduced oestrogen (van Nes et al., 2012). Approximately half of the women in this study experienced insomnia up to seven years. Women who received exemestane had worse insomnia vs. those who received tamoxifen. Sexual problems were more highlighted with exemestane in the form of vaginal atrophy (vaginal dryness and dyspareunia) than with tamoxifen. Tamoxifen is linked to thromboembolic complications and impaired sexual function due to low libido and a diminished ability to become aroused and experience orgasm (van Nes et al., 2012). These side effects undoubtedly impair the QoL of these women. Moreover, a 2008 report associated tamoxifen with an increased incidence of benign endometrial lesions and an increased risk of endometrial cancer in postmenopausal patients (Nasu, Takai, Nishida, & Narahara, 2008).

SOCIAL SUPPORT AND QoL

Social Support: Partners, Family Members, and Friends

Documented studies show that social support is a well-recognized factor of health and well-being. Inadequate social support is correlated with significant increase of breast cancer-related morbidity and mortality (Jeong et al., 2010). In the Nurses' Health Study that prospectively investigated social network and support and survival among 2,835 patients diagnosed with breast cancer (stages I to IV), multivariate-adjusted analyses revealed that social isolation before diagnosis resulted in a 66% elevation in risk of all-cause mortality (HR = 1.66; 95% CI, 1.04-2.65) and a 114% increased risk of breast cancer mortality (HR = 2.14; 95% CI, 1.11-4.12) compared with counterparts who experienced social integration (Kroenke et al., 2006). In a similar study of a large cohort of breast cancer patients with median follow-up of 5.6 years, a larger social network and interaction with friends and family, as well as participation in community activities and religious services, was associated with decreased (15-25%) all-cause mortality rather than breast cancer-specific mortality (Beasley et al., 2010). In the Life After Cancer Epidemiology study of females diagnosed with early-stage, invasive breast cancer, multivariate-adjusted analyses demonstrated that women who were socially isolated had a 34% increased risk of all-cause mortality (HR = 1.34; 95% CI, 1.03-1.73). Those who experienced low levels of social support from family and friends and low social/religious attendance and participation had a significant 58% increase in all-cause mortality (HR = 1.58; 95% CI, 1.07-2.36; Kroenke et al., 2013). Importantly, women with significant social support (i.e., informational and emotional support from partner and a larger social network with family and friends) reported significantly better physical and mental HRQL and fewer breast cancer symptoms (Leung, Pachana & McLaughlin, 2014).

The attentiveness and responsiveness of spouses as primary caregivers, communication involving the openness to share one's emotions, relationship satisfaction, and marital support are found to be significantly associated with the psychosocial outcomes of breast cancer patients (Manne et al., 2004). Conversely, criticism and spouse withdrawal, unwillingness to respond constructively to the patient's multifaceted needs, and negative advice affect breast cancer patients' ability to cope and, by extension, QoL (Manne et al., 2006). Some studies show that feelings of inadequacy or guilt, depression, increased demand on time, role strain, increased support of children, multiple roles, apprehension regarding sexual intimacy, and fear of partner loss contribute to male partners experiencing emotional stress. This may reduce their capacity to be good caregivers (Fekih-Romdhane, Henchiri, Ridha, Labbane, & Cheour, 2019). This highlights the need for couple-focused psychosocial and psychological interventions, especially for young couples who are more susceptible to suffering and poor QoL (Regan et al., 2015).

Conventional and Online Support Programs/Networks

Conventional couples' intervention has been useful in reducing psychological stress and improving QoL for breast cancer patients (Anderson et al., 2008). In a pilot study by Baucom et al. (2009), a couples'-based relationship enhancement intervention program improved positive functioning for couples and minimized the negative effects of breast cancer. A later study examined the effectiveness of a supportive group vs. a skill-based couple-focused group intervention on couples' relationship and psychological functioning. It revealed an improved well-being for couples in both groups, as well as a decrease in anxiety, cancer-specific distress, and depressive symptoms. The results also indicated that the couples'-focused skill-based supportive intervention was more operative for less distress breast cancer patients; the supportive group therapy gave better results for patients faced with more distress (Manne, Siegel, Heckman, & Kashy, 2016).

There is growing evidence to demonstrate the efficacy of conventional psychosocial and psychological interventions to reduce emotional stress and promote adaptation to breast cancer. However, these may not be realistic options for young couples due to challenges in enrolling patients and partners in these interventions. Conventional counseling interventions may not sufficiently address the distinct, complex needs of young breast cancer patients and their partners. Therefore, there is a growing participation in online-based support networks and programs (Mendes-Santos, Weiderpass, Santana, & Andersson, 2019). Some studies show that participation in online-based support offers advantages like reductions in depression, social isolation and breast cancer-related trauma. It also shows enhancements to decision making, social support, personal empowerment, and self-esteem (Winzelberg et al., 2003).

Cancer Chat Canada is a collaborative initiative that utilizes a secure online platform to offer professionally facilitated group support to patients and family caregivers. Findings from the study show good satisfaction, social bonding, improved self-care and mood, and meaningful communication between patients and caregivers regarding the disease (Stephen et al., 2013). Another successful online support program, Comprehensive Health Enhancement Support System (CHESS), is designed for low-income women with breast cancer. This electronic health system provides patients with decision-making and health monitoring tools. Using the network, patients can connect with health professionals on cancer-specific information to aid with treatment-related decisions, as well as receive emotional support from survivors (Namkoong et al., 2013). The popularity and use of online interactive cancer communication systems for patients with breast cancer will continue to grow as they offer better access to social and professional support, allow patients and caregivers flexibility in terms of time, and add benefits on overcoming barriers associated with transportation and childcare (Villani et al., 2018).

REHABILITATION INTERVENTION AND QoL

Psychosocial and Psychoeducational Interventions

Psychosocial interventions are organized psychological or social interventions generally useful to address social disorders and cessation of drug abuse or to prevent relapse. They are wide and include cognitive behavioral therapy, psychoeducation support, and expression of emotion (Inan & Ustun, 2019). Healthcare professionals, including medical practitioners and nurses, can offer psychoeducational programs to breast cancer patients with the aim of supporting them to adjust to the diagnosis, optimizing their behavior and to address distress and emotional concerns (Dastan & Buzlu, 2012).

Stress-related psychosocial factors may have adverse effects on the outcomes of breast cancer patients (Dastan & Buzlu, 2012). Rottman, Dalton, Christensen, Frederiksen, and Johansen (2010) conducted a longitudinal study in which they found a significant correlation between self-efficacy and education, with the former a significant predictor of emotional well-being and active style of adjustments in breast cancer patients. Matsuda examined the efficacy of psycho-educational and psychosocial support interventions to improve the QoL for early stage breast cancer patients. The study found improved breast cancer-related symptoms and increased emotional well-being. It did not show improved global QoL six months post-intervention (Matsuda, Yamaoka, Tango, Matsuda, & Nishimoto, 2014). The results of Cochrane Review were similar, with improvement in QoL using cancer-specific measures and general psychological distress (Galway et al., 2012).

Some studies have demonstrated that adjuvant chemotherapy may cause cognitive impairment due to neural damage in patients with breast cancer (Apple et al., 2018; van der Willik et al., 2018). Therefore, the management of this side effect and others are important to improve the QoL in breast cancer patients (Inagaki et al., 2006). Optimal rehabilitation for women with breast cancer involves intervention and contributions from numerous healthcare professionals to help remediate and re-establish diminished physical, emotional, psychosocial, and occupational functioning during and posttreatment (Juvet et al., 2009).

Cognitive behavioral therapy is a short-term, goal-orientated psychosocial intervention. It is extensively used for improving mental health by altering behavior or thinking, causing challenges to individuals (Musiat & Tarrier, 2014). Cognitive behavioral therapy uses the straightforward principles of cognitive and behavioral psychology. The specific model for insomnia has been found to improve cognitive and global dimensions of the QoL, general mood, and physical fatigue 12-months post-intervention in breast cancer patients (Aricò, Raggi, & Ferri, 2016). In the meta-analysis of randomized control trials by Xiao et al. (2017), cognitive behavioral therapy showed significant effectiveness in decreasing depression in breast cancer patients post-surgery. In addition, mindfulness-based cognitive therapy significantly reduced the intensity of posttreatment pain, signifying that this type of cognitive therapy may be an effective pain rehabilitation therapy for breast cancer (Johannsen et al., 2016). This psychological intervention also improved survival and reduced psychological symptoms 12-months posttreatment in women with metastatic breast cancer (Mustafa et al., 2013). It had favorable effects on depression, mood disturbance, and anxiety in women with non-metastatic breast cancer (Hickey, & Carter, 2015).

PHYSICAL ACTIVITY AND QoL

Physical Activity and HRQL

Epidemiological studies have confirmed that physical activity among females reduces the risk of breast cancer incidence and overall mortality while improving breast-cancer specific survival (Sternfeld et al., 2009). A review by Friedenreich & Cust (2008) consisted of 34 case-control and 28 cohort studies designed to examine the possible biological mechanisms whereby physical activity impacted breast cancer risk among females. The authors found an estimated risk reduction of 25-30% associated with improved physical activity (Friedenreich & Cust, 2008). To accomplish such an effect, females are encouraged to engage in a physical exercise regime of moderate to vigorous intensity (Kushi et al., 2012).

Breast cancer survivors are encouraged to embrace a healthy lifestyle post-diagnosis. The Cochrane Review confirmed that physical exercise may have valuable effects on the HRQL, including social functioning, body image/self-esteem, sexuality, fatigue, anxiety, sleep disturbance, pain, emotional well-being, and cancer-specific concerns at varying follow-up periods (Lahart, Metsios, Nevill, & Carmichael, 2015). Irwin et al. (2003) assessed self-reported physical activity levels in terms of household and sports activities among 806 breast cancer patients. They found that 32% attained recommended levels of physical activity defined by moderate to vigorous intensity of 150 minutes per week (Irwin et al., 2003). In their earlier study entitled Health, Eating, Activity, and Lifestyle (HEAL), there was an 11% reduction in total physical exercise among breast cancer patients equivalent to an estimated two hours per week post-diagnosis compared with pre-diagnosis (Irwin et al., 2003).

A systematic and meta-analysis review of 22 prospective cohort studies by Lahart et al. (2015) found that breast cancer patients who engaged in pre-diagnosed high levels of recreational physical activities had significantly lower risk of recurrence, breast cancer-related death (HR = 0.73; 95% CI, 0.54-0.98) and all-cause (HR = 0.82; 95% CI, 0.70-0.96; Lahart et al., 2015). A similar study published by Ibrahim et al. (2011) demonstrated that pre-diagnosis physical activity decreased breast cancer-specific deaths by 18%. However, it had no significant effect on breast cancer-related mortality. Conversely, pre-diagnosis physical activity significantly decreased breast cancer-specific deaths by 34% (HR = 0.66; 95% CI, 0.57-0.77) and all-cause mortality by 41% (HR = 0.59; 95% CI, 0.53-0.65). Disease recurrence decreased by 24% (HR = 0.76; 95% CI, 0.66-0.87; Ibrahim & Al-Homaidh, 2011). In a Norwegian population-based survival study of 1,364 breast cancer patients, obese women (BMI > or = 30 kg/m^2) had a 47% increase (HR = 1.47; 95% CI, 1.08-1.99). Those of normal weight and 55 years or older at diagnosis had a 66% (HR = 0.34; 95% CI, 0.16-0.71) decrease in overall mortality if they engaged in pre-diagnosis regular physical activity (compared with sedentary women; Emaus et al., 2010).

Physical Activity and Therapy

Breast cancer treatments (i.e., surgery, radiation, endocrine therapy, and chemotherapy) can induce injuries and impairments in the locomotor systems. This includes a decrease in motion of the shoulder and muscle strength, lymphedema, pain, and other disabilities which negatively affect the ability to adequately perform daily living activities and reduce HRQL (O'Toole et al., 2015). The impact of these side effects may be felt many years posttreatment. They may negatively affect self-esteem and well-being, as well as decrease the QoL of breast cancer patients (Carpender, 1998; Lash & Silliman, 2002). The use of aromatase inhibitors in the treatment of breast cancer has become the standard adjuvant therapy of postmenopausal patients. Although there are constant improvements in disease-free survival, it threatens many aspects of health-related quality. This includes osteoporosis, depression, anxiety, low self-esteem, pain, fatigue, reduced physical fitness, and increased fat mass (Amir, Seruga, Niraula, Carlsson, & Ocaña, 2011).

A number of studies have evaluated the impact of exercise programs on the HRQL of breast cancer survivors undergoing different modalities of treatment (Lahart et al., 2018). Observational evidence in the literature proposes that physical activity reduces side effects like fatigue related to chemotherapy or musculoskeletal syndrome induced by the aromatase inhibitor, thus improving HRQL (Peterson & Ligibel, 2018). In the randomized control trial by Paulo et al. (2019), there were potential benefits of improved social functioning, physical health and functioning, and general health perception. It also reduced fatigue and sleep disturbance in postmenopausal breast cancer patients (stages I-II) undergoing aromatase inhibitor therapy who performed resistance and aerobic training three times per week (Paulo et al., 2019). Their findings were similar to the hormones and physical exercise study in which Thomas et al. (2016) observed the effects of 12 months of combined resistance and aerobic exercise intervention compared with standard care in postmenopausal breast cancer survivors treated with aromatase inhibitors. They found improvements in body composition, alleviation of negative side effects, and improved health outcomes (Thomas et al., 2016). Aromatase inhibitors-associated arthralgia was diminished in postmenopausal breast cancer patients undergoing approximately 120 minutes of moderate-intensity aerobic exercise (Arem et al., 2016). Reduced aromatase inhibitors-associated arthralgia and depressive symptoms and improved QoL and functional performance were observed in breast cancer patients on adjuvant therapy who participated in an eight-week home-based exercise program of combined aerobic and resistance exercises (DeNysschen et al., 2014). Supporting evidence was observed in the study by Hojan, Molińska-Glura, and Milecki (2013) where aerobic and resistance training improved QoL and decreased adverse effects of endocrine therapy in premenopausal breast cancer patients.

Types of Physical Activity and QoL

Physical exercise is a critical component of cancer rehabilitation. A six-month community-based exercise intervention demonstrated significantly improved areas of QoL, including pain, vitality, mental health, physical function, emotional function, social function, and reduced pain in breast cancer survivors (Knob, Thompson, Fennie, & Erdos, 2014). Findings from two systematic and meta-analysis studies demonstrated that exercise intervention of longer duration (greater than 12 weeks) during and posttreatment in breast cancer patients may enable enhanced QoL and fitness and decreased fatigue (Ferrer, Huedo-Medina, Johnson, Ryan, & Pescatello, 2011; Meneses-Echávez, González-Jiménez, & Ramírez-Vélez, 2015). Studies have shown that tai chi exercises for a 12-week duration improved HRQL, social functioning, vitality, memory, cognitive functions, and musculature while decreasing pain and fatigue in breast cancer patients (Janelsins et al., 2011). The improved HRQL could be due to the regulation of biomarkers (insulin-like growth factor and interleukin-8) and inflammatory responses (Janelsins et al., 2011).

Pilates exercise is commonly accepted as a fitness activity. A systematic review and meta-analysis studies have demonstrated that they improve QoL, self-reported upper extremity function, motion of the shoulder, and improvements in social appearance (Pinto-Carral, Molina, de Pedro, & Ayán, 2018). In another study, there was reduction in severity of lymphedema pain and pain severity, as well as improved functional status (Şener, Malkoç, Ergin, Karadibak, & Yavuzşen, 2017). The authors in the latter study suggested that Pilates-based exercises appear to be an operative method of rehabilitation of upper extremity disorders related with breast cancer treatment (Şener et al., 2017). Yoga is a meditative physical activity. In a study by Sudarshan et al. (2013), 12 one-hour weekly yoga sessions significantly improved physical function in Stage I-III postoperative breast cancer patients (Sudarshan et al., 2013; Table 1). Other studies have demonstrated significant improvements in QoL and significant lowering of depressive symptoms (El-Hashimi & Gorey, 2019).

CONCLUSION

This review examined the literature to highlight the persistent and important effects of breast cancer and its treatment modalities on long-term survival. It reviewed the interconnectedness of the physical, social, psychological, and psychosocial aspects of the QoL in breast cancer survivors. There is strong evidence that the regular practice of physical exercise after diagnosis positively influences QoL, morbidity, mortality, and prognosis of survivors of breast cancer. Combined resistance and aerobic exercises have potential benefits on the QoL of breast cancer survivors undergoing treatments like aromatase inhibitor therapy. These are important approaches to minimize the effects of treatment and improve health. Clinicians and researchers should select the most appropriate treatments, using validated instruments to assess changes in QoL. This will provide valuable data and improve the overall QoL of breast cancer survivors.

There continues to be a growth in the use of Internet interventions. There are suggestions that e-health interventions should become part of regular psychosocial care of breast cancer survivors. A tiered model of care may present a challenge because care should be tailored to meet individual patient needs.

Table 1. Outcome of exercise intervention on breast cancer patients before and after therapy

Studies	Study Population	Type(s) of Physical Exercise	Outcome of Exercise Intervention
Irwin et al. (2003)	Eight-hundred and twelve patients with incident breast carcinoma (from in situ to Stage IIIa)	Types of sports and household activities pre- and postdiagnosis	Physical activity significantly decreased after patients were diagnosed with breast cancer.
Lahart et al. (2015)	Meta-analysis of 22 prospective cohort studies (123,574 participants)	Recreational physical activity pre- and post diagnosis	An inverse relationship was found between physical activity and all-cause, breast cancer-related death and breast cancer events.
Ibrahim and Al-Homaidh (2011)	Meta-analysis of six studies (12,108 patients with breast cancer)	Physical activity pre- and post diagnosis	Post diagnosis physical activity reduced breast cancer deaths by 34%, all causes mortality by 41%, and disease recurrence by 24%.
Sprod et al. (2012)	Twenty-one breast cancer survivors	Tai chi chuan exercise	Tai chi chuan exercise improved total health-related QoL, physical and social functioning, and general mental health.
Pinto-Carral et al. (2018)	Meta-analysis of five randomized controlled trials and two un-controlled studies	Pilates exercises	Pilates exercises relieved the impact of breast cancer-related symptoms with improved functional status, fitness, and mood.
Şener et al. (2017)	Sixty female breast cancer patients who developed lymphedema posttreatment	Clinical Pilates exercises	Reductions were found in the severity of lymphedema accompanied by improved social appearance, anxiety, QoL, and upper extremity functions scores.
Sudarshan et al. (2013)	One-hour weekly yoga exercise sessions	Fourteen stage I-III postoperative breast cancer patients	Improved physical functions like right and left shoulder abduction flexibility with amelioration in anxiety, depression, and pain symptoms post-yoga intervention.
El-Hashimi et al. (2019)	Meta-analysis of eight randomized controlled trials with 545 participants	Yoga and aerobic exercises	Both interventions were associated with clinically significant improvements in QoL.

REFERENCES

Abu-helalah, M., Al-hanaqta, M., Alshraideh, H., & Hijazeen, J. (2014). Quality of life and psychological well-being of breast cancer survivors in Jordan. *Asian Pacific Journal of Cancer Prevention, 15*(14), 5927–5936. doi:10.7314/APJCP.2014.15.14.5927 PMID:25081724

Ahmed, A. E., Almuzaini, A. S., Alsadhan, M. A., Alharbi, A. G., Almuzaini, H. S., Ali, Y. Z., & Jazieh, A.-R. (2018). Health-related predictors of quality of life in cancer patients in Saudi Arabia. *Journal of Cancer Education, 33*(5), 1011–1019. doi:10.100713187-017-1198-3 PMID:28271388

Amir, E., Seruga, B., Niraula, S., Carlsson, L., & Ocaña, A. (2011). Toxicity of adjuvant endocrine therapy in postmenopausal breast cancer patients: A systematic review and meta-analysis. *JNCI: Journal of the National Cancer Institute, 103*(17), 1299–1309. doi:10.1093/jnci/djr242 PMID:21743022

Andersen, B. L., Yang, H. C., Farrar, W. B., Golden-Kreutz, D. M., Emery, C. F., Thornton, L. M., & Carson, W. E. (2008). Psychologic intervention improves survival for breast cancer patients: A randomized clinical trial. *Cancer, 113*(12), 3450–3458. doi:10.1002/cncr.23969 PMID:19016270

Andrzejczak, E., Markocka-Mączka, K., & Lewandowski, A. (2013). Partner relationships after mastectomy in women not offered breast reconstruction. *Psycho-Oncology, 22*(7), 1653–1657. doi:10.1002/pon.3197 PMID:23045167

Apple, A. C., Schroeder, M. P., Ryals, A. J., Wagner, L. I., Cella, D., Shih, P.-A., ... Wang, L. (2018). Hippocampal functional connectivity is related to self-reported cognitive concerns in breast cancer patients undergoing adjuvant therapy. *NeuroImage. Clinical, 20*(7), 110–118. doi:10.1016/j.nicl.2018.07.010 PMID:30094161

Arem, H., Sorkin, M., Cartmel, B., Fiellin, M., Capozza, S., Harrigan, M., ... Irwin, M. L. (2016). Exercise adherence in a randomized trial of exercise on aromatase inhibitor arthralgias in breast cancer survivors: The Hormones and Physical Exercise (HOPE) study. *Journal of Cancer Survivorship: Research and Practice, 10*(4), 654–662. doi:10.100711764-015-0511-6 PMID:26782031

Aricò, D., Raggi, A., & Ferri, R. (2016). Cognitive behavioral therapy for insomnia in breast cancer survivors: A review of the literature. *Frontiers in Psychology, 7*(4), 654–662. doi:10.3389/fpsyg.2016.01162 PMID:27536265

Avis, N. E., Ip, E., & Foley, K. L. (2006). Evaluation of the Quality of Life in Adult Cancer Survivors (QLACS) scale for long-term cancer survivors in a sample of breast cancer survivors. *Health and Quality of Life Outcomes*, *4*(1), 92. doi:10.1186/1477-7525-4-92 PMID:17140438

Avis, N. E., Smith, K. W., McGraw, S., Smith, R. G., Petronis, V. M., & Carver, C. S. (2005). Assessing quality of life in adult cancer survivors (QLACS). *Quality of Life Research: An International Journal of Quality of Life Aspects of Treatment, Care and Rehabilitation*, *14*(4), 1007–1023. doi:10.100711136-004-2147-2 PMID:16041897

Baucom, D. H., Porter, L. S., Kirby, J. S., Gremore, T. M., Wiesenthal, N., Aldridge, W., ... Keefe, F. J. (2009). A couple-based intervention for female breast cancer. *Psycho-Oncology*, *18*(3), 276–283. doi:10.1002/pon.1395 PMID:18702064

Baumgartner, R., Baumgartner, K., Irwin, M. L., McTiernan, A., Bernstein, L., Gilliland, F. D., ... Ballard-Barbash, R. (2004). Physical activity levels among breast cancer survivors. *Medicine and Science in Sports and Exercise, 36*(9), 1484-1491. Retrieved from http://www.ncbi.nlm.nih.gov/pmc/articles/PMC3000611/

Beasley, J. M., Newcomb, P. A., Trentham-Dietz, A., Hampton, J. M., Ceballos, R. M., Titus-Ernstoff, L., ... Holmes, M. D. (2010). Social networks and survival after breast cancer diagnosis. *Journal of Cancer Survivorship: Research and Practice*, *4*(4), 372–380. doi:10.100711764-010-0139-5 PMID:20652435

Bloom, J. R. (2002). Surviving and thriving? *Psycho-Oncology*, *11*(2), 89–92. doi:10.1002/pon.606 PMID:11921324

Bray, F., Ferlay, J., Soerjomataram, I., Siegel, R. L., Torre, L. A., & Jemal, A. (2018). Global cancer statistics 2018: GLOBOCAN estimates of incidence and mortality worldwide for 36 cancers in 185 countries. *CA: a Cancer Journal for Clinicians*, *68*(6), 394–424. doi:10.3322/caac.21492 PMID:30207593

Campbell-Enns, H., & Woodgate, R. (2015). The psychosocial experiences of women with breast cancer across the lifespan: A systematic review protocol. *JBI Database of Systematic Reviews and Implementation Reports*, *13*(1), 112–121. doi:10.11124/jbisrir-2015-1795 PMID:26447012

Cheung, Y. B., Luo, N., Ng, R., & Lee, C. F. (2014). Mapping the functional assessment of cancer therapy - Breast (FACT-B) to the 5-level EuroQoL group's 5-dimension questionnaire (EQ-5D-5L) utility index in a multi-ethnic Asian population. *Health and Quality of Life Outcomes*, *12*(1), 180. doi:10.118612955-014-0180-6 PMID:25495840

Dastan, N. B., & Buzlu, S. (2012). Psychoeducation intervention to improve adjustment to cancer among Turkish stage I-II breast cancer patients: A randomized controlled trial. *Asian Pacific Journal of Cancer Prevention, 13*(10), 5313–5318. doi:10.7314/APJCP.2012.13.10.5313 PMID:23244155

DeNysschen, C. A., Burton, H., Ademuyiwa, F., Levine, E., Tetewsky, S., & O'Connor, T. (2014). Exercise intervention in breast cancer patients with aromatase inhibitor-associated arthralgia: A pilot study. *European Journal of Cancer Care, 23*(4), 493–501. doi:10.1111/ecc.12155 PMID:24289215

DeSantis, C. E., Ma, J., Goding Sauer, A., Newman, L. A., & Jemal, A. (2017). Breast cancer statistics, 2017, racial disparity in mortality by state. *CA: a Cancer Journal for Clinicians, 67*(6), 439–448. doi:10.3322/caac.21412 PMID:28972651

Di Bella, O., Cocchiara, R. A., De Luca, A., Frusone, F., Aceti, V., Sestili, C., D'Egidio, V., Mannocci, … Torre, G.L (2018). Functional Assessment of Cancer Therapy Questionnaire for Breast Cancer (FACT-B+4): Italianversion validation. *Clin. Ter., 169*(4), e151-e154. doi:10.7417/T.2018.2071

Dieli-Conwright, C. M., Mortimer, J. E., Schroeder, E. T., Courneya, K., Demark-Wahnefried, W., Buchanan, T. A., ... Bernstein, L. (2014). Randomized controlled trial to evaluate the effects of combined progressive exercise on metabolic syndrome in breast cancer survivors: Rationale, design, and methods. *BMC Cancer, 14*(1), 238. doi:10.1186/1471-2407-14-238 PMID:24708832

Edwards, E., & Maxwell, M. (2002). Psychological interventions for women with metastatic breast cancer. Cochrane Database of Systematic Reviews, 44, 3137-3150. doi:10.1002/14651858.CD004253

El-Hashimi, D., & Gorey, K. M. (2019). Yoga-specific enhancement of quality of life among women with breast cancer: Systematic review and exploratory meta-analysis of randomized controlled trials. *Journal of Evidence-Based Integrative Medicine, 24*(6). doi:10.1177/2515690X19828325 PMID:30791697

Emaus, A., Veierod, M. B., Tretli, S., Finstad, S. E., Selmer, R., Furberg, A.-S., ... Thune, I. (2010). Metabolic profile, physical activity, and mortality in breast cancer patients. *Breast Cancer Research and Treatment, 121*(3), 651–660. doi:10.100710549-009-0603-y PMID:19882245

Escobar, A., Trujillo-Martín Mdel, M., Rueda, A., Pérez-Ruiz, E., Avis, N. E., & Bilbao, A. (2015). Cross-cultural adaptation, reliability and validity of the Spanish version of the Quality of Life in Adult Cancer Survivors (QLACS) questionnaire: application in a sample of short-term survivors. *Health Qual Life Outcomes, 13,* 182. doi:10.118612955-015-0378-2

Fekih-Romdhane, F., Henchiri, H., Ridha, R., Labbane, R., & Cheour, M. (2019). Niveau de détresse psychologique et de fardeau perçu chez les conjoints de femmes atteintes d'un cancer du sein. *L'Encéphale*, *45*(2), 190–192. doi:10.1016/j.encep.2018.09.003 PMID:30428997

Ferrer, R. A., Huedo-Medina, T. B., Johnson, B. T., Ryan, S., & Pescatello, L. S. (2011). Exercise interventions for cancer survivors: A meta-analysis of quality of life outcomes. *Annals of Behavioral Medicine*, *41*(1), 32–47. doi:10.100712160-010-9225-1 PMID:20931309

Friedenreich, C. M., & Cust, A. E. (2008). Physical activity and breast cancer risk: Impact of timing, type and dose of activity and population subgroup effects. *British Journal of Sports Medicine*, *42*(8), 636–647. doi:10.1136/bjsm.2006.029132 PMID:18487249

Galalae, R. M., Michel, J., Siebmann, J. U., Küchler, T., Eilf, K., & Kimmig, B. (2005). Significant negative impact of adjuvant chemotherapy on health-related quality of life (HR-QoL) in women with breast cancer treated by conserving surgery and postoperative 3-D radiotherapy. *Strahlentherapie und Onkologie*, *181*(10), 645–651. doi:10.100700066-005-1403-x PMID:16220403

Galway, K., Black, A., Cantwell, M., Cardwell, C. R., Mills, M., & Donnelly, M. (2012). Psychosocial interventions to improve quality of life and emotional wellbeing for recently diagnosed cancer patients. *Cochrane Database of Systematic Reviews*, *181*(10), 645–651. doi:10.1002/14651858.CD007064.pub2 PMID:23152241

Ganesh, S., Lye, M.-S., & Lau, F. N. (2016). Quality of life among breast cancer patients in Malaysia. *Asian Pacific Journal of Cancer Prevention*, *17*(4), 1677–1684. doi:10.7314/APJCP.2016.17.4.1677 PMID:27221837

Ganz, P. (2002). Quality of life in long-term, disease-free survivors of breast cancer: A follow-up study. *CancerSpectrum Knowledge Environment*, *94*(1), 39–49. PMID:11773281

Gordon, N. H., & Siminoff, L. A. (2010). Measuring quality of life of long-term breast cancer survivors: The long term quality of life - breast cancer (LTQOL-BC) scale. *Journal of Psychosocial Oncology*, *28*(6), 589–609. doi:10.1080/07347332.2010.516806 PMID:21058158

Goyal, N. G., Levine, B. J., Van Zee, K. J., Naftalis, E., & Avis, N. E. (2018). Trajectories of quality of life following breast cancer diagnosis. *Breast Cancer Res Treat.*, *169*(1), 163-173. doi:10.100710549-018-4677-2

Grimison, P. S., & Stockler, M. R. (2007). Quality of life and adjuvant systemic therapy for early-stage breast cancer. *Expert Review of Anticancer Therapy*, *7*(8), 1123–1134. doi:10.1586/14737140.7.8.1123 PMID:18028021

Hahn, E. A., Segawa, E., Kaiser, K., Cella, D., & Smith, B. D. (2015). Validation of the Functional Assessment of Cancer Therapy-Breast (FACT-B) quality of life instrument. *Journal of Clinical Oncology*, *33*(15suppl), e17753–e17753. doi:10.1200/jco.2015.33.15_suppl.e17753

Hojan, K., Molińska-Glura, M., & Milecki, P. (2013). Physical activity and body composition, body physique, and quality of life in premenopausal breast cancer patients during endocrine therapy: A feasibility study. *Acta Oncologica*, *52*(2), 319–326. doi:10.3109/0284186X.2012.744468 PMID:23193959

Hopwood, P., Haviland, J., Mills, J., Sumo, G., & Bliss, J. (2007). The impact of age and clinical factors on quality of life in early breast cancer: An analysis of 2208 women recruited to the UK START Trial (Standardisation of Breast Radiotherapy Trial). *The Breast*, *16*(3), 241–251. doi:10.1016/j.breast.2006.11.003 PMID:17236771

Hwang, S. Y., Chang, S. J., & Park, B.-W. (2013). Does chemotherapy really affect the quality of life of women with breast cancer? *Journal of Breast Cancer*, *16*(2), 229. doi:10.4048/jbc.2013.16.2.229 PMID:23843858

Ibrahim, E. M., & Al-Homaidh, A. (2011). Physical activity and survival after breast cancer diagnosis: Meta-analysis of published studies. *Medical Oncology (Northwood, London, England)*, *28*(3), 753–765. doi:10.100712032-010-9536-x PMID:20411366

Inagaki, M., Yoshikawa, E., Matsuoka, Y., Sugawara, Y., Nakano, T., Akechi, T., ... Uchitomi, Y. (2006). Smaller regional volumes of brain gray and white matter demonstrated in breast cancer survivors exposed to adjuvant chemotherapy. *Cancer*, *109*(1), 146–156. doi:10.1002/cncr.22368 PMID:17131349

Inan, F. S., & Ustun, B. (2019). After the pychoeducational intervention: Turkish breast cancer survivors' experiences. *European Journal of Breast Health*, *15*(1), 37–42. doi:10.5152/ejbh.2018.4255 PMID:30816352

Irwin, M. L., Crumley, D., McTiernan, A., Bernstein, L., Baumgartner, R., Gilliland, F. D., ... Ballard-Barbash, R. (2003). Physical activity levels before and after a diagnosis of breast carcinoma. *Cancer*, *97*(7), 1746–1757. doi:10.1002/cncr.11227 PMID:12655532

Jafari, N., Farajzadegan, Z., Zamani, A., Bahrami, F., Emami, H., & Loghmani, A. (2013). Spiritual well-being and quality of life in Iranian women with breast cancer undergoing radiation therapy. *Support Care Cancer, 21*(5), 1219-1225. doi:10.100700520-012-1650-1

Janelsins, M. C., Davis, P. G., Wideman, L., Katula, J. A., Sprod, L. K., Peppone, L. J., ... Mustian, K. M. (2011). Effects of tai chi chuan on insulin and cytokine levels in a randomized controlled pilot study on breast cancer survivors. *Clinical Breast Cancer, 11*(3), 161–170. doi:10.1016/j.clbc.2011.03.013 PMID:21665136

Jeong, Y., Kim, J. Y., Ryu, J. S., Lee, K. E., Ha, E. H., & Park, H. (2010). The associations between social support, health-related behaviors, socioeconomic status and depression in medical students. *Epidemiology and Health, 32*, e2010009. doi:10.4178/epih/e2010009 PMID:21191462

Johannsen, M., O'Connor, M., O'Toole, M. S., Jensen, A. B., Hojris, I., & Zachariae, R. (2016). Efficacy of mindfulness-based cognitive therapy on late post-treatment pain in women treated for primary breast cancer: A randomized controlled trial. *Journal of Clinical Oncology, 34*(28), 3390–3399. doi:10.1200/JCO.2015.65.0770 PMID:27325850

Jong, M. C., Boers, I., Schouten van der Velden, A. P., van der Meij, S., Göker, E., Timmer-Bonte, A. N. J. H., & van Wietmarschen, H. A. (2018). A randomized study of yoga for fatigue and quality of life in women with breast cancer undergoing (neo) adjuvant chemotherapy. *Journal of Alternative and Complementary Medicine (New York, N.Y.), 24*(9-10), 942–953. doi:10.1089/acm.2018.0191 PMID:30247961

Juvet, L. K., Elvsaas, I.-K. Ø., Leivseth, G., Anker, G., Bertheussen, G. F., Falkmer, U., … Norderhaug, I. N. (2009). Rehabilitation of breast cancer patients. *Rehabilitation of Breast Cancer Patients*. Retrieved from http://www.ncbi.nlm.nih.gov/pubmed/29319956

Kara, B., & Kaya, G. (2017). Functional status and associated factors in patients with colon cancer receiving chemotherapy. *Journal of Archives in Military Medicine*, 372-380. doi:10.5812/jamm.11882

Knobf, M. T., Thompson, A. S., Fennie, K., & Erdos, D. (2014). The effect of a community-based exercise intervention on symptoms and quality of life. *Cancer Nursing, 37*(2), E43–E50. doi:10.1097/NCC.0b013e318288d40e PMID:23519041

Kroenke, C. H., Kubzansky, L. D., Schernhammer, E. S., Holmes, M. D., & Kawachi, I. (2006). Social networks, social support, and survival after breast cancer diagnosis. *Journal of Clinical Oncology, 24*(7), 1105–1111. doi:10.1200/JCO.2005.04.2846 PMID:16505430

Kroenke, C. H., Quesenberry, C., Kwan, M. L., Sweeney, C., Castillo, A., & Caan, B. J. (2013). Social networks, social support, and burden in relationships, and mortality after breast cancer diagnosis in the Life After Breast Cancer Epidemiology (LACE) study. *Breast Cancer Research and Treatment*, *137*(1), 261–271. doi:10.100710549-012-2253-8 PMID:23143212

Kushi, L. H., Doyle, C., McCullough, M., Rock, C. L., Demark-Wahnefried, W., Bandera, E. V., ... Gansler, T. (2012). American Cancer Society guidelines on nutrition and physical activity for cancer prevention. *CA: a Cancer Journal for Clinicians*, *62*(1), 30–67. doi:10.3322/caac.20140 PMID:22237782

Lahart, I. M., Metsios, G. S., Nevill, A. M., & Carmichael, A. R. (2015). Physical activity, risk of death and recurrence in breast cancer survivors: A systematic review and meta-analysis of epidemiological studies. *Acta Oncologica*, *54*(5), 635–654. doi:10.3109/0284186X.2014.998275 PMID:25752971

Lahart, I. M., Metsios, G. S., Nevill, A. M., & Carmichael, A. R. (2018). Physical activity for women with breast cancer after adjuvant therapy. *Cochrane Database of Systematic Reviews*, *1*(1), CD011292. doi:10.1002/14651858.CD011292.pub2 PMID:29376559

Lash, T. L., & Silliman, R. A. (2002). Long-term follow-up of upper-body function among breast cancer survivors. *The Breast Journal*, *8*(1), 28–33. doi:10.1046/j.1524-4741.2002.08006.x PMID:11856158

Leung, J., Pachana, N. A., & McLaughlin, D. (2014). Social support and health-related quality of life in women with breast cancer: A longitudinal study. *Psycho-Oncology*, *23*(9), 1014–1020. doi:10.1002/pon.3523 PMID:24700668

Loftus, L. S., Sokol, G. H., & Laronga, C. (2017). Breast cancer survivorship: Patient characteristics and plans for high-quality care. *Southern Medical Journal*, *110*(10), 673–677. doi:10.14423/SMJ.0000000000000701 PMID:28973710

Manne, S., Ostroff, J., Rini, C., Fox, K., Goldstein, L., & Grana, G. (2004). The interpersonal process model of intimacy: The role of self-disclosure, partner disclosure, and partner responsiveness in interactions between breast cancer patients and their partners. *Journal of Family Psychology*, *18*(4), 589–599. doi:10.1037/0893-3200.18.4.589 PMID:15598164

Manne, S. L., Ostroff, J. S., Norton, T. R., Fox, K., Goldstein, L., & Grana, G. (2006). Cancer-related relationship communication in couples coping with early stage breast cancer. *Psycho-Oncology*, *15*(3), 234–247. doi:10.1002/pon.941 PMID:15926198

Manne, S. L., Siegel, S. D., Heckman, C. J., & Kashy, D. A. (2016). A randomized clinical trial of a supportive versus a skill-based couple-focused group intervention for breast cancer patients. *Journal of Consulting and Clinical Psychology*, *84*(8), 668–681. doi:10.1037/ccp0000110 PMID:27228264

Matsuda, A., Yamaoka, K., Tango, T., Matsuda, T., & Nishimoto, H. (2014). Effectiveness of psychoeducational support on quality of life in early-stage breast cancer patients: A systematic review and meta-analysis of randomized controlled trials. *Quality of Life Research: An International Journal of Quality of Life Aspects of Treatment, Care and Rehabilitation*, *23*(1), 21–30. doi:10.100711136-013-0460-3 PMID:23881515

Mendes-Santos, C., Weiderpass, E., Santana, R., & Andersson, G. (2019). A guided internet-delivered individually-tailored ACT-influenced cognitive behavioural intervention to improve psychosocial outcomes in breast cancer survivors (iNNOVBC): Study protocol. *Internet Interventions*, *17*(1), 100236. doi:10.1016/j.invent.2019.01.004 PMID:30949435

Meneses-Echávez, J. F., González-Jiménez, E., & Ramírez-Vélez, R. (2015). Effects of supervised exercise on cancer-related fatigue in breast cancer survivors: A systematic review and meta-analysis. *BMC Cancer*, *15*(1), 77. doi:10.118612885-015-1069-4 PMID:25885168

Montazeri, A. (2008). Health-related quality of life in breast cancer patients: A bibliographic review of the literature from 1974 to 2007. *Journal of Experimental & Clinical Cancer Research*, *27*(1), 32. doi:10.1186/1756-9966-27-32 PMID:18759983

Musiat, P., & Tarrier, N. (2014). Collateral outcomes in e-mental health: A systematic review of the evidence for added benefits of computerized cognitive behavior therapy interventions for mental health. *Psychological Medicine*, *44*(15), 3137–3150. doi:10.1017/S0033291714000245 PMID:25065947

Mustafa, M., Carson-Stevens, A., Gillespie, D., & Edwards, A. G. (2013). Psychological interventions for women with metastatic breast cancer. *Cochrane Database of Systematic Reviews*, *4*(6), CD004253. doi:10.1002/14651858.CD004253.pub4 PMID:23737397

Muszalik, M., Kołucka-Pluta, M., Kędziora-Kornatowska, K., & Robaczewska, J. (2016). Quality of life of women with breast cancer undergoing radiotherapy using the Functional Assessment of Chronic Illness Therapy-Fatigue questionnaire. *Clinical Interventions in Aging*, *11*, 1489–1494. doi:10.2147/CIA.S113530 PMID:27799754

Namkoong, K., McLaughlin, B., Yoo, W., Hull, S. J., Shah, D. V., Kim, S. C., ... Gustafson, D. H. (2013). … Gustafson, D. H. (2013). The effects of expression: How providing emotional support online improves cancer patients' coping strategies. *Journal of the National Cancer Institute. Monographs*, *2013*(47), 169–174. doi:10.1093/jncimonographs/lgt033 PMID:24395987

Nguyen, J., Popovic, M., Chow, E., Cella, D., Beaumont, J. L., Chu, D., ... Bottomley, A. (2015). EORTC QLQ-BR23 and FACT-B for the assessment of quality of life in patients with breast cancer: A literature review. *Journal of Comparative Effectiveness Research*, *4*(2), 157–166. doi:10.2217/cer.14.76 PMID:25825844

O'Toole, J. A., Ferguson, C. M., Swaroop, M. N., Horick, N., Skolny, M. N., Brunelle, C. L., ... Taghian, A. G. (2015). The impact of breast cancer-related lymphedema on the ability to perform upper extremity activities of daily living. *Breast Cancer Research and Treatment*, *150*(2), 381–388. doi:10.100710549-015-3325-3 PMID:25749734

Paterson, C. L., Lengacher, C. A., Donovan, K. A., Kip, K. E., & Tofthagen, C. S. (2015). Body image in younger breast cancer survivors. *Cancer Nursing*, *31*(2), 1. doi:10.1097/NCC.0000000000000251 PMID:25881807

Paulo, T. R. S., Rossi, F. E., Viezel, J., Tosello, G. T., Seidinger, S. C., Simões, R. R., ... Freitas, I. F. (2019). The impact of an exercise program on quality of life in older breast cancer survivors undergoing aromatase inhibitor therapy: A randomized controlled trial. *Health and Quality of Life Outcomes*, *17*(1), 17. doi:10.118612955-019-1090-4 PMID:30658629

Peterson, L. L., & Ligibel, J. A. (2018). Physical activity and breast cancer: An opportunity to improve outcomes. *Current Oncology Reports*, *20*(7), 50. doi:10.100711912-018-0702-1 PMID:29713835

Pinto-Carral, A., Molina, A. J., de Pedro, Á., & Ayán, C. (2018). Pilates for women with breast cancer: A systematic review and meta-analysis. *Complementary Therapies in Medicine*, *41*(7), 130–140. doi:10.1016/j.ctim.2018.09.011 PMID:30477829

Regan, T., Levesque, J. V., Lambert, S. D., & Kelly, B. (2015). A qualitative investigation of health care professionals', patients' and partners' views on psychosocial issues and related interventions for couples coping with cancer. *PLoS One*, *10*(7), e0133837. doi:10.1371/journal.pone.0133837 PMID:26222890

Rietman, J. S., Dijkstra, P. U., Debreczeni, R., Geertzen, J. H., Robinson, D. P., & de Vries, J. (2004). Impairments, disabilities and health related quality of life after treatment for breast cancer: A follow-up study 2.7 years after surgery. *Disability and Rehabilitation*, *26*(2), 78–84. doi:10.1080/09638280310001629642 PMID:14668143

Rottmann, N., Dalton, S. O., Christensen, J., Frederiksen, K., & Johansen, C. (2010). Self-efficacy, adjustment style and well-being in breast cancer patients: A longitudinal study. *Quality of Life Research: An International Journal of Quality of Life Aspects of Treatment, Care and Rehabilitation, 19*(6), 827–836. doi:10.100711136-010-9653-1 PMID:20401551

Saki, A., Ebrahim, H., & Tehranian, N. (2011, January 1). Evaluating the risk factors of breast cancer using the analysis of tree models. *OFOGH-E-DANESH, 17*(2), 61-68. Retrieved from https://www.sid.ir/en/journal/ViewPaper.aspx?id=196820

Şener, H. Ö., Malkoç, M., Ergin, G., Karadibak, D., & Yavuzşen, T. (2017). Effects of clinical Pilates exercises on patients Developing lymphedema after breast cancer treatment: A randomized clinical trial. *The Journal of Breast Health, 13*(1), 16–22. doi:10.5152/tjbh.2016.3136 PMID:28331763

Simpionato De Paula, É., Castanheira Nascimento, L., Melani, S., & Rocha, M. (n.d.). *The influence of social support on strengthening families of children with chronic renal failure.* Retrieved from www.eerp.usp.br/rlae

Sohl, S. J., Levine, B., & Avis, N. E. (2015). Evaluation of the quality of life in adult cancer survivors (QLACS) scale for early post-treatment breast cancer survivors. *Quality of Life Research: An International Journal of Quality of Life Aspects of Treatment, Care and Rehabilitation, 24*(1), 205–212. doi:10.100711136-014-0749-x PMID:24996392

Spatuzzi, R., Vespa, A., Lorenzi, P., Miccinesi, G., Ricciuti, M., Cifarelli, W., ... Aieta, M. (2016). Evaluation of social support, quality of life, and body image in women with breast cancer. *Breast Care (Basel, Switzerland), 11*(1), 28–32. doi:10.1159/000443493 PMID:27051393

Stephen, J., Rojubally, A., Macgregor, K., McLeod, D., Speca, M., Taylor-Brown, J., ... Mackenzie, G. (2013). Evaluation of CancerChatCanada: A program of online support for Canadians affected by cancer. *Current Oncology (Toronto, Ont.), 20*(1), 39–47. doi:10.3747/co.20.1210 PMID:23443892

Sternfeld, B., Weltzien, E., Quesenberry, C. P. Jr, Castillo, A. L., Kwan, M., Slattery, M. L., & Caan, B. J. (2009). Physical activity and risk of recurrence and mortality in breast cancer survivors: Findings from the LACE study. *Cancer Epidemiology, Biomarkers & Prevention, 18*(1), 87–95. doi:10.1158/1055-9965.EPI-08-0595 PMID:19124485

Sudarshan, M., Petrucci, A., Dumitra, S., Duplisea, J., Wexler, S., & Meterissian, S. (2013). Yoga therapy for breast cancer patients: A prospective cohort study. *Complementary Therapies in Clinical Practice*, *19*(4), 227–229. doi:10.1016/j.ctcp.2013.06.004 PMID:24199978

Tan, M. L., Idris, D. B., Teo, L. W., Loh, S. Y., Seow, G. C., Chia, Y. Y., & Tin, A. S. (2014). Validation of EORTC QLQ-C30 and QLQ-BR23 questionnaires in the measurement of quality of life of breast cancer patients in Singapore. *Asia-Pacific Journal of Oncology Nursing*, *1*(1), 22-32. doi:10.4103/2347-5625.135817

Tao, Z., Shi, A., Lu, C., Song, T., Zhang, Z., & Zhao, J. (2015). Breast cancer: Epidemiology and etiology. *Cell Biochemistry and Biophysics*, *72*(2), 333–338. doi:10.100712013-014-0459-6 PMID:25543329

Teven, C. M., Schmid, D. B., Sisco, M., Ward, J., & Howard, M. A. (2017). Systemic therapy for early-stage breast cancer: What the plastic surgeon should know. *Eplasty*, *17*, e7. PMID:28293332

Thomas, G. A., Cartmel, B., Harrigan, M., Fiellin, M., Capozza, S., Zhou, Y., ... Irwin, M. L. (2016). The effect of exercise on body composition and bone mineral density in breast Cancer survivors taking aromatase inhibitors. *The Observatory Journal*, *1*, 1–6. PMID:28026901

Traore, B. M., El Fakir, S., Charaka, H., Benaicha, N., Najdi, A., Zidouh, A., . . . Nejjari, C. (2018). Evolution of quality of life in patients with breast cancer during the first year of follow-up in Morocco. *BMC Cancer*, *18*(1), 109. doi:10.118612885-018-4008-3

van der Willik, K. D., Koppelmans, V., Hauptmann, M., Compter, A., Ikram, M. A., & Schagen, S. B. (2018). Inflammation markers and cognitive performance in breast cancer survivors 20 years after completion of chemotherapy: A cohort study. *Breast Cancer Research: BCR*, *20*(1), 135. doi:10.118613058-018-1062-3 PMID:30442190

van Londen, G. J., Perera, S., Vujevich, K., Rastogi, P., Lembersky, B., Brufsky, A., ... Greenspan, S. L. (2011). The impact of an aromatase inhibitor on body composition and gonadal hormone levels in women with breast cancer. *Breast Cancer Research and Treatment*, *125*(2), 441–446. doi:10.100710549-010-1223-2 PMID:21046232

van Nes, J. G. H., Fontein, D. B. Y., Hille, E. T. M., Voskuil, D. W., van Leeuwen, F. E., de Haes, J. C. J. M., ... van de Velde, C. J. H. (2012). Quality of life in relation to tamoxifen or exemestane treatment in postmenopausal breast cancer patients: A Tamoxifen Exemestane Adjuvant Multinational (TEAM) trial side study. *Breast Cancer Research and Treatment*, *134*(1), 267–276. doi:10.100710549-012-2028-2 PMID:22453754 van Vulpen, J. K., Peeters, P. H. M., Velthuis, M. J., van der Wall, E., & May, A. M. (2016). Effects of physical exercise during adjuvant breast cancer treatment on physical and psychosocial dimensions of cancer-related fatigue: A meta-analysis. *Maturitas*, *85*(4), 104–111. doi:10.1016/j.maturitas.2015.12.007 PMID:26857888

Whelan, T. J., Levine, M., Julian, J., Kirkbride, P., & Skingley, P. (2000). The effects of radiation therapy on quality of life of women with breast carcinoma: Results of a randomized trial. Ontario Clinical Oncology Group. *Cancer*, *88*(10), 2260–2266. doi:10.1002/(SICI)1097-0142(20000515)88:10<2260::AID-CNCR9>3.0.CO;2-M PMID:10820347

WHO. (2018). Breast cancer. *WHO*. Retrieved from https://www.who.int/cancer/prevention/diagnosis-screening/breast-cancer/en/

Winzelberg, A. J., Classen, C., Alpers, G. W., Roberts, H., Koopman, C., Adams, R. E., ... Taylor, C. B. (2003). Evaluation of an internet support group for women with primary breast cancer. *Cancer*, *97*(5), 1164–1173. doi:10.1002/cncr.11174 PMID:12599221

Xiao, C., Miller, A. H., Felger, J., Mister, D., Liu, T., & Torres, M. A. (2016). A prospective study of quality of life in breast cancer patients undergoing radiation therapy. *Adv Radiat Oncol.*, *1*(1), 10–16. doi:10.1016/j.adro.2016.01.003 PMID:27453954

Xiao, F., Song, X., Chen, Q., Dai, Y., Xu, R., Qiu, C., & Guo, Q. (2017). Effectiveness of psychological interventions on depression in patients after breast cancer surgery: A meta-analysis of randomized controlled trials. *Clinical Breast Cancer*, *17*(3), 171–179. doi:10.1016/j.clbc.2016.11.003 PMID:28040415

Yan, B., Yang, L. M., Hao, L. P., Yang, C., Quan, L., Wang, L. H., . . . Yuan, J. M. (2016). Determinants of quality of life for breast cancer patients in Shanghai, China. *PLoS One*, *11*(4), e0153714. doi:10.1371/journal.pone.0153714

Yucel, B., Akkaş, E. A., Okur, Y., Eren, A. A., Eren, M. F., Karapinar, H., . . . Kiliçkap, S. (2014). The impact of radiotherapy on quality of life for cancer patients: a longitudinal study. *Support Care Cancer, 22*(9), 2479-2487. doi:10.100700520-014-2235-y

Zhang, H., Zhao, Q., Cao, P., & Ren, G. (2017). Resilience and quality of life: Exploring the mediator role of social support in patients with breast cancer. *Medical Science Monitor: International Medical Journal of Experimental and Clinical Research, 23*, 5969-5979. doi:10.12659/msm.907730

Chapter 5
Autism Spectrum Disorders:
A Systematic Review From the Perspective of Computer-Assisted Developments

Vikas Khullar
https://orcid.org/0000-0002-0404-3652
CT Institute of Engineering, Management, and Technology, Jalandhar, India

Harjit Pal Singh
CT Institute of Engineering, Management, and Technology, Jalandhar, India

Manju Bala
Khalsa College of Engineering and Technology, Amritsar, India

ABSTRACT

In the area of psychosis, autism spectrum disorder (ASD) is a mental disorder included with the major deficits associated with social interaction, communication, and repetitive or stereotypical behavior. A large number of computer-assisted approaches have been developed over the last few decades to improve the lifestyle of the subject with ASD. The aim of this study is to provide a detailed review of computational advancements for ASD interventions. This chapter summarizes the basic theories in autism and also discusses the technological developments of autism in the present era. With the enrichment in technological developments, researchers and experts focused on the monitoring and improvement of the skills (social, communication, and behavioral) in individuals with autism-related disorders. In conclusion, the work presented in this chapter summarizes that the evolutionary computational interventions have a remarkable possibility for the monitoring and basic skills enhancement in ASD.

DOI: 10.4018/978-1-7998-1185-5.ch005

INTRODUCTION

In the area of psychosis, Autism Spectrum Disorder (ASD) is a complex and fascinating mental disorder. It included the major deficits associated with social interaction, communication, and repetitive or stereotypical behavior (Diagnostic and Statistical Manual of Mental Disorders -Fifth Edition, 2013). Throughout their life, considerable challenges are there to both the individual with autism and their family. In 1943, Dr. Leo Kanner was the first author that phrased the Autistic disorder as a distinct entity (Kanner, 1943). Since then, the dramatic increase (from 4-5 in 10000 to 1 in 59) has been recorded in Autistic cases in various geographical locations across the world (Baio et al., 2018; Bonnet-Brilhault, 2017; Loucas et al., 2008; Ratajczak, 2011). Initially, the prevalence associated with autism was in the range of 3.3 to 16 per 10,000 (Wing, 1993). The recent report presented by Autism and Developmental Disabilities Monitoring Network in America, the percentage of ASD affected children is 1 in 59 ("Data & Statistics on Autism Spectrum Disorder," 2019). The statistics provided by the Rehabilitation Council of India (Barua & Daley, 2001) stated the prevalence rate in India can be 1 in 500 people or more than 2,160,000 people. The low awareness about autism diagnosis in India is a major cause of the low prevalence rate in India.

In the present era, computer-assisted technological research for autism has been divided into several interlinked and inter-trade chapters. Some studies were related to enhancing the knowledge of autistics, where others were dealing with autistic behavioral improvement along with its techniques. This age had highly favored for the use of advanced technological tools for supporting ASD's such as augmented systems, sensor technologies, artificial intelligence, virtual reality, etc. The utilization of interventions for ASD has been highly recommended by the authors. The year 2011 onwards, advance and evolutionary computation dependent areas (such as software development, robotics, video modeling, internetworking, artificial intelligence, virtual reality, etc.) are now highly being used as a part of ASD intervention. As per present trends, automated environments are the first preference of researchers.

The main objective of this chapter is to present the technology-wise computer-assisted developments from the early stages of computer technology in evolutionary computational development. During this era, internet-connected systems; intelligent systems and robotic systems have been playing a vital role in the communication and behavior improvement of ASD's. This chapter is organized into different sections based on the types of computer-assistive technologies. In the initial sections, a detailed explanation about autism and its behavioral issues has discussed. Then the role of computer-assisted technologies has presented in proceeding section. Further sections are detailing for computer-assisted interventions starting from the initial understanding till the presently using evolutionary computer-assisted interventions.

BEHAVIORAL CHARACTERISTICS OF ASD

Typical or normally developing children are behaving normally as they are socially interactive; gazing at faces; respond on the voices; replying gestures; immediate react of events; have an attachment to caregivers; can do physically normal activities; attract or enjoying socially towards other children, etc (Bentenuto, De Falco, & Venuti, 2016; Must et al., 2014; Rutgers et al., 2007). However in the case of ASD, children are socially inactive, slow motor skills, the deficit in formal or informal language, behave repetitively/ stereotypically actions or communications, etc. The detailed symptoms of autism have included lack of eye contact, lack of social responses, no attachment to caregivers, delayed motor skills, poor response to calling, failure to respond gestures, language delay, unusual physical control/ coordination, unusual attachment with object, lack of imaginative/pretend play, not interested in playing with other children, absence of nonverbal communication, anxious behavior, repetitive responses, etc (Dawson, Meltzoff, Osterling, & Rinaldi, 2006; Diagnostic and Statistical Manual of Mental Disorders (Fifth Edition), 2013; Diagnostic and Statistical Manual of Mental Disorders (Fourth Edition), 1994; Hazen, Stornelli, O'Rourke, Koesterer, & McDougle, 2014; Klin, Jones, Schultz, & Volkmar, 2003; Seltzer et al., 2003; Wing & Gould, 1979). As other correlating impairments, ASD has also identified as attached with unpredictable behavior, tantrum, meltdown, intellectual disability, seizures, attention-deficit/hyperactivity disorder, anxiety, etc (Ames & Fletcher-Watson, 2010; Klin et al., 2003; Rutherford, Pennington, & Rogers, 2006; Wing & Gould, 1979). With the help of above-surveyed literature, Table 1 had drawn to define some major syndromes related to ASD and its characteristics as discussed by DSM-V in detail.

ROLE OF COMPUTER ASSISTED TECHNOLOGIES IN ASD

The computer-assisted technologies are working with the broadening scope in comparison to the manual or other technological methods. Some individual with autism never developed their communication & other behavioral skills and they require continues support which is difficult for a human caretaker or professional. ASD persons have too much reserved behavior during interaction with other humans which leads to difficulty in therapy or other treatments. But children with autism are having a keen interest in objects like display screens, mobile instruments, and other personalized objects, etc.

Manual card or mechanical/ electrical machine based instruments have a very limited scope of operation, such as in 1961, the electrically connected automatic controlled environment was utilized (Ferster & Demyer, 1961) for measuring the

Table 1. Syndromes related to ASD and its Characteristics as discussed by DSM-V

Impairment	Responses
Lack of social interaction	Eye to eye gaze
	Unusual facial expression
	Inappropriate body posture
	Lack of gestures for social interaction
	Pear relationship development failure
	Lack of share enjoyment and interests
	Lack of social & emotional reciprocity
Lack of communication	Delay in the development of spoken language
	Disability to maintain a conversation with others
Repetitive and stereotypic behavior	Idiotic activities
	Pretend/ imaginative play
	Inflexible rituals
	Stereotyped, restricted and repetitive motor movements

Source: Diagnostic and Statistical Manual of Mental Disorders -Fifth Edition (2013)

performance of autistics. The experiments were operated on the basis of electrically controlled machines such as candy vending machines, phonograph, colorful kaleidoscope, pinball machine. The lacks in such machines are that they are not easy to operate or maintain and also not precise enough. Another author had worked to identify the verbal ability of the autistic children by using a manual paper printed "Peabody Picture Vocabulary Test" (Aurnhammer-frith, 1969). The paper-based systems are difficult to preserve and recollect. The significance of initial screening is core to conduct the detailed diagnostic procedure to ascertain the concrete and concerned information. With manual screening tools and diagnostic criteria, it is very difficult to differentiate between different psychoses issues by non-professionals. The professional automated ASD screening and diagnostic tools are highly required for identifying the correct signs and symptoms through the behavioral observation and assessment questionnaires or tests, which also reduces the risk of human error. Manual printed card-based Picture Exchange Communication System (PECS) was utilized for identifying the relationship between different parameters of verbal communication (Carr & Felce, 2007; Jennifer B. Ganz & Simpson, 2004).

To overcome the problems governed by manual or electromechanical systems, the computer-assisted technologies have presently opened the door of the new acceptable world of interventions. In earlier phases of computer-assisted interventions, Colby had incorporated computer-controlled equipment for teaching nonspeaking children. As compared to non-computer interventions for behavioral improvement, the computer-controlled environment had been reflected the significant change in lesser intervention time (Colby, 1967). Due to logical, non-frightening, highest tolerance and steady nature, the computer had suggested as an approved entry in the environment of Autism that provides accurate responses (Panyan, 1984; Plienis & Romanczyk, 1985). Autistics reacted more comfortably during interaction with a computer than a human. The result of computer-based learning systems had also enhanced the response in autistics (Frost, 1981; Goldenberg, 1979). Authors had also made a positive view to utilizing computer-based instructions is been potentially reduced the learning insufficiency in the autistic students. In other theories, autistics had enjoyed the use of the internet and also had been shown their improved interest in social connections through social websites (Gillespie-Lynch, Kapp, Shane-Simpson, Smith, & Hutman, 2014).

Traditionally computer has been reflected as a desktop or laptop device, but today computers represent any electronic device that works with high-speed data like smart-phones, smart-watches, tablets, other data processing, and internet-connected devices, etc. in ASD, the use of computers for enhancing the academic, behavioral, and social outcomes is a relatively new area of research with great potential. Initially, authors had worked to identify the positive impacts of the clinical utilization of computer-assisted interventions for treating ASD patients. In the present era, computing and related technological interventions are playing a vital role to understand the psychosis and cognition allied complications, where ASD is the fastest-growing neurodevelopmental disorder across the world (Ardhanareeswarana & Volkmar, 2015; Bonnet-Brilhault, 2017).

At present, machines are able to interact with humans through their audio emotions, video expressions, physiological expressions, etc. That emerging area in computing technologies said to be effective by improvising with the psychology and cognition related theories. In the affective computing machine adapts the human state and respond accordingly may be in real-time. There some features are mentioned that promoted the utilization of Computer-Assisted technologies for helping ASD are highlighted as follows (Begoli, DeFalco, & Ogle, 2016; Gillespie-Lynch et al., 2014; Plienis & Romanczyk, 1985):

1. Logical, accurate, non-frightening, highest tolerance and steady in responses.
2. Controllable due to governing by predefined rules.
3. High-speed data storage and processing.
4. Handheld and wearable devices those are easy to carry.
5. Artificially intelligent machines are able to make decisions and also can work as assistive-devices.
6. Able to create a virtual scenario.
7. Real-time communication with the internet

8. ASDs are feeling comfortable during interaction with electronic devices.
9. Co-tropical interaction with individuals with ASD

COMPUTER-ASSISTED DEVELOPMENTS IN ASD

This section has focused on the initial understanding of the computer-assisted intervention in autism to the evolutionary interventions has been summarized in the present work. This chapter is further divided into computer-assisted technology-wise developments in autism, such as early Computer-Assisted Multimedia & Multidimensional Technologies, Computer-Assisted Handheld & Wearable Technologies, Computer-Assisted Games, Humanoids & Robots, Computer-Assisted Online Systems & Internet Connected Devices, etc.

Computer-Assisted Multimedia and Multidimensional Video Technologies

Multimedia systems potentially have an important role to work on skill enhancement of subjects with autism. A lot of tasks for the multimedia interventions had accomplished by authors, but still, it has been largely unexplored. During the initial phases, the basic graphics designing and graphics programming languages had an important role in the area of autism. Goldenberg in 1979 had used LOGO which was a graphics-oriented computer language for children and provided playful for the serious treatment of language manipulation (Goldenberg, 1987). In 1987, Interactive boards had impacted positively for improving the language, behavior, and participation in the social community. The author had raised 25% improvement in Autistic responses in comparison to the defined baseline. In the boon era of computation, Higgins and Boone had suggested guidelines for the development of different software for Autistics in consideration for cognitive ability, task variation, over selectivity, multiple cues, etc (Higgins & Boone, 1996). For functional living skills, Instruction with video modeling methods has been utilized to train the autistics. Here improvement in autistics had been observed as the number of correct replies related to skill acquisition (Shipley-Benamou, Lutzker, & Taubman, 2002). The augmentative and alternative system of communication (AAC) is playing a major role in the improvement of verbal and non-verbal communication. In enhancement, experiments had been conducted for analyzing the impact on their learning using aided and non-aided devices (such as electronic voice-based output communication aids, miniature objects, communication boards, manual signs, natural gestures) (Sigafoos & Drasgow, 2001). Autistics had more interest in software utilization as sensory support in comparison to the traditional supports (Bernard-Opitz,

Figure 1. Component of computer training procedure
Source: Kinney et al. (2003)

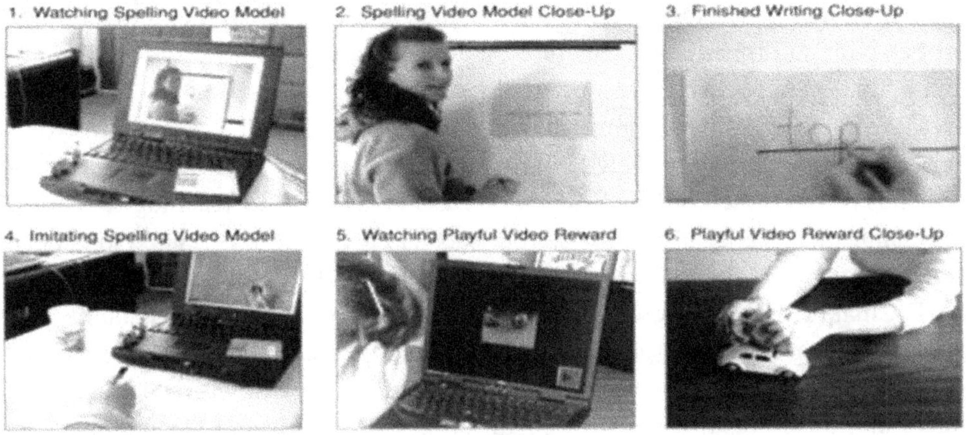
1. Watching Spelling Video Model
2. Spelling Video Model Close-Up
3. Finished Writing Close-Up
4. Imitating Spelling Video Model
5. Watching Playful Video Reward
6. Playful Video Reward Close-Up

Sriram, & Nakhoda-Sapuan, 2001). For removing the communicative barriers, a computer-based software intervention including constructed or unconstructed tasks was developed. Improvement in functional communicative skills of the Autistics had also been recorded during conducted training on computer-based interventions (Hetzroni & Tannous, 2004).

Corbett, 2003 had used video modeling to enhance the socio-emotions, sensitivity and observation skills of the Autistic children. The results highlighted that the autistics had gained 51% in case of social-emotional reorganization. By incorporating facial emotion included photographs, 18% of the audio tone had also improved in autistics (Corbett, 2003). Using photographs of toys or other objects in video, authors had worked on "how to spell and reward video" for the writing of correct spelling which had resulted in the significant improvement in autistics (Kinney, Vedora, & Stromer, 2003). In 2003, Kinney had also used computerized video training models for the improvement of spelling learning capabilities in Autistics as presented in Figure 1.

By adding live-prompting in video modeling for making correct replies, the motor and vocal responses of Autistic children had also improved (LeBlanc et al., 2003). Further by adding video with self-modeling technique, improvement in the frequency of spontaneous requests and replies had been observed(Wert & Neisworth, 2003). Further, computer-based structural visual biases or spatiotemporal contingency tasks had also used for measuring response time or performance of autistics (Iarocci, Burack, Shore, Mottron, & Enns, 2006). Here, a computer screen was used to display the combinations of two black and two white dots to represent local (Black-White-Black-White) and global level (Black-Black-White-White). The findings suggested that the Autistics were able to perform well during structural visual like images and figures. But ASD had performed poorly in the case of difficult and changeable objects included faces, emotions, etc. Other researchers had designed some computer-based social stories and simulative environment for rectification in the behavior and functional skills of each autistic participant (Sansosti & Powell-Smith, 2008) (Ayres, Maguire, & McClimon, 2009).

The enhanced milieu teaching (manipulated stimuli) included prerecorded voice messages in VOCA that reflected improvements in the communication behavior of Autistics (Olive et al., 2007). AAC based PECS was used for teaching functional communication ability of Autistics. Four sets had used that was related to people, objects, action, and sequence containing ten familiar and unfamiliar pictures in each (D. F. Cihak, 2007). The author used an AAC-based five-step instructional method for the teaching of reading pictures through visual literacy. The given instructional sets were sequenced on the basis of content, complexity, response, and language. According to the results, autistics enhanced about 68% mean of comprehension skills with experimental picture sets. TeachTown, a computer-assisted instruction system was used by (Whalen et al., 2010) to enhance the expressive language, play, imitation, social interaction, motor, and daily living skills of autistics. The training was conducted by computer lessons and natural environmental activities in which motivations of 15 to 30 seconds of animated video as a reward. An automated data collection and reporting system were also included to identify the effectiveness of the system. In comparison to the standardized tools, the training of ASD children on the TeachTown program for 2 months (20 minutes per day) had identified with improvement in the skills.

A Computer-based program also played a vital role had observed that the slow biological movements were more impactful for teaching students for reproducing facial expressions & body movements in autism. This was done using a computer-based program and attached hardware. With advancements in computer vision and artificial intelligence technologies, Bimbrahw, 2012 had implemented self-care applications for tracking children with ASD where different modules contained activity tracking, decision-making, prompting, and graphical interface. It was also highlighted that ASD impaired children were able to achieve independence during self-care activities by following simple verbal instructions (Bimbrahw, Boger, & Mihailidis, 2012). Ashburner, 2012 applied the keyboarding in place of handwriting to reduce communication barriers in ASD's affected children. Typing speed on a portable word processor of two composition tasks was measured as compared to handwriting where tests had shown improved motivation in ASDs (Ashburner, Ziviani, & Pennington, 2012). For finding the impact for enhancing social collaboration and conversational behavior in Autistics, two computer programs *Join-In* and *No-Problem* were developed and evaluated by (Bauminger-Zviely, Eden, Zancanaro, Weiss, & Gal, 2013). The author identified that by using computer-based technologies along with other collaborative technologies had helped for improving social interaction ability, social problem solving, and social cognition in ASD. Han, 2014 worked on effective human-computer communication with emotional dialogues by extraction and recognition of emotional dialogue information of Autistics. Studies conducted in the area of the face, speech, gesture, and posture recognition were found suitable for promoting the positive emotional exchanges and development in Autistics (Han & Li, 2014).

With the advancements in three dimension technologies, 'FakeSpace' environment had confirmed the existence of complex motor alterations with different motor dysfunctions in Autistic syndrome. It had generated 3D cave images of 1,280 x 1,024 pixels resolution on three 8 x 8 x 8 canvas walls with the help of Marquee Ultra 8500 projectors. Precise measurements of postural activities had monitored through implanted magnetic motion sensor or tracker system. Physical movements of 16 children with ASD were analyzed also through a video camera with automatic physical motion analyzer (Nobile et al., 2011). Three Dimensional-Social Understanding (3D-SU) virtual environment systems had used to improve the verbal and nonverbal communication, social initiation and cognition behavior. A Head Mounted Display (HMD) was used by Autistics to project 3D-SU virtual videos with reduced external environmental interference. The implemented environment had reflected the improved performance with non-verbal communication, social initiations and social cognition in ASD's subject (Cheng, Huang, & Yang, 2015). Electronic text software had included with different font types, sizes, text-to-speech, graphical representations, vocabulary, hyperlink connectivity, that help to improve the learning capabilities of ASD. Training sessions had involved with interactive material and a survey questionnaire to be filled by users and the interactive experimental results have been revealed a positive impact on the learning skills of ASDs(Knight, Wood, Spooner, Browder, & O'Brien, 2015)(Omar & Bidin, 2015)(Van Der Aa, Pollmann, Plaat, & Van Der Gaag, 2016).

Generally, children are very attracted towards Interactive social stories; authors had used social stories with the features of pleasant, interesting, engaging and user-friendly. It helped to raise the social and other behavioral skills in individuals with autism (Acar, Tekin-iftar, & Yikmis, 2016; Chen, 2018; Mccoy, Holloway, Healy, Rispoli, & Neely, 2016; Ngar, Yuan, Ho, & Ip, 2018; Sani-bozkurt, Vuran, & Akbulut, 2017). Elementary education in autism is the task of high responsibility, where multimedia and virtual reality related technologies are playing a successful role ((Kang & Chang, 2018; Rivera, Garc, Mart, Alarcos, & Ana, 2019)

Computer-Assisted Handheld and Wearable Technologies

Other than the personal computer (PC), handheld and wearable technology-based systems have done great initialization in the area of autism. With the intervention of portable technologies, the use of computational technology is being simplified. A portable handheld intervention was employed for video modeling or simulations to enhance the independent transition of Autistic children. Here, 10 videos were individually created based on positive self-modeling. The personal point of view of children was utilized for the transitioning from one place to other such as; from the bus to the classroom, from the classroom to the music room, from the music room to the bathroom, from the bathroom to the classroom, and from the classroom to the cafeteria and so on. Without intervention Autistics independent transition was only 7%, however, with handheld intervention, it has been improved to 70% of overall independent transitions (D. Cihak, Fahrenkrog, Ayres, & Smith, 2010).

Personal Digital Assistant (PDA), Video and TEACHH based multi-task had deployed for ASDs. The evaluated resultants had depicted with the positive effects of intervention for ASD children on the basis of dependent variables (Mechling & Savidge, 2011). iPod based speech-generating device was examined as a communication intervention program (Achmadi et al., 2012). A number of visual icons including snacks and toys were programmed as preferred stimuli to produce corresponding speech output on touching. During the initial session, no successful independent request was occurring, but after continuous sessions using intervention had been resulted in improved independent communication responses. Ganz, 2014 had developed an iPad based application as shown in figure 2 and observed the supported usage of visual script applications on handheld electronic devices for enhancing communication skills by varying levels of prompting.

The improved independent communication was observed for prompted as well as unprompted speech (J B Ganz et al., 2014). Further conducted experiments reflected that the iPad worked better due to the touch screen-based application in tests [47].In a survey related to treating the behavior of autistics, the parents and professionals of ASD's had also shown a keen interest in the uses of iPad and related applications (Clark, Austin, & Craike, 2014). In another study, the iPad had been identified as a preferred choice as a therapist (Lee et al., 2015).

The wearable stress sensor had used to generate alert to caregivers for higher stress level (Northrup, Lantz, Hamlin, & Case, 2016). The Internet of Things (IoT) based framework named "WearSense" had designed and implemented to detect the stereotypic behavior by extracting features from a three-dimensional accelerometer of the wristband. The conducted experiments had resulted in 94.6% accurate identification related to stereotypic behavior (Amiri et al., 2017). The Wearable Virtual Reality (WVR) with wearable bio-sensors for continues monitoring is an

Figure 2. iPad application screen
Source: Ganz et al. (2014)

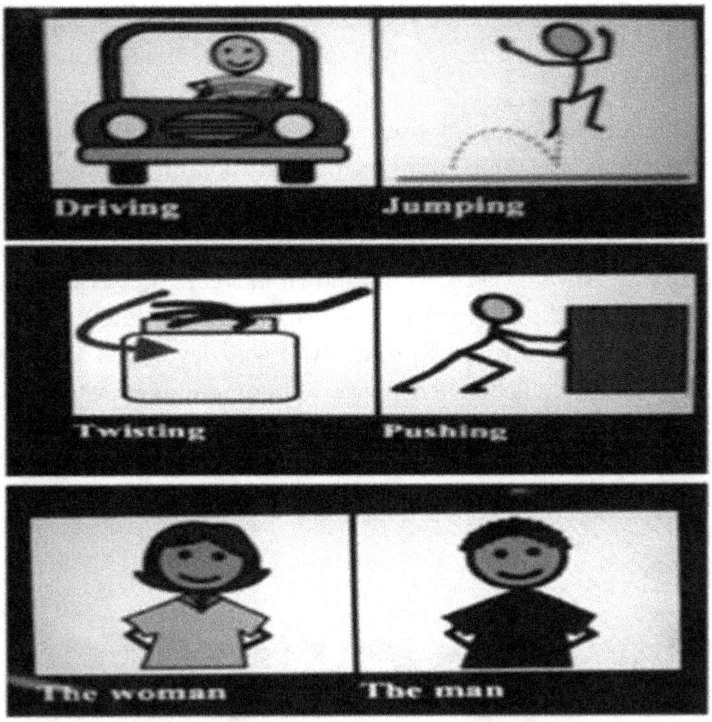

evolutionary powerful approach in the treatment of subjects with autism-like disorders (Benssassi, Gomez, Boyd, Hayes, & Ye, 2018; Garzotto et al., 2018; Koo, Gaul, Rivera, Pan, & Fong, 2018; Weenk, Goor, Frietman, & Engelen, 2017).

Computer-Assisted Games, Humanoid and Robotic Systems

Computer games are an effective tool for children on the autism spectrum because they are consistent and predictable, may involve limited social factors, and allow children to take control and determine the pace of the activity. Different experimental findings with computer-based games are enhancing the level of interaction in autistics. In earlier literature, (Enea & Colby, 1973) using hypothesis regarding attraction among machines, the computer games-based linguistic research had conducted for the treatment of language skills in non-speaking autistic patients. The experimental findings with computer-based games had enhanced the level of interaction in autistics.

Humanoid and Robotic systems are developing as interactive devices that have been used for children with autism and could provide feedback on performance during in specific sessions. These systems can have human-like abilities to interact with autistics. (Pioggia et al., 2007) had developed an android prototype, named as FACE, which had artificial skin, the servomotors, and an Artificial Neural Network which also able to express six basic emotions (happiness, sadness, surprise, anger, disgust, fear). Through a computer program and the audio system, FACE was capable of interacting predefined facial emotions with Autistics. After training the autistics for facial emotions using FACE, improvement in social behavior was noted. The image of the FACE is shown in figure 3.

In another experiment, a discrete trail with interactive simulation software-based virtual kid, namely "SIMon (DTKid)" as shown in figure 4, was developed for the improvement in trainer skills (Randell, Hall, Bizo, & Remington, 2007).

A child-sized humanoid (namely KASPAR) was developed and tested for the enhancement in social behavior and nonverbal communication in autistics. This humanoid was acted as social mediators between Teacher and Autistic with its three-dimensional physical availability, moving head, arms, hands, and interactive

Figure 3. FACE
Source: Pioggia et al. (2007)

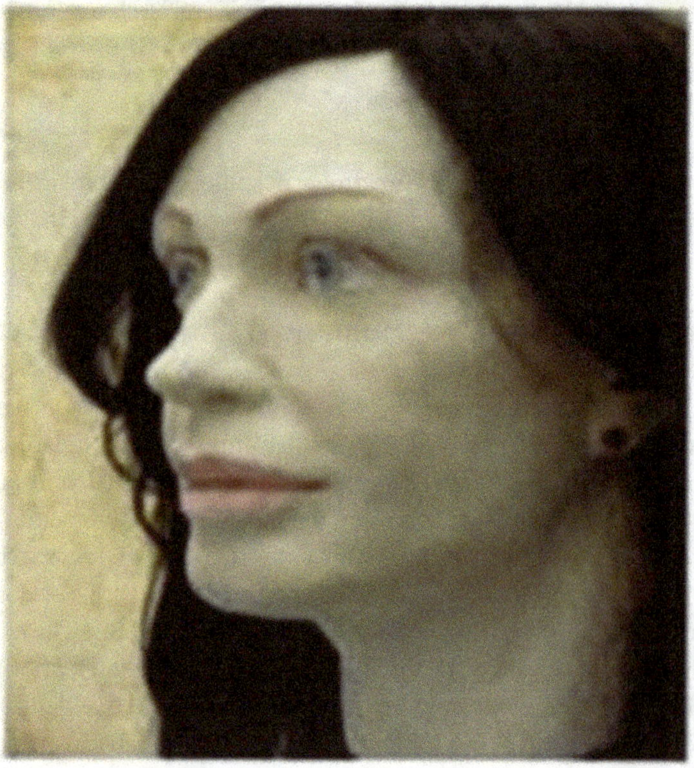

Figure 4. SIMon-DTKid
Source: Randell et al. (2007)

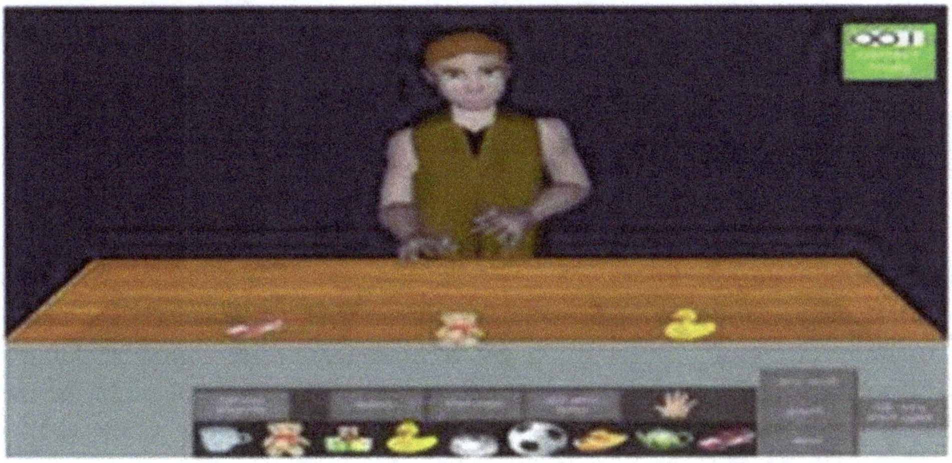

facial expressions/gestures. Autistic children started interacting with humanoid and showed less hesitation with co-presenter or stranger adult body touch and gaze of deficit children also had found reduced in later sessions. Interaction of autistic children with virtual child had also enhanced the confidence and knowledge of a teacher to handle such children (Robins, Dautenhahn, & Dickerson, 2009).

The experimental findings with computer-based games had enhanced the level of interaction in autistics. For learning & motivation for autistic children, (Frutos, Bustos, Zapirain, & Zorrilla, 2011) developed a computer-based game, which includes voice recognition and detection system and the efficient development was observed in autistics. The video clips had incorporated with toy pictures which had utilized to improve games play dialogues. For the improvement of social, behavioral skills in Autistics (such as eye gaze, facial emotions, facial expressions, social interaction),

Figure 5. FaceSay game screen shots
Source: Rice et al. (2015)

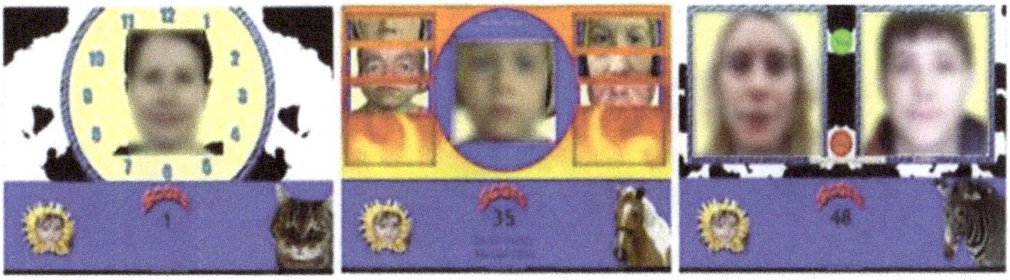

Figure 6. Faces with different emotional intensity
Source: Bekele et al. (2014)

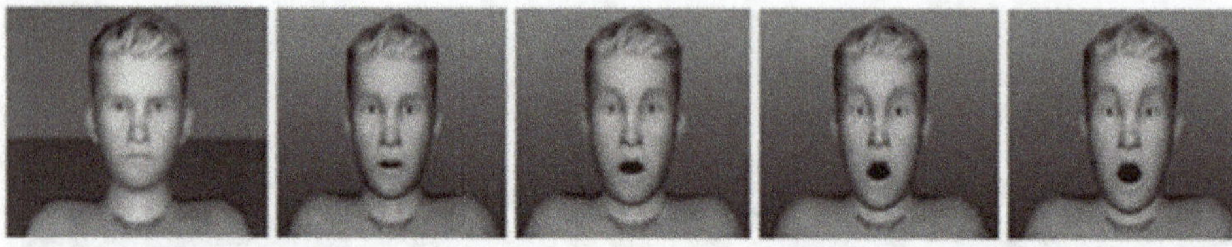

the “FaceSay” software was used by Hopkins, 2011 as shown in figure 5 (Hopkins et al., 2011). FaceSay had contained realistic avatars based three different games (“Amazing Gazing” for eye gaze, “Band-Aid Click” for facial recognition, “Follow the Leader”). “FaceSay” was capable of emotion and face recognition. In the continuation, “FaceSay” game was also used by (Rice, Wall, Fogel, & Shic, 2015) for improving the ASDs with eye-gaze, metalizing, attention, affect reorganization and face reorganization skills.

It was evident that the virtual reality avatars have the capability to produce a variety of facial emotions with the level of intensity (Bekele et al., 2014).

The Virtual Reality (VR) based social communication platform was proposed to improve the core deficits in social communication by applying virtual peers to

Figure 7. Pleo
Source: Kim et al. (2013)

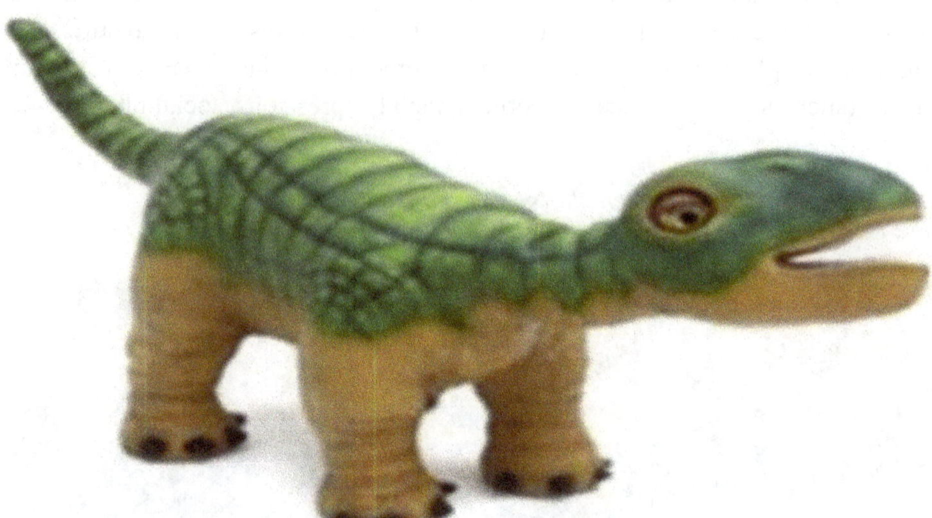

Figure 8. Robotic assistance for an individual with ASD
Source: Lewis et al. (2016)

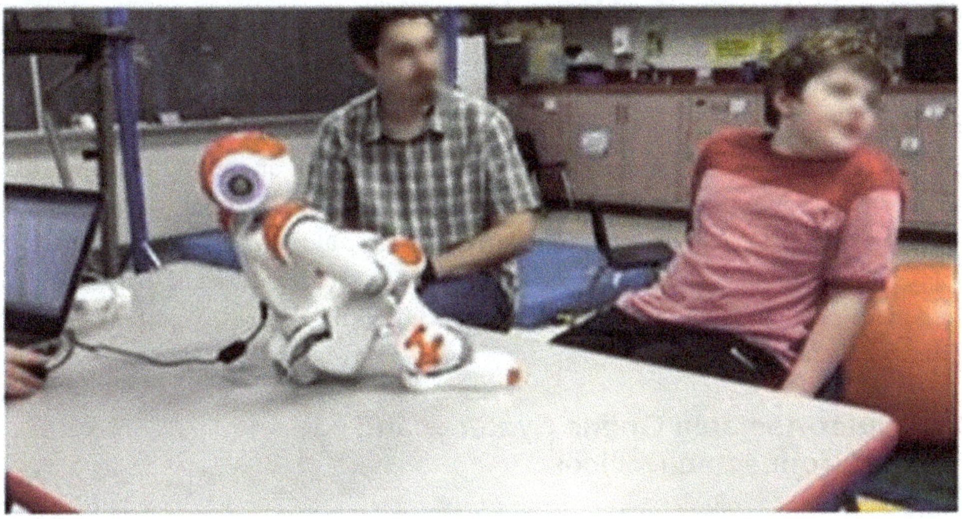

narrating social stories. This system had also utilized real-time physiological signals as markers such as anxiety, meltdown, etc (Kuriakose & Lahiri, 2015).

Autistic social deficits and interaction responses were compared with (Kim et al., 2013) in two different environments, i.e. in first the autistic are interacting with other normal adult and in second the autistic are interacting with the robot. The emotionally and intentionally expressible social toy dinosaur robot "Pleo" as shown in figure 7 is able to express his interest, disinterest, happiness, disappointment, agreement, and disagreement by using sounds and physical movements. During interacting with "Pleo", autistics had found social improvements for enhancing interaction and speech skills.

A multi-model behavior-related information of ASD's was gathered using the socially assistive robotic system (Petric et al., 2014) and improved objective diagnosis for ASD's was developed. Robots are also able to work as co-partner of therapist for improving the behavioral skills of ASDs is represented in figure 8 (Lewis, Charron, Clamp, & Craig, 2016). As per discussed literature, authors concluded that the assistance through robotic environment had a great role in the identification and improvement of autistic behavior.

Authors had also defended the emotions of autistic faces using Fisher faces algorithm and other traditional algorithms (Khullar, Singh, & Bala, 2017). Authors had worked to develop serious games (Grossard et al., 2017; Tanaka et al., 2012). Han, 2014 had proposed a man-machine interactive system based emotion calculation model. It had features of the face, speech, emotion, gesture, and posture for calculating defined emotions such as surprise, fear, disgust, anger, joy, grief. The studies were conducted on 56 subjects that reflected the man-machine dialogue had improved emotional reactions, cognitive, behavioral, communication, etc. It had also improved the ability of understanding using specified games and virtual environment (Han & Li, 2014). (Grossard et al., 2017) had suggested that the serious game developers should work on more adapted games for ASD's along with the clinical approval by experts in the future. In recent research, patterns of joint attention had identified during human-robot interaction, and it highlights that the robotic structures are more beneficial to improve attention in ASD's (Anzalone et al., 2018). Another study had Developed a Semi-Autonomous Robotic System to assist individuals with autism for raising their Visual Perspective-Taking Skills (Zaraki, Wood, Robins, & Dautenhahn, 2018).

Computer-Assisted Online Systems and Internet Connected Devices

According to the present era, online systems and Internet Connected Devices were advantageous as systematic approaches with easily assessable to available information and also had cost-effective results for the clinicians and caregivers. According to this fact, the impact of the secured online support group was evaluated by the author for analyzing the symptoms of stress, anxiety, and depression in autistic parents(Clifford & Minnes, 2013). This secure system is included with a chatting module and an online discussion board for posting online comments or questions had used. Online monitoring was implemented for physical self-awareness for ASD's which was explaining their actions and memory by conducting the squares arranging task. It was noted that when ASD control their own actions on the computer then they were easily able to find the right block rather than controlled by the experimenter(Grainger, Williams, & Lind, 2014). The Internet of Things (IoT), peer to peer (P2P), web and sensor-based technological systems (shown in figure 9) had used for creating one to one communication system between the autistics and caregivers for their monitoring (Sula et al., 2013).

Various significant benefits of the Internet like easy access, social networks, etc had highlighted in concern to the computer-mediated community (Gillespie-Lynch et al., 2014). The Internet-based service delivery method for improvement in the communication skills of children with autism had implemented and results shown the positive impact on autistics (Meadan et al., 2016). Internet-based reward system for individuals with autism had developed which results in server-based data access and recording (Constantin, Johnson, Smith, Lengyel, & Brosnan, 2017). With the easiness in interaction graphical interfaces, even non-technical professionals are able to access the internet or robotic at its user level (B & Kolesi, 2017). Application

Figure 9. Smart Box Device
Source: Sula et al. (2013)

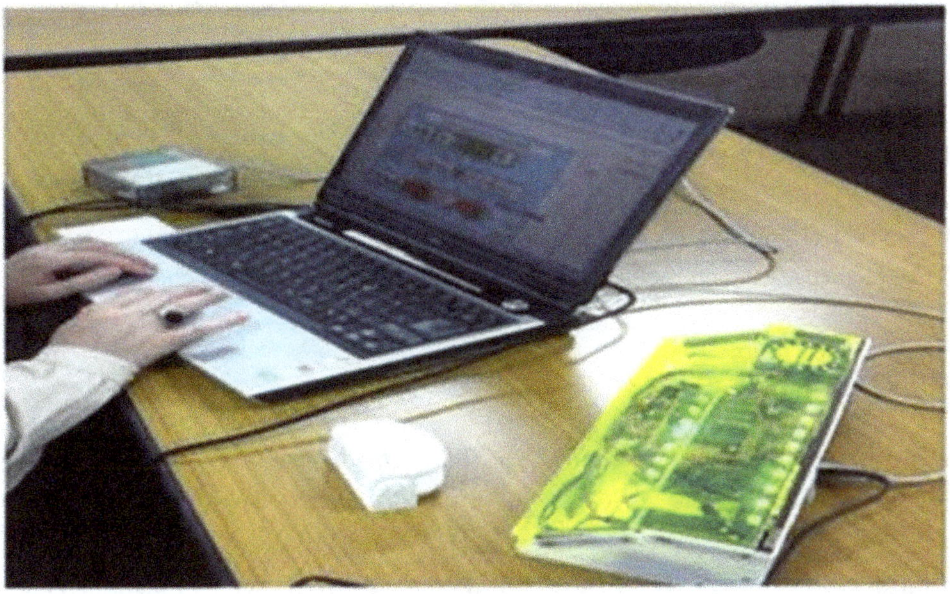

is available on iHealth care having refined tie-ups with the Internet of Things based sensing devices, which is capable to provide remote access to physiological monitoring (Pandia Rajan & Edward Rajan, 2018). The Internet of Toys is another booming area with a combination of Internet, Artificial Intelligence and Big Data related technologies. Authors had started utilizing this in concern of Autism (Peter, Kühne, Barco, Jong, & Straten, 2016; Rivera et al., 2019).

CONCLUSION

In recent years, there has been an increased interest of researchers to improve the life of an individual with autism. An appreciative position of ASD and technology relevant research has achieved since the examiners are still improving the present technologies for making the easier everyday life of ASD's. This study had provided detailed base regarding the developments for computer-assisted advancements as technological interventions for ASD. The work in the present paper had different computer-assisted technological developments of autism for skill enhancements had been reviewed. The possibility of digital signal processing, internet controlled devices, Internet of Things (IoT), artificial intelligence, handheld digital devices and robotic controlled machines as technological interventions in autism had been highlighted. However, this study can act as a significant base review in the context of future technologies for autism-like deep learning-based diagnosis; big data-based huge data management; cloud computing-based software as service; robotics-based humanoid interventions; etc.

ACKNOWLEDGMENT

We are thankful for the I.K.G. Punjab Technical University, India and CT Institute of Engineering, Management and Technology, India for made this chapter possible.

REFERENCES

Acar, C., Tekin-iftar, E., & Yikmis, A. (2016). *Effects of Mother-Delivered Social Stories and Video Modeling in Teaching Social Skills to Children With Autism Spectrum Disorders*. doi:10.1177/0022466916649164

Achmadi, D., Kagohara, D. M., Van Der Meer, L., O'Reilly, M. F., Lancioni, G. E., Sutherland, D., ... Sigafoos, J. (2012). Teaching advanced operation of an iPod-based speech-generating device to two students with autism spectrum disorders. *Research in Autism Spectrum Disorders*, *6*(4), 1258–1264. doi:10.1016/j.rasd.2012.05.005

Ames, C., & Fletcher-Watson, S. (2010). *A review of methods in the study of attention in autism. Developmental Review*. Elsevier Inc. doi:10.1016/j.dr.2009.12.003

Amiri, A. M., Peltier, N., Goldberg, C., Sun, Y., Nathan, A., Hiremath, S. V., & Mankodiya, K. (2017). WearSense: Detecting Autism Stereotypic Behaviors through Smartwatches. *Journal of Healthcare*, *5*(11), 2017. PMID:28264474

Anzalone, S. M., Xavier, J., Boucenna, S., Billeci, L., Narzisi, A., & Muratori, F. … Chetouani, M. (2018). Quantifying patterns of joint attention during human-robot interactions: An application for autism spectrum disorder assessment. *Pattern Recognition Letters*. doi:10.1016/j.patrec.2018.03.007

Ardhanareeswarana, K., & Volkmar, F. (2015). Focus: Austism Spectrum Disorders. *Medicine*, *88*(1), 3–4. doi:10.1002/ddrr.75

Ashburner, J., Ziviani, J., & Pennington, A. (2012). The Introduction of Keyboarding to Children With Autism Spectrum Disorders With Handwriting Difficulties: A Help or a Hindrance? *Australasian Journal of Special Education*, *36*(01), 32–61. doi:10.1017/jse.2012.6

Aurnhammer-frith, U. T. A. (1969). Emphasis and meaning in recall in normal and autistic children. *Journal of Language and Speech*, *12*(1), 29–38. doi:10.1177/002383096901200103 PMID:5789294

Ayres, K. M., Maguire, A., & McClimon, D. (2009). Acquisition and Generalization of Chained Tasks Taught with Computer Based Video Instruction to Children with Autism. *Education and Training in Developmental Disabilities*, *44*(4), 493–508.

Baio, J., Wiggins, L., Christensen, D. L., Maenner, M. J., Daniels, J., Warren, Z., … Dowling, N. F. (2018). *Prevalence of Autism Spectrum Disorder Among Children Aged 8 Years* (Vol. 67). Academic Press.

Bauminger-Zviely, N., Eden, S., Zancanaro, M., Weiss, P. L., & Gal, E. (2013). Increasing social engagement in children with high-functioning autism spectrum disorder using collaborative technologies in the school environment. *Autism*, *17*(3), 317–339. doi:10.1177/1362361312472989 PMID:23614935

Begoli, E., DeFalco, J., & Ogle, C. (2016). The Promise and Relevance of Emerging Technologies in the Education of Children with Autism Spectrum Disorder. In *Advances in Early Childhood and K-12 Education (AECKE)* (pp. 184–203). Hershey, PA: IGI Global. doi:10.4018/978-1-5225-0816-8

Bekele, E., Crittendon, J., Zheng, Z., Swanson, A., Weitlauf, A., Warren, Z., & Sarkar, N. (2014). Assessing the utility of a virtual environment for enhancing facial affect recognition in adolescents with autism. *Journal of Autism and Developmental Disorders*, *44*(7), 1641–1650. doi:10.100710803-014-2035-8 PMID:24419871

Benssassi, E. M., Gomez, J.-C., Boyd, L. E., Hayes, G. R., & Ye, J. (2018). Wearable Assistive Technologies for Autism: Opportunities and Challenges. *IEEE Pervasive Computing*, *17*(2), 11–21. doi:10.1109/MPRV.2018.022511239

Bentenuto, A., De Falco, S., & Venuti, P. (2016). Mother-child play: A comparison of autism spectrum disorder, down syndrome, and typical development. *Frontiers in Psychology*, *7*, 1–9. doi:10.3389/fpsyg.2016.01829 PMID:27920745

Bernard-Opitz, V., Sriram, N., & Nakhoda-Sapuan, S. (2001). Enhancing social problem solving in children with autism and normal children through computer-assisted instruction. *Journal of Autism and Developmental Disorders*, *31*(4), 377–384. doi:10.1023/A:1010660502130 PMID:11569584

Bimbrahw, J., Boger, J., & Mihailidis, A. (2012). Investigating the efficacy of a computerized prompting device to assist children with autism spectrum disorder with activities of daily living. *Assistive Technology*, *24*(4), 286–298. doi:10.1080/10400435.2012.680661

Bonnet-Brilhault, F. (2017). Autism: An early neurodevelopmental disorder. *Archives de Pediatrie*, *24*(4), 384–390. doi:10.1016/j.arcped.2017.01.014 PMID:28256376

Carr, D., & Felce, J. (2007). The effects of PECS teaching to phase III on the communicative interactions between children with autism and their teachers. *Journal of Autism and Developmental Disorders*, *37*(4), 724–737. doi:10.100710803-006-0203-1 PMID:17006780

Chen, K. H. (2018). Effects of multimedia teaching integrated social story on autistic children ' s social interaction. *Quality & Quantity*, *52*(S2), 1399–1408. doi:10.100711135-018-0731-8

Cheng, Y., Huang, C.-L., & Yang, C.-S. (2015). Using a 3D Immersive Virtual Environment System to Enhance Social Understanding and Social Skills for Children With Autism Spectrum Disorders. *Focus on Autism and Other Developmental Disabilities*, *30*(4), 222–236. doi:10.1177/1088357615583473

Cihak, D., Fahrenkrog, C., Ayres, K. M., & Smith, C. (2010). The Use of Video Modeling via a Video iPod and a System of Least Prompts to Improve Transitional Behaviors for Students with Autism Spectrum Disorders in the General Education Classroom. *Journal of Positive Behavior Interventions*, *12*(2), 103–115. doi:10.1177/1098300709332346

Cihak, D. F. (2007). Teaching students with autism to read pictures. *Research in Autism Spectrum Disorders*, *1*(4), 318–329. doi:10.1016/j.rasd.2006.12.002

Clark, M. L. E., Austin, D. W., & Craike, M. J. (2014). Professional and Parental Attitudes Toward iPad Application Use in Autism Spectrum Disorder. *Focus on Autism and Other Developmental Disabilities*. doi:10.1177/1088357614537353

Clifford, T., & Minnes, P. (2013). Logging on: Evaluating an online support group for parents of children with autism spectrum disorders. *Journal of Autism and Developmental Disorders*, *43*(7), 1662–1675. doi:10.100710803-012-1714-6 PMID:23143075

Colby, K. M. (1967). Computer simulation of change in personal belief systems. *Journal of Systems Research and Behavioral Science*, *12*(3), 248–253. PMID:6059766

Constantin, A., Johnson, H., Smith, E., Lengyel, D., & Brosnan, M. (2017). Designing computer-based rewards with and for children with Autism Spectrum Disorder and/or Intellectual Disability. *Computers in Human Behavior*, *75*, 404–414. doi:10.1016/j.chb.2017.05.030

Corbett, B. A. (2003). Video modeling: A window into the world of autism. *The Behavior Analyst Today*, *4*(3), 88–96. doi:10.1037/h0100025

Data & Statistics on Autism Spectrum Disorder. (2019). Retrieved from https://www.cdc.gov/ncbddd/autism/data.html

Dawson, G., Meltzoff, A. N., Osterling, J., & Rinaldi, J. (2006). Neuropsychological Correlates of Early Symptoms of Autism. *Child Development*, *69*(5), 1276–1285. doi:10.1111/j.1467-8624.1998.tb06211.x PMID:9839415

Diagnostic and Statistical Manual of Mental Disorders. (1994). (4th ed.). Washington, DC: American Psychiatric Association.

Diagnostic and Statistical Manual of Mental Disorders. (2013). (5th ed.). Arlington, VA: American Psychiatric Association.

Enea, H., & Colby, K. M. (1973). Idiolectic language-analysis for understanding doctor-patient dialogues. In *3rd International Joint Conference on Artificial Intelligence* (pp. 278–290). Academic Press.

Ferster, C. B., & Demyer, M. K. (1961). The development of performances in autistic children in an automatically controlled environment. *Journal of Chronic Diseases*, *13*(4), 312–345. doi:10.1016/0021-9681(61)90059-5 PMID:13699188

Frost, R. E. (1981). An interactive computer environment for autistic children. In *The Johns Hopkins First National Search for Applications of Personal Computing to Aid the Handicapped* (p. 1981). Los Angeles, CA: IEEE Computer Society.

Frutos, M., Bustos, I., Zapirain, B. G., & Zorrilla, A. M. (2011). Computer game to learn and enhance speech problems for children with autism. *Proceedings of CGAMES'2011 USA - 16th International Conference on Computer Games: AI, Animation, Mobile, Interactive Multimedia, Educational and Serious Games*, 209–216. 10.1109/CGAMES.2011.6000340

Ganz, J. B., Boles, M. B., Goodwyn, F. D., & Flores, M. M. (2014). Efficacy of Handheld Electronic Visual Supports to Enhance Vocabulary in Children With ASD. *Focus on Autism and Other Developmental Disabilities*, *29*(1), 3–12. doi:10.1177/1088357613504991

Ganz, J. B., & Simpson, R. L. (2004). Effects on communicative requesting and speech development of the picture exchange communication system in children with characteristics of autism. *Journal of Autism and Developmental Disorders*, *34*(4), 395–409. doi:10.1023/B:JADD.0000037416.59095.d7 PMID:15449515

Garzotto, F., Messina, N., Matarazzo, V., Moskwa, L., Oliva, G., & Facchini, R. (2018). Empowering Interventions for Persons with Neurodevelopmental Disorders through Wearable Virtual Reality and Bio-sensors. *Conference on Human Factors in Computing Systems - CHI '18*, 1–6. 10.1145/3170427.3188636

Gillespie-Lynch, K., Kapp, S. K., Shane-Simpson, C., Smith, D. S., & Hutman, T. (2014). Intersections between the autism spectrum and the internet: Perceived benefits and preferred functions of computer-mediated communication. *Intellectual and Developmental Disabilities*, *52*(6), 456–469. doi:10.1352/1934-9556-52.6.456 PMID:25409132

Goldenberg, E. P. (1979). *Special technology for special children*. Academic Press.

Goldenberg, E. P. (1987). *Exploring Language with Logo*. The MIT Press.

Grainger, C., Williams, D. M., & Lind, S. E. (2014). Online action monitoring and memory for self-performed actions in autism spectrum disorder. *Journal of Autism and Developmental Disorders*, *44*(5), 1193–1206. doi:10.100710803-013-1987-4 PMID:24193578

Grossard, C., Grynspan, O., Serret, S., Jouen, A. L., Bailly, K., & Cohen, D. (2017). Serious games to teach social interactions and emotions to individuals with autism spectrum disorders (ASD). *Computers & Education*, *113*, 195–211. doi:10.1016/j.compedu.2017.05.002

Han, L., & Li, X. (2014). The appliance of affective computing in man-machine dialogue: Assisting therapy of having autism. In *4th International Conference on Communication Systems and Network Technologies, CSNT 2014* (pp. 1093–1096). 10.1109/CSNT.2014.223

Hazen, E. P., Stornelli, J. L., O'Rourke, J. A., Koesterer, K., & McDougle, C. J. (2014). Sensory symptoms in autism spectrum disorders. *Harvard Review of Psychiatry*, *22*(2), 112–124. doi:10.1097/01.HRP.0000445143.08773.58 PMID:24614766

Hetzroni, O. E., & Tannous, J. (2004). Effects of a computer-based intervention program on the communicative functions of children with autism. *Journal of Autism and Developmental Disorders*, *34*(2), 95–113. doi:10.1023/B:JADD.0000022602.40506.bf PMID:15162930

Higgins, K., & Boone, R. (1996). Creating individualized computer-assisted instruction for students with autism using multimedia. *Focus on Autism and Other Developmental Disabilities*, *11*(2), 69–78. doi:10.1177/108835769601100202

Hopkins, I. M., Gower, M. W., Perez, T. A., Smith, D. S., Amthor, F. R., Casey Wimsatt, F., & Biasini, F. J. (2011). Avatar assistant: Improving social skills in students with an asd through a computer-based intervention. *Journal of Autism and Developmental Disorders*, *41*(11), 1543–1555. doi:10.100710803-011-1179-z PMID:21287255

Iarocci, G., Burack, J. A., Shore, D. I., Mottron, L., & Enns, J. T. (2006). Global-local visual processing in high functioning children with autism: Structural vs. implicit task biases. *Journal of Autism and Developmental Disorders*, *36*(1), 117–129. doi:10.100710803-005-0045-2 PMID:16397823

Kang, Y., & Chang, Y. (2018). Using game technology to teach six elementary school children with autism to take a shower independently. *Developmental Neurorehabilitation*, *00*(00), 1–9. doi:10.1080/17518423.2018.1501778 PMID:30060690

Kanner, L. (1943). *Autistic Disturbances of Affective Contact*. Academic Press.

Khullar, V., Singh, H. P., & Bala, M. (2017). ASD Faces are Less Explainable. *Autism - Open Access Research*, *7*(3), 3–7. doi:10.4172/2165-7890.1000210

Kim, E. S., Berkovits, L. D., Bernier, E. P., Leyzberg, D., Shic, F., Paul, R., & Scassellati, B. (2013). Social robots as embedded reinforcers of social behavior in children with autism. *Journal of Autism and Developmental Disorders*, *43*(5), 1038–1049. doi:10.100710803-012-1645-2 PMID:23111617

Kinney, E. M., Vedora, J., & Stromer, R. (2003). Computer-Presented Video Models to Teach Generative Spelling to a Child with an Autism Spectrum Disorder. *Journal of Positive Behavior Interventions*, *5*(1), 22–29. doi:10.1177/10983007030050010301

Klin, A., Jones, W., Schultz, R., & Volkmar, F. (2003). The enactive mind, or from actions to cognition : Lessons from autism. *Philosophical Transactions of the Royal Society*, *358*(1430), 345–360. doi:10.1098/rstb.2002.1202 PMID:12639332

Knight, V. F., Wood, C. L., Spooner, F., Browder, D. M., & O'Brien, C. P. (2015). An Exploratory Study Using Science eTexts With Students With Autism Spectrum Disorder. *Focus on Autism and Other Developmental Disabilities*, *30*(2), 86–99. doi:10.1177/1088357614559214

Koo, S. H., Gaul, K., Rivera, S., Pan, T., & Fong, D. (2018). Wearable Technology Design for Autism Spectrum Disorders. *Archives of Design Research*, *31*(1), 37–55. doi:10.15187/adr.2018.02.31.1.37

Kuriakose, S., & Lahiri, U. (2015). Understanding the Psycho-Physiological Implications of Interaction with a Virtual Reality-Based System in Adolescents with Autism: A Feasibility Study. *IEEE Transactions on Neural Systems and Rehabilitation Engineering, 23*(4), 665–675. doi:10.1109/TNSRE.2015.2393891 PMID:25643409

LeBlanc, L. A., Coates, A. M., Daneshvar, S., Charlop-Christy, M. H., Morris, C., & Lancaster, B. M. (2003). Using video modeling and reinforcement to teach perspective-taking skills to children with autism. *Journal of Applied Behavior Analysis, 36*(2), 253–257. doi:10.1901/jaba.2003.36-253 PMID:12858990

Lee, A., Lang, R., Davenport, K., Moore, M., Rispoli, M., Van Der Meer, L., ... Chung, C. (2015). Comparison of therapist implemented and iPad-assisted interventions for children with autism. *Developmental Neurorehabilitation, 18*(2), 97–103. doi: 10.3109/17518423.2013.830231 PMID:24088050

Lewis, L., Charron, N., Clamp, C., & Craig, M. (2016). Soft systems methodology as a tool to aid a pilot study in robot-assisted therapy. *ACM/IEEE International Conference on Human-Robot Interaction*, 467–468. 10.1109/HRI.2016.7451809

Loucas, T., Charman, T., Pickles, A., Simonoff, E., Chandler, S., Meldrum, D., & Baird, G. (2008). Autistic symptomatology and language ability in autism spectrum disorder and specific language impairment. *Journal of Child Psychology and Psychiatry, 49*(11), 1184–1192. doi:10.1111/j.1469-7610.2008.01951.x

Mccoy, A., Holloway, J., Healy, O., Rispoli, M., & Neely, L. (2016). *A Systematic Review and Evaluation of Video Modeling, Role-Play and Computer-Based Instruction as Social Skills Interventions for Children and Adolescents with High-Functioning Autism*. doi:10.100740489-015-0065-6

Meadan, H., Snodgrass, M. R., Meyer, L. E., Fisher, K. W., Chung, M. Y., & Halle, J. W. (2016). Internet-Based Parent-Implemented Intervention for Young Children With Autism. *Journal of Early Intervention, 38*(1), 3–23. doi:10.1177/1053815116630327

Mechling, L. C., & Savidge, E. J. (2011). Using a personal digital assistant to increase completion of novel tasks and independent transitioning by students with autism spectrum disorder. *Journal of Autism and Developmental Disorders, 41*(6), 687–704. doi:10.100710803-010-1088-6 PMID:20714798

Must, A., Phillips, S. M., Curtin, C., Anderson, S. E., Maslin, M., Lividini, K., & Bandini, L. G. (2014). Comparison of sedentary behaviors between children with autism spectrum disorders and typically developing children. *Autism, 18*(4), 376–384. doi:10.1177/1362361313479039 PMID:24113339

Ngar, S., Yuan, V., Ho, H., & Ip, S. (2018). Using virtual reality to train emotional and social skills in children with autism spectrum disorder. *London Journal of Primary Care*, *1472*, 1–3. doi:10.1080/17571472.2018.1483000 PMID:30083244

Nobile, M., Perego, P., Piccinini, L., Mani, E., Rossi, A., Bellina, M., & Molteni, M. (2011). Further evidence of complex motor dysfunction in drug naïve children with autism using automatic motion analysis of gait. *Autism*, *15*(3), 263–283. doi:10.1177/1362361309356929 PMID:21478224

Northrup, C. M., Lantz, J., Hamlin, T., & Case, N. (2016). *Wearable Stress Sensors for Children with Autism Spectrum Disorder with In Situ Alerts to Caregivers via a Mobile Phone*. Academic Press.

Olive, M. L., De La Cruz, B., Davis, T. N., Chan, J. M., Lang, R. B., O'Reilly, M. F., & Dickson, S. M. (2007). The effects of enhanced milieu teaching and a voice output communication aid on the requesting of three children with autism. *Journal of Autism and Developmental Disorders*, *37*(8), 1505–1513. doi:10.100710803-006-0243-6 PMID:17066309

Omar, S., & Bidin, A. (2015). The Impact of Multimedia Graphic and Text with Autistic Learners in Reading. *Universal Journal of Educational Research*, *3*(12), 989–996. doi:10.13189/ujer.2015.031206

Pandia Rajan, J., & Edward Rajan, S. (2018). An Internet of Things based physiological signal monitoring and receiving system for virtual enhanced health care network. *Technology and Health Care*, *26*(2), 379–385. doi:10.3233/THC-171173 PMID:29526864

Panyan, M. V. (1984). Computer technology for autistic students. *Journal of Autism and Developmental Disorders*, *14*(4), 375–382. doi:10.1007/BF02409828 PMID:6549182

Peter, J., Kühne, R., Barco, A., Jong, C. De, & Straten, C. L. Van. (2016). Asking Today the Crucial Questions of Tomorrow: Social Robots and the Internet of Toys. *Studies in Childhood and Youth*, 25–46. doi:10.1007/978-3-030-10898-4

Petric, F., Hrvatini, K., Babic, A., Malovan, L., Miklic, D., Kovacic, Z., … Simlesa, S. (2014). Four tasks of a robot-assisted autism spectrum disorder diagnostic protocol: First clinical tests. *Proceedings of the 4th IEEE Global Humanitarian Technology Conference, GHTC 2014*, 510–517. 10.1109/GHTC.2014.6970331

Pioggia, G., Sica, M. L., Ferro, M., Igliozzi, R., Muratori, F., Ahluwalia, A., & De Rossi, D. (2007). Human-robot interaction in autism: FACE, an android-based social therapy. *Proceedings - IEEE International Workshop on Robot and Human Interactive Communication*, 605–612. 10.1109/ROMAN.2007.4415156

Plienis, A. J., & Romanczyk, R. G. (1985). Analyses of performance, behavior, and predictors for severely disturbed children: A comparison of adult vs. computer instruction. *Analysis and Intervention In Developmental Disablities*, *5*(4), 345–356. doi:10.1016/0270-4684(85)90004-7

Randell, T., Hall, M., Bizo, L., & Remington, B. (2007). DTkid: Interactive simulation software for training tutors of children with autism. *Journal of Autism and Developmental Disorders*, *37*(4), 637–647. doi:10.100710803-006-0193-z PMID:17019627

Ratajczak, H. V. (2011). Theoretical aspects of autism: Causes—A review. *Journal of Immunotoxicology*, *8*(1), 68–79. doi:10.3109/1547691X.2010.545086 PMID:21299355

Rice, L. M., Wall, C. A., Fogel, A., & Shic, F. (2015). Computer-Assisted Face Processing Instruction Improves Emotion Recognition, Mentalizing, and Social Skills in Students with ASD. *Journal of Autism and Developmental Disorders*, *45*(7), 2176–2186. doi:10.100710803-015-2380-2 PMID:25694364

Rivera, D., Garc, A., Mart, L., Alarcos, B., & Ana, G. (2019). Secure Communications and Protected Data for a Internet of Things Smart Toy Platform. *Journal of IEEE Internet of Things*, *4662*, 1–11. doi:10.1109/JIOT.2019.2891103

Robins, B., Dautenhahn, K., & Dickerson, P. (2009). From isolation to communication: A case study evaluation of robot assisted play for children with autism with a minimally expressive humanoid robot. *Proceedings of the 2nd International Conferences on Advances in Computer-Human Interactions, ACHI 2009*, 205–211. 10.1109/ACHI.2009.32

Rutgers, A. H., Van IJzendoorn, M. H., Bakermans-Kranenburg, M. J., Swinkels, S. H. N., Van Daalen, E., Dietz, C., ... Van Engeland, H. (2007). Autism, attachment and parenting: A comparison of children with autism spectrum disorder, mental retardation, language disorder, and non-clinical children. *Journal of Abnormal Child Psychology*, *35*(5), 859–870. doi:10.100710802-007-9139-y PMID:17505877

Rutherford, M. D., Pennington, B. F., & Rogers, S. J. (2006). The perception of animacy in young children with autism. *Journal of Autism and Developmental Disorders*, *36*(8), 983–992. doi:10.100710803-006-0136-8 PMID:16897392

Sani-bozkurt, S., Vuran, S., & Akbulut, Y. (2017). *Design and Use of Interactive Social Stories for Children with Autism Spectrum Disorder*. Academic Press.

Sansosti, F. J., & Powell-Smith, K. (2008). Using Computer-Presented Social Stories and Video Models to Increase the Social Communication Skills of Children With High-Functioning Autism Spectrum Disorders. *Journal of Positive Behavior Interventions*, *10*(3), 162–178. doi:10.1177/1098300708316259

Seltzer, M. M., Krauss, M. W., Shattuck, P. T., Orsmond, G., Swe, A., & Lord, C. (2003). The symptoms of autism spectrum disorders. *Journal of Autism and Developmental Disorders*, *33*(6), 565–581. doi:10.1023/B:JADD.0000005995.02453.0b PMID:14714927

Shipley-Benamou, R., Lutzker, J. R., & Taubman, M. (2002). Teaching Daily Living Skills to Children with Autism Through Instructional Video Modeling. *Journal of Positive Behavior Interventions*, *4*(3), 166–177. doi:10.1177/109830070200400305 01

Sigafoos, J., & Drasgow, E. (2001). Conditional Use of Aided and Unaided AAC: A Review and Clinical Case Demonstration. *Focus on Autism and Other Developmental Disabilities*, *16*(3), 152–161. doi:10.1177/108835760101600303

Sula, A., Spaho, E., Matsuo, K., Barolli, L., Miho, R., & Xhafa, F. (2013). An IoT-based System for Supporting Children with Autism Spectrum Disorder. In *8th International Conference on Automatic Face and Gesture Recognition International Conference on Broadband, Wireless Computing, Communication and Applications* (pp. 282–289). 10.1109/BWCCA.2013.51

Tanaka, J. W., Wolf, J. M., Klaiman, C., Koenig, K., Cockburn, J., Herlihy, L., ... Schultz, R. T. (2012). The perception and identification of facial emotions in individuals with autism spectrum disorders using the Let's Face It! Emotion Skills Battery. *Journal of Child Psychology and Psychiatry, and Allied Disciplines*, *53*(12), 1259–1267. doi:10.1111/j.1469-7610.2012.02571.x PMID:22780332

Van Der Aa, C., Pollmann, M. M. H., Plaat, A., & Van Der Gaag, R. J. (2016). Computer-mediated communication in adults with high-functioning autism spectrum disorders and controls. *Research in Autism Spectrum Disorders*, *23*, 15–27. doi:10.1016/j.rasd.2015.11.007

Weenk, M., Van Goor, H., Frietman, B., & Engelen, L. J. (2017). Continuous Monitoring of Vital Signs Using Wearable Devices on the General Ward. *Pilot Study Corresponding Author*, *5*(7), 1–14. doi:10.2196/mhealth.7208 PMID:28679490

Wert, B. Y., & Neisworth, J. T. (2003). Effects of Video Self-Modeling on Spontaneous Requesting in Children with Autism. *Journal of Positive Behavior Interventions*, *5*(1), 30–34. doi:10.1177/10983007030050010501

Whalen, C., Moss, D., Ilan, A. B., Vaupel, M., Fielding, P., Macdonald, K., ... Symon, J. (2010). Efficacy of TeachTown: Basics computer-assisted intervention for the Intensive Comprehensive Autism Program in Los Angeles Unified School District. *Autism*, *14*(3), 179–197. doi:10.1177/1362361310363282 PMID:20484002

Wing, L. (1993). The definition and prevalence of autism: A review. *European Child & Adolescent Psychiatry*, *2*(2), 61–74. doi:10.1007/BF02098832 PMID:21590530

Wing, L., & Gould, J. (1979). Severe impairments of social interaction and associated abnormalities in children: Epidemiology and classification. *Journal of Autism and Developmental Disorders*, *9*(1), 11–29. doi:10.1007/BF01531288 PMID:155684

Zaraki, A., Wood, L., Robins, B., & Dautenhahn, K. (2018). Development of a Semi-Autonomous Robotic System to Assist Children with Autism in Developing Visual Perspective Taking Skills. *2018 27th IEEE International Symposium on Robot and Human Interactive Communication (RO-MAN)*, 969–976.

Chapter 6
Understanding Psychological Distress Among Female Caregivers of the Patients With Mental Illness

Abhijit Pathak
https://orcid.org/0000-0003-3134-9523
Department of Humanities and Social Sciences, National Institute of Technology, Rourkela, India

Chittaranjan Subudhi
Department of Social Work, Central University of Tamil Nadu, India

ABSTRACT

The present study aims to find the level of psychological distress in female caregivers of patients with mental illness in the context of Jharkhand and its relations with the socio-demographic variable. The sample was drawn from five blocks of Hazaribagh districts of Jharkhand and the respondents were 200 relatives of the patients with mental illness. A socio-demographic data sheet used for recording the socio-demographic characteristics and Kessler Psychological Distress Scale version 10 (K10) used for assessing their psychological distress. The result shows that female gender is having more psychological distress than male and may lead to common mental disorder under persistent condition. The mean score of female was higher than male (i.e., 26.36 [SD= 9.44] and 22.23 [SD= 8.86], respectively). The difference between both the genders found to be significant at less than 0.001 p values in Man Whitney U test.

DOI: 10.4018/978-1-7998-1185-5.ch006

INTRODUCTION

Psychological distress which encompasses of worthlessness, hopelessness, sadness leads to gradual loss of interest to socialize and to work triggered by unfriendly socio, economic and cultural environment (Mirowsky& Rose, 2002; Kleinman, 199; Kirmayer, 1989). This didn't stop only to emotional disturbance but can cause to neurotic and mental disorder in the absence of proper support (Phillips, 2009; Watson, 2009). Relatives or the caregiver of the patients with mental or physical illness are not spared of its influences. Relatives or caregivers staying with their patients live in the same social, cultural and economic environment exhibit tremendous stress due to handling the symptoms of patient with financial insufficiency and stigmatized attitude of the society with less cooperation from the neighbors (Eag, 2014; Lesselo, Kajula & Malema, 2016;Raj, Shiri & Jangam, 2016;Chadda, 2014). In such environment, women who look after the family members, kids and old parents get additional workload to look after her man who has met with mental illness who was earlier the bread earner of the family. The noncooperation of other members of the family, expressed emotion of the other member on her husband, critical comments by in laws, physical abuse, domestic violence done by irresponsible alcoholic and substance abused husband, guilt of not able to sustain financially, concern of the suicidal behavior of the patient, over load of roles and responsibilities towards the family, recapitulation of the memories of the leisure and its gradual decrease in frequency and poor physical health in addition to the earning pressure mounting on the shoulder of the women can put her under the high level of psychological distress leading her to suffer from common to severe mental disorder (Ramiro, Hassan, Peedicayil, 2004; Vizcarra et al., 2004; Kingston, McDonald, Austin, Tough, 2015; Jungbauer et al., 2004). Therefore, bringing the symptoms into the notice and their management seems necessary (Kessler et al., 2003). Being one of the least developed states of India, Jharkhand has very poor health facilities. Adequate medical facilities are mostly confined to capital and other important towns. Underutilization of medical care and naxalite activities which sometimes corners transportation and reluctant attitude of medical staff to move into the remote rural areas and cultural practices and unawareness of medical schemes among local residents make the existing scenario more complicated (Saxena, 2009; Statistcal Profile, 2013; Gosh, 2014). There are few studies on prevalence and comparison of psychological distress and its correlates exist in India and hardly any studies is there which talk about psychological distress of caregivers of mentally ill patients and especially the comparison among gender.

Therefore, the present study is trying to find out the distress level among gender with the significant association with education, occupation and income.

METHODOLOGY

The current study is a community based cross- sectional study conducted at Hazaribagh district between July 2014 and February 2016. The studycover 200 individuals living with mental illness. The sample size was calculated on the basis of population of adult i.e. 12 lacks in Hazariagh district (mention the State) with an expected 20% prevalence of mental illness as reported by the previous studies with an 95% confidence level and 0.05 confidence interval [18–20]. Respondents were either had blood relations or marriage, living for more than 2 years were included in the study. Any person having physical or mental retardation, illness or age below 18 years and above 60 years has been excluded from the study. Nav Bharat Jagriti Kendra (NBJK), a nonprofit organization serving community with psychiatric program in Hazaribagh District extending their support by providing the lists of 1200 patients with mental illness which facilitated to find out the relatives of mentally ill patients. To strictly follow the inclusion and exclusion criteria, the study used purposive sampling technique. The data was collected door to door and informed written consent was taken from respondents. A semi- structured socio-demographic data sheet was used to record socio- demographic details of the respondents. To collect distress score, Kessler Psychological Distress Scale (KPDS) version 10 was used. This scale is consists of 10 questions with emotional responses ranging to 5 different levels for each questions from "none of the time" to "all the time". The score ranges between 10 and 50. Lower score indicate "nil, mild, moderate" and higher score meant "severe" distress. The 2001 Victorian Population Health Sur-vey adopted a set of cut off scores which guided to screen Distress level, a score between 10-19 means ' likely to be well', 20-24 'likely to have a mild disorder', 25-29 'likely to have a moderate disorder and 30-50 indicated 'severe dis-order' (Victorian Population Health Survey, 2001). The scale was in English, therefore, who were unable to read or comprehend were assisted by the train volunteers consist of post graduate students. Frequency and percentiles were used for comparing socio-demographic variables; Man Whitney U test was used for comparing distress among genders.

RESULTS

The table 1 shows the presence of psychological distress among gender at different levels. The table clearly shows that females are less "likely to be well" i.e. 28.1% than male who accounts to 46.2% in this category. Females have been reported to develop "severe disorder" i.e. 40.6% al-most half of the population falls under this category whereasfigures for male for the same category accounts to 20.2% only. The difference in distress score among gender has been found statistically significant

Table 1. Showing the presence and comparison of psychological distress among the Gender (N=200)

Group	Likely to be well n(%)	Likely to have a mild disorder n(%)	Likely to have a moderate disorder n(%)	Likely to have a severe disorder n(%)	Mean score± SD	Mann Whitney U	P
Male	48(46.2)	21(20.2)	14(13.5)	21(20.2)	22.23±8.86	3680.000	0.001***
Female	27(28.1)	14(14.6)	16(16.7)	39(40.6)	26.36±9.44		

Note- ***significant at 0.001 level.

Table 2. Socio demographic profile of male and female (N=200)

Variable		Male=104/ (%)	Female=96/ (%)
Educational status	Illiterate	5 (4.8)	36 (37.5)
	Below 10th	39 (37.5)	43 (44.8)
	10th pass	21 (20.2)	10 (10.4)
	Intermediate	16 (15.4)	4 (4.2)
	Graduate and above	23 (22.1)	3 (3.1)
Occupational status	Unemployed	12 (11.5)	55 (57.3)
	Daily wagers	27 (26.0)	16 (16.7)
	Farmers/ self-employed	34 (32.7)	15 (15.6)
	Govt./Private Jobs	31 (29.8)	10 (10.4)
Income in Indian rupees (Annually)	Less than 25000	17 (16.3)	58 (60.4)
	25000 to 1 lakh	61 (58.7)	28 (29.2)
	1 lakh and above	26 (25.0)	10 (10.4)

at p- value less than 0.001 levels in Mann Whitney U Test.*Table 1. Showing the presence and comparison of psychological distress among the Gender (N=200)*

The table 2 talks about the socio- demographic variable of genders, where in terms of education, there has been a significant difference in education level where majority of respondents are having low level of education but high number of women are illiterate and below matriculation of education i.e. 37.5% and 44.8% whereas in male, despite high number of middle school educated i.e. 37.5% still there are significant number of males in graduation category 22.1%. When it comes to occupation, male population show significant participation in daily wagers, farmers or self-employed and professional or regular jobs i.e. 26% 32.7% and 29.8%. But figures in female show totally opposite picture where 57.3% of females are unemployed, 16.7% are daily wagers,15.6% are farmers/self- employed and 10.4% are professional or in regular jobs. Due to this, income also varies in both the group where significant population of male lies between 25,000 to 1 lakh and above i.e. 58.7% and 25% respectively. In female, significant number of women earns below 25,000 rupees annually i.e. 60.4% and moderate amount of women lies be-tween 25000 and 1 lakh i.e. 29.2% and only 10.4% of the female income is above 1 lakh category. The difference in all categories has been found significant in chi- square test at 0.001 levels.

DISCUSSION

The finding of the study presents the prevalence of mild to severe psychological distress. Despite male population of 46.2% are "well". Still, aggregate percentage of male population is between "mild to severe" distresses in which 20.2% falls in "severe" categories. In female, 28.1% of female are "well" but aggregate of female population 71.9% lies be-tween "mild to severe" categories. It is important to note that half of the male respondents are well and majority of female are in distress. The current study used Kessler Psychological Distress scale for measuring psychological distress. The scale has wide acclamation and acceptance across globe to identify Common Mental Disorder (CMD) with minimum biases and high reliability validity. Higher score indicate presence of mental illness (Baillie, 2005).

Relatives suffer from Common Mental Disorder (CMD) which deepens their distress level. They feel mental illness has brought disgrace to the family in short, stigma of being a relative of mentally ill. Subjective and objective burden, social discrimination by society concertize the "taboo" (Hoeing & Hamilton, 1966; Cousineau, McDowell, Hotz, &Hebert, 2003; Ptaznik& Nelson, 1984). Being in the early adulthood and lacking experience of handling the patient increases the distress level causes expressed emotion, quarrel leading to unhealthy relationship between patient and his/her caregiver (Kumar et al., 2009; Lazzarino et al., 2014; Liebana-Pressa et al., 2014; Link & Phelan, 2001; Magana, et al., 2007; Martin, 1992).

Female as per the current study has more psychological distress which has been corroborated with the other studies (Natalie, Ian, Steve, & Paul, 2003; Math &Srinivasanraju, 2010; Mirowsky& Ross, 2002). Female, especially the spouse has to look after the family members, her morbid husband and has to earn for the sustenance of the self and other members of the family resulting in greater distress, burden and strain on health (Natalie, et a., 2003; Nwanze, 2011; Ostman, &Kjelin, 2002; Perlick et al., 1999;Phillips, 2009; Pits, &Sansen, 2015). However several studies contradicted with the argument and didn't find differences in stress and burden among genders (Prasad, Abraham, Akila, Joseph, &Jocob, 2003; Ptaznik& Nelson, 1984; Ramiro, Hassan, &Peedicayil, 204); Rauktis, Koeske, &Tereshko, 2004).

The association of socio-demographic factors gives the complete picture of differences in distress level. As per the figures, women are more illiterate and under educated as comparison to males which supports the facts of ignorance and poor understanding of mental illness, sluggish coping skills, more expressed emotion, domestic violence, burnout and fear of any step leading to injury or death of the patient. Often these women are mostly engaged in low paid jobs and most of the time unemployed and take substantial risk in jobs which results in illness, injury and spending on treatment thus, low saving and low income. So the mounting distress and burden confirms the presence of unidentifiable disorder (Reinares et al., 2006; Sakuma et al., 2015; Sanuade&Boatemaa, 2015).

Males as per study are under educated and moderately lies in matriculation, intermediate and graduate category and fairly distributed across different categories of occupation and relatively have better income level than female and hence have less psychological distress. Studies indicated males having "managerial style" help them to stay away with patients leading to less stressful situation by disseminating task (Saxena, 2009). Therefore, many studies across continents have proved lower education, low paid & uncertain occupation and low income are associated positively with psycho-logical distress irrespective of gender(Schulz&Williamson, 1991; Shah, Wadoo&Latoo, 2010; Sharma, Chakraborti, & Grover, 2016; Sintayehu et al., 2015; Sreeja, Sandhya, Rakesh & Singh, 2009; Vijayalakshmi et al., 2013).

It is interesting to note that socio- economic indicator has given the perfect clue to researchers and policy-makers exactly where to intervene. Jharkhand where basic infrastructure is sluggish is needed to improve. Proper educational and primary health facilities need revision and so as psycho-education is needed across community and gender to improve mental health of both patient and relative. Strategies are required to empower women by providing training on different trades, to make them social entrepreneur and independent and financial aids to the women and family of the mentally ill should be incorporated by the policymakers through different social schemes (Vizcarraeial, 2004; Waris&Viraktamath, 2013; Watson, 2009; Yusuf &Nuha, 2011; Zendjidjan et al., 2012).

CONCLUSION

Due to small sample size and purposive sampling technique without incorporating all the districts of Jharkhand it is hard to generalize the study. So it would be beneficial for the researchers and policymakers if they replicate the same for the entire Jharkhand and plan policy accordingly. The study despite limitations is able to reveal the unidentified psychological disorder the relatives of patient with mental illness are facing, vulnerability of women of being caregiver of the mentally ill and

Table 3. Difference in distress level along with socio- demographic variable between two group (N=200)

Variable	Group	Category	Well	Mild	Moderate	Severe	Total	Chi-square	P value
Education	Male	Below 10th	14(35.9)	6(15.4)	6(15.4)	13(33.3)	39(100)	20.016	.067
		10th Pass	10(47.6)	6(28.6)	3(14.3)	02(09.5)	21(100)		
		Intermediate	13(81.2)	1(06.2)	0(00.0)	02(12.5)	16(100)		
		Graduate	10(43.5)	7(30.4)	4(17.4)	02(08.7)	23(100)		
		Illiterate	01(20.0)	1(20.0)	1(20.0)	02(40.0)	05(100)		
	Female	Below 10th	14(32.6)	11(25.6)	05(11.6)	13(30.2)	43(100)	32.017	.001***
		10th Pass	05(50.0)	01(10.0)	02(20.6)	02(20.0)	10(100)		
		Intermediate	03(75.0)	00(00.0)	00(00.0)	01(25.0)	04(100)		
		Graduate	02(66.7)	01(33.3)	00(00.0)	00(00.0)	03(100)		
		Illiterate	03(08.3)	01(02.8)	09(25.0)	23(63.9)	36(100)		
Occupation	Male	Unemployed	05(41.7)	03(25.0)	02(16.7)	02(16.7)	12(100)	4.565	.870
		Daily wager	13(48.1)	06(22.2)	04(14.8)	04(14.8)	27(100)		
		Farmer & self Employed	19(55.9)	04(11.8)	04(11.8)	07(20.6)	34(100)		
		Govt/Private Jobs	11(35.5)	08(25.8)	04(12.9)	08(25.8)	31(100)		
	Female	Unemployed	06(10.9)	06(10.9)	14(25.5)	29(52.7)	55(100)	28.933	.001***
		Daily wager	07(43.8)	03(18.8)	00(00.0)	06(37.5)	16(100)		
		Farmer & self Employed	09(60.0)	02(13.3)	01(06.7)	03(20.0)	15(100)		
		Govt/Private Jobs	05(50.0)	03(30.6)	01(10.0)	01(10.0)	10(100)		
Annual Income	Male	<25000	08(47.1)	03(17.6)	02(11.8)	04(23.5)	17(100)	8.334	.215
		25001-100000	29(47.5)	08(13.1)	10(16.4)	14(23.0)	61(100)		
		>100001	11(42.3)	10(38.5)	02(07.7)	03(11.5)	26(100)		
	Female	<25000	06(10.3)	08(13.8)	15(25.9)	29(50.0)	58(100)	27.599	.000***
		25001-100000	15(53.6)	04(14.3)	01(03.6)	08(28.6)	28(100)		
		>100001	06(60.0)	02(20.0)	00(00.0)	02(20.0)	10(100)		

the areas of intervention which could lift the socioeconomic condition of female caregiver of mentally ill patient.

ACKNOWLEDGMENT

I would like to express my gratitude to my participants of the study and Nav Bharat Jagriti Kendra (A NGO, based in Hazaribagh, Jharkhand) for supporting and cooperating in the study. A special thanks to Dr. Ronald C. Kessler for granting me the permission to use 'Kessler Psychological Distress Scale - Version -10' for current research paper.

REFERENCES

Ae-Ngibise, K. A., Doku, V. C. K., Asante, K. P., & Owusu-Agyei, S. (2015). The experience of caregivers of people living with serious mental disorders: A study from rural Ghana. *Global Health Action, 8*(1), 10. doi:10.3402/gha.v8.26957 PMID:25967587

Al-Gamal, E., & Yorke, J. (2014, March). Perceived breathlessness and psychological distress among patients with chronic obstructive pulmonary disease and their spouses. *Nursing & Health Sciences, 16*(1), 103–111. doi:10.1111/nhs.12073 PMID:23692348

Baillie, A. J. (2005). Predictive gender and education bias in Kessler's psychological distress Scale (k10). *Social Psychiatry and Psychiatric Epidemiology, 40*(9), 743–748. doi:10.100700127-005-0935-9 PMID:16142511

Barman, N., & Chakaravorty, P. (2012). A descriptive study to assess the level of stress among family members of selected mentally ill clients attending psychiatry OPD of a tertiary care teaching hospital. *Open Journal of Psychiatry& Allied Sciences., 3*, 65–73.

Belek, I. (2000). Social class, income, education, area of residence and psychological distress: Does social class have an independent effect on psychological distress in Antalya, Turkey? *Social Psychiatry and Psychiatric Epidemiology, 35*(2), 94–101. doi:10.1007001270050013 PMID:10784372

Cadieux, N., & Marchand, A. (2014). Psychological distress in the workforce: a multilevel and longitudinal analysis of the cases of regulated occupation in Canada. *BMC Public Health.* Retrieved from www.ncbi.nlm.nih.gov/pubmed/25099686

Caron, J., & Liu, A. (2011). Factors associated with psychological distress in the Canadian Population: a comparison of low- income and non-income sub groups. *Community Mental Health Journal, 47*(3), 318-30.

Census Organisation of India. (2011). *Population Census 2011*. Available at: http://www.census2011.co.in/census/district/102-hazaribagh.html

Chadda, R. K. (2014). Caring for the family caregivers of persons with mental illness. *Indian Journal of Psychiatry, 56*(3), 221. doi:10.4103/0019-5545.140616 PMID:25316932

Chien, W. T., Chan, S. W., & Thompson, D. R. (2006). Effects of a mutual support group for families of Chinese people with schizophrenia: 18- month follow-up. *The British Journal of Psychiatry, 189*(1), 41–49. doi:10.1192/bjp.bp.105.008375 PMID:16816305

Clyburn, L. D., Stones, M. J., Hadjistavropoulos, T., & Tuokko, H. (2000). Predicting caregiver burden and depression in Alzheimer's disease. *The Journals of Gerontology. Series B, Psychological Sciences and Social Sciences*, *55*(1), S2–S13. doi:10.1093/geronb/55.1.S2 PMID:10728125

Diwakar, N., & Ahamad, T. (2015). Skill development of women through vocational training. *International Journal of Applied Research.*, *1*(6), 79–83.

Draper, B. (2004). *Dealing with Dementia: A guide to Alzheimer's Disease and Depression in Caregivers of Patients with Dementia*. Academic Press.

Election Commission of India. (2014). *Systematic Voters' Education and Electoral Participation*. State Sveep Plan 2014, Jharkhand, Office of the Chief Electoral Officer, Jharkhand. Available at: http://eci.nic.in/eci_main1/SVEEP/statesweepplan2014/JHARKHAND.pdf

Farina, A. (1982). The stigma of mental disorders. In A. Miller (Ed.), *The Eye of the Beholder* (pp. 305–363). New York: Praeger.

Gosh, S. (2014). Equity in the utilization of healthcare services in India: Evidence from National Sample Survey. *International Journal of Health Policy and Management*, *2*(1), 29–38. doi:10.15171/ijhpm.2014.06 PMID:24596902

Gruetzner, H. (2001). *Alzheimer's: A caregiver's guide and sourcebook*. New York: John Wiley.

Hoeing, J., & Hamilton, M. W. (1966). The schizophrenia patients in the community and is effect on the household. *The International Journal of Social Psychiatry*, *12*(3), 165–176. doi:10.1177/002076406601200301 PMID:5964677

Iseselo, M. K., Kajula, L., & Yahya-Malima, K. I. (2016). The psychosocial problems of families caring for relatives with mental illnesses and their coping strategies: A qualitative urban based study in Dar es Salaam, Tanzania. *BMC Psychiatry*, *16*(1), 146. doi:10.118612888-016-0857-y PMID:27177934

Jungbauer, J., Wittmund, B., Dietrich, S., & Angermeyer, M. C. (2004). The disregarded caregivers: Subjective burden in spouses of schizophrenia patients. *Schizophrenia Bulletin*, *30*(3), 665–675. doi:10.1093/oxfordjournals.schbul.a007114 PMID:15631259

Kammath, R., Robin, S., & Chandrasekaran, V. (2014). Common mental disorder: A challenge among people living with Human Immuno Deficiency virus infection/acquired immunodeficiency syndrome in Udupi, India. *Annals of Medical and Health Sciences Research*, *4*(2), 242–247. doi:10.4103/2141-9248.129051 PMID:24761246

Kaushik, P., & Bhatia, M. S. (2013). Burden and quality of life in spouses of patients with schizophrenia and bipolar disorders. *Delhi Psychiatry Journal.*, *16*, 83–88.

Kessler, R. C., Barker, P. R., Colpe, L. J., Epstein, J. F., Gfroerer, J. C., Hiripi, E., & Zaslavaky, A. M. (2003). Screening for serious mental illness in the general population. *Archives of General Psychiatry*, *60*(2), 184–189. doi:10.1001/archpsyc.60.2.184 PMID:12578436

Kingston, D., McDonald, S., Austin, M. P., & Tough, S. (2015). *Association between Prenatal and Postnatal Psychological Distress and Toddler Cognitive Development: A Systematic Review*. Released on 21/5/015. Retrieved from www.ncbi.nlm.nih.gov/pubmed/?term=maternal+psychological+distress+and+todler+cognitive+development

Kirmayer, L. J. (1989). Cultural variations in the response to psychiatric disorders and psychological distress. *Social Science & Medicine*, *29*(3), 327–339. doi:10.1016/0277-9536(89)90281-5 PMID:2669146

Kleinman, A. (1991). *Rethinking Psychiatry. From Cultural Category to Personal Experience*. New York: The Free Press.

Kumar, D., Kumar, P., Singh, A. R., & Bhandari, S. S. (2012). Knowledge and attitude towards mental illness of key informants and general population: A comparative study. *Dysphrenia*, *3*(1), 57–64.

Kumar, S., & Mohanty, S. (2007). Spousal burden of care in schizophrenia. *Journal of the Indian Academy of Applied Psychology*, *33*, 189–194.

Kumar, S., Singh, A. R., Verma, A. N., Verma, P. K., & Chaudhary, S. (2009). Subjective burden on spouses of schizophrenia patients. *Industrial Psychiatry Journal*, *18*(2), 97–100. doi:10.4103/0972-6748.62268 PMID:21180485

Lazzarino, A. L., Yiengpruqsawan, V., Seubsman, S. A., Steptoe, A., & Sleigh, A. C. (2014). The association between unhealthy behaviors, mental stress and low socio economic status in an international comparison of representative samples from Thailand and England. *Globalization and Health*, *10*(10).

Liebana-Pressa, C., Fernandez-Martinez, M. E., Gandara, A. R., Muñoz-Villanueva, M. C., Vázquez-Casares, A. M., & Rodríguez-Borrego, M. A. (2014). Psychological distress in health science college students and its relationship with academic engagement. [PubMed]. *Revista da Escola de Enfermagem da U S P.*, *48*(4), 715–722.

Link, B., & Phelan, J. (2001). Conceptualizing stigma. *Annual Review of Sociology*, *27*(1), 363–385. doi:10.1146/annurev.soc.27.1.363

Martin-Yellow, I. S. (1992). The burden of schizophrenia on the family. A study from Nigeria. *The British Journal of Psychiatry*, *161*, 779–782.

Math, S. B., & Srinivasaraju, R. (2010). Indian psychiatric epidemiological studies: Learning from the past. *Indian Journal of Psychiatry*, *52*(7), S95–S103. doi:10.4103/0019-5545.69220 PMID:21836725

Mirowsky, J., & Ross, C. E. (2002). Selecting outcomes for the sociology of mental health: Issues of measurement and dimensionality. *Journal of Health and Social Behavior*, (43), 152–170. doi:10.2307/3090194 PMID:12096697

Natalie, C., Ian, M.D., Steve, H., & Paul, H. (2003). Measuring chronic patient's feelings of being a burden to their caregivers: Development and preliminary validation of a scale. *Official Journal of Medical Care Section, American Public Health Association*, *41*(1), 110-118.

Nwanze, K. (2011) *Closing the gender gap in rural development.* President, International Fund for Agriculture Development. Retrieved from http://www.intracen.org/Closing-the-gender-gap-in-ruraldevelopment/#sthash.F2p63fz1.dpuf

Ostman, M., & Kjelin, L. (2002). Stigma by association: Psychological factors in relatives of people with mental illness. *The British Journal of Psychiatry*, *181*(6), 494–498. doi:10.1192/bjp.181.6.494 PMID:12456519

Perlick, D., Clarkin, J.F., Sirey, J., Raue, P., Greenfield, S., Struening, E., & Rosenheck, R. (1999). Burden experienced by caregiver of persons with bipolar affective disorders. *The British Journal of Psychiatry Journal*, *175*, 56-62.

Phillips, M. R. (2009). Is distress a symptom of mental disorders, a marker of impairment, both or neither? *World Psychiatry; Official Journal of the World Psychiatric Association (WPA)*, (8), 91–92. PMID:19516930

Pits, S., & Hansen, V. (2015). The relationship between lifestyle, occupational health and work related factors with presenteeism among general practitioners. *Archives of Environmental & Occupational Health*. Retrieved from www.ncbi.nlm.nih.gov/pubmed/25892305

Prasad, J., Abraham, S., Akila, B., Joseph, A., & Jacaob, K. S. (2003). Symptoms related to the reproductive tract and mental health among women in rural southern India. *The National Medical Journal of India*, *16*(6), 303–308. PMID:14765620

Ptaznik, H., & Nelson, G. (1984). Stress and Social Support: The burden experienced by the family of a mentally ill person. *American Journal of Community Psychology*, *12*, 589–607. PMID:6496414

Raj, E. A., Shiri, S., & Jangam, K. V. (2016). Subjective burden, psychological distress, and perceived social support among caregivers of persons with schizophrenia. *Indian Journal of Social Psychiatry*, *32*(1), 42. doi:10.4103/0971-9962.176767

Ramiro, S. L., Hassan, F., & Peedicayil, A. (2004). Risk markers of severe psychological violence against women: A world safe multi- country study. *Injury Control and Safety Promotion*, *11*(2), 131–137. doi:10.1080/15660970412331292360 PMID:15370350

Rauktis, M., Koeske, G. F., & Tereshko, O. (1995). Negative social interactions, distress & depression among those caring for a seriously and persistently mentally ill relative. *American Journal of Community Psychology*, *23*(2), 279–299. doi:10.1007/BF02506939 PMID:7572833

Reinares, M., Vieta, E., Colom, F., Martinez-Aran, A., Torrent, C., Comes, M., ... Sanchezmoreno, J. (2006). What really matters to bipolar patients' caregivers: Sources of family burden. *Journal of Affective Disorders*, *94*(1-3), 157–163. doi:10.1016/j.jad.2006.04.022 PMID:16737741

Sakuma, A., Takahashi, Y., Veda, I., Sato, H., Ketsura, M., Abe, M., ... Matsumoto, K. (2015). Post–Traumatic Stress Disorder and Depression prevalence and associated risk factors among local disaster relief and reconstruction worker fourteen months after the Great East Japan Earthquake: A cross sectional study. *BMC Psychiatry*, *15*(1), 58. doi:10.118612888-015-0440-y PMID:25879546

Sanuade, O. A., & Boatemaa, S. (2015). Caregiver profiles and determinants of caregiving burden in Ghana. *Public Health*, *129*(7), 941–947. doi:10.1016/j.puhe.2015.05.016 PMID:26115592

Saxena, K. B. (2009). The naxalite movement and the crisis of governance: Reform measures for regaining people's trust. *Social Change*, *39*(4), 475–503.

Schulz, R., & Williamson, G. (1991). A Two-year longitudinal study of depression among Alzheimer's caregivers. *Psychology and Aging*, *6*(4), 569–578. doi:10.1037/0882-7974.6.4.569 PMID:1777145

Shah, J.A., Wadoo, O., & Latoo, J. (2010). Psychological Distress in Carers with Mental Disorders. *British Journal of Medical Practitioners, 3*(3), 327.

Sharma, N., Chakrabarti, S., & Grover, S. (2016). Gender differences in care giving among family-caregivers of people with mental illness. *World Journal of Psychiatry*, *6*(1), 7–17. doi:10.5498/wjp.v6.i1.7 PMID:27014594

Sintayehu, M., Mulat, H., Yohannis, Z., Adera, T., & Fekade, M. (2015). Prevalence of mental distress and associated factors among caregivers of patients with severe mental illness in the outpatient unit of Amanuel Hospital, Addis Ababa, Ethiopia, 2013: Cross-sectional study. *Journal of Molecular Psychiatry*, *3*(1), 9. doi:10.118640303-015-0014-4 PMID:26457184

Sreeja, I., Sandhya, G., Rakesh, L., & Singh, M. (2009). Comparison of burden between family caregivers of patients having schizophrenia and epilepsy. *International Journal of Epidemiology*, *6*, 2.

Vijaylakshmi, P., Reddy, D., Math, S. B., & Thimmaiah, R. (2013). Attitudes of undergraduates towards mental illness: A comparison between the nursing and business managements students in India. *South African Journal of Psychology. Suid-Afrikaanse Tydskrif vir Sielkunde*, *19*(3), 66–73.

Vizcarra, B., Hassan, F., Wanda, M., Hunter, Munroz, R.S., Ramiro, L., & Paula De, S.C. (2004). Partner violence as a risk factor for mental health among women from communities in the Philippines, Egypt, Chile & India. *Injury Control & Safety Promotion. Journal, 11*(2), 125-129.

Waris, A., & Viraktamath, B. C. (2013). Gender gap and Women's empowerment in India- Issues & Strategies. *International Journal of Scientific and Research Publications*, *3*(9). Retrieved from http://www.ijsrp.org/research-paper-0913/ijsrp-p21116.pdf

Watson, D. (2009). Differentiating the mood and anxiety disorders: A quadripartite model. *Annual Review of Clinical Psychology*, *5*(5), 221–247. doi:10.1146/annurev.clinpsy.032408.153510 PMID:19327030

Yusuf, A. J., & Nuhu, F. T. (2011). Factors associated with emotional distress among caregivers of patients with schizophrenia in Katsina, Nigeria. *Social Psychiatry and Psychiatric Epidemiology*, *46*(1), 11–16. doi:10.100700127-009-0166-6 PMID:19907909

Zendjidjian, X., Richieri, R., Adida, M., Limousin, S., Gaubert, N., Parola, N., ... Boyer, L. (2012). Quality of life among caregivers of individuals with affective disorders. *Journal of Affective Disorders*, *136*(3), 660–665. doi:10.1016/j.jad.2011.10.011 PMID:22100129

Chapter 7
Health and Well-Being Among the Jats of Western Uttar Pradesh:
An Anthropological Life Cycle Approach

Dhananjay Kumar
https://orcid.org/0000-0002-7799-4344
Centre for Culture and Development, Vadodara, India

ABSTRACT

The chapter interrogates the explicit and implicit perception of health and well-being among the Jats of Western Uttar Pradesh by using anthropological life cycle approach. The research combined village ethnography and empirical field work to discuss their behavioural choices that they make to maintain good spiritual, mental and physical well-being. For the purpose of the study, both primary and secondary data have been used. Taking a village as a unit is a generally accepted way of the doing research in the social anthropology, and the author has used this approach to gain the overview of health, well-being, wellness, and belief pattern as perceived by the villagers.

INTRODUCTION

In general, health and well-being are typically viewed in only biomedical context, so that the life cycle are often considered only in terms of body biology hence narrowed defined. This ethnocentric view disregards the intricate interrelationship of biology, psychology, social interaction and cultural dimensions. Thus modes of maintaining

DOI: 10.4018/978-1-7998-1185-5.ch007

health and well-being are framed in terms of regimens imposed on body only. However, this chapter take a cultural view of Jats to view of the human life cycle to evaluate factors that appear to contribute to health and well-being as well as those that appear to cause illness. To find an answer, this chapter presents a novel approach to see health, well-being and wellness from an anthropological life-cycle perspective. Based on these questions, the chapter has been organized in two sections. The first section deals with an extensive conceptual and methodological conversation on the existing literature on health and well-being. It provides the theoretical dimension that make some suggestions on understanding about the use of the terms 'health', 'well-being' and 'wellness' in terms of this holistic paradigm. It also studies how life-cycle approach is well placed to give a crucial insights understanding of health and belief pattern of particular community. The second section vividly provide an ethnographic account of how Jats overview health through systematic life-cycle or stages of human life.

METHODOLOGY

The chapter is based on an empirical research conducted while carrying out author's fieldwork among the Jats of Meerut district of western Uttar Pradesh during 2012-2013 and 2014-2015 as part of his PhD thesis. For the purpose of the study both primary and secondary data have been used. Primary data were gathered through ethnographic field work from one village, in Mawana block of Meerut. By taking a village as a unit is generally accepted way of the doing research in the social anthropology, and author has used this approach to gain the overview of health, well-being, wellness, and belief pattern as perceived the by the villagers. To generate primary data a primary census conducted in the village. Followed by this, in-depth interviews conducted using interview guidelines. Interview schedule, interview guidelines, focused group discussion and observation research technique were used in the field. The structured and open ended questionnaire are prepared and used for the study. The data related to life cycle ritual and practices were conducted generally elderly persons. Few case studies aimed to present in people actual behaviour at the different phases. These data were supported by the various secondary literature collected during and after field work.

CONCEPTUAL FRAMEWORK

The chapter examines the health, well-being and belief perception among the Jats from the life- cycle approach. Obviously time is important component in any society.

Every culture defines time in its own way. Medical anthropology and life cycle approach used to provide the analytic framework of the study. Attempts have been made to understand the relations, linkages, and patterns between the health and well-being in Jats and their life-stages. How they perceive health and wellbeing at the different stages of life-cycle. It was observed that concept of tradition and modern health system are inadequate to deal with the Jats' perception of health and well-being. Although medical anthropologist study the health concepts, but health and well-being from life cycle approach a novel study in more contemporary literature. It tries to answer a few questions, such as what is health and well-being, how culture is related to it, how culture perceive this, what are the main medical anthropological approach relevant to study this perceptions and how relevant the anthropological informed life-cycle approach is relevant to document this perception.

PART I: THEORETICAL DIMENSION

The Health

The meaning of the term health has outgrown Eurocentric words implying 'whole', 'hale' and 'holy'. It destined to refer the wholeness of a person. Health, thus, has strong association with holiness, happiness, hygiene, cleanliness, sanity and real-self. Many of these aspects of health are usually emphasized in vernacular health system, apart from biomedical model, such as Ayurveda, Tao and also Hippocratic system.

In the biomedical perspective, early definitions of health focused on the theme of the body's ability to function; health was seen as a state of normal function that could be disrupted from time to time by disease. But biomedical model also consist several other approaches to understand health. As Capra (1982:340), noted that Hippocratic theory also accounted for ecological factors, but this aspect has been neglected with the rise of Cartesian (rationalistic) science. One of the books in the Hippocratic Corpus, Capra pointed, entitled *Airs, Waters and Places*, could be clubbed in sub-discipline of human ecology. It shows, how the well-being of individuals is influenced by environmental factors such as the quality of air, water and food, the topography of the land and general living habits. As Capra writes: "the Hippocratic tradition, with its emphasis on the fundamental interrelation of body, mind, and environment, represents a high point in Western medical philosophy that is as strong in its appeal for our time as it was twenty-five hundred years ago" (Capra 1982:341). Capra (1982:336) also concluded, however, that Western medical practitioners, in following the biomedical model, seem to have lost this holistic view of health and healing. Thus, most traditional health systems acknowledged that of a close symbiotic relationship between physical body with its immediate environment, so also mind and body.

It is clear from above discussion that health cannot merely defined with prevalent narrow window of illness. It is more than and beyond the absence or presences of illness. In this regard, the much relevant definition given by the (World Health Organization, 1978) has correctly said health as, "the state of complete physical, mental, and social well-being, and not merely an absence of disease or infirmity". As a result, it focuses not only on reducing mortality and morbidity, but on the impact of health determinants, the economic, environmental and social conditions, on health and well-being at various stages in life.

The following definition is not critic proof. This definition is not entirely satisfactory, in that the 'complete state' as it does not include the spiritual dimension of human life (Myers, Sweeney, & Witmer, 2000). Critic said, it still fall in purview of western Eurocentric definition of health without considering the parts of non-western ideology where health closely related to other aspect of life, like spirituality or religion. In January, 1998, the Executive Board of WHO adopted a resolution recommending that the World Health Assembly should add the word 'spiritual' to the definition of health, but the resolution is still pending (Dalal, 2016:8). Thus health has dynamic definition. The present revised definition used by Dalal (2016) is like "Health is a dynamic balance of physical, mental, social and moral modes of being aspiring for higher existence; not just the absence of evil, illness of infirmity".

The Health and Well Being

Through an extensive survey of various dictionary meaning, it came to different interpretation of the health and wellbeing. *The New Oxford Dictionary of English* (1998:864) still provides us with a biomedical and mechanistic 'definition' of health. It sees 'health' briefly as 'the state of being free from illness or injury'. This definition seems more concerned with the absence of certain conditions than the presence of others. It also does not mention the notions of well-being and wellness. Opposite to this, the Collins Concise Dictionary (Sinclair, 1998:662) offers a relativist-functionalist perspective. It expands the meaning of 'health' somewhat by stating that health is the state of being bodily and mentally vigorous and free from disease. The another, the Oxford Advanced Learner's Dictionary (Wehmeier, 2002:551), resonates with both a relativist-functionalist and a homocentric view in that it defines health as the condition of a person's body or mind, the state of being physically and mentally healthy, and able to function optimally within all of these dimensions. Its definition is based on the conviction that the well-being of people and the living systems of the planet which they inhabit come first (Van & Neves, 2004:9-3). The Cambridge International Dictionary of English (Procter, 2002:655) provides us with an 'idealistic' perspective on health, one which philosophically seems to resonate with an eco-centric paradigm, i.e. the assumption that all things in nature are related to one another in a complex but systematic way (Meyer, Moore, & Viljoen, 2002:464). It broadens the meaning of health by also using the term 'well-being' in its definition: the condition of the body and the degree to which it is free from illness, or the state of being well.

Interrelationships of 'Health', 'Well-Being' and 'Wellness'

Our literature survey indicated that 'health', 'well-being' and 'wellness' tend to be used interchangeably, much as we have done so far in this discussion. Green & Shellenberger (1991:15, 18-19) use the combined term 'health and wellness' for their holistic orientation (with 'health' referring to an objective biomedical condition and 'wellness' to a more emotional condition, i.e. feeling well or unwell). Wass (2000:47), in turn, points out that many people may identify themselves as healthy more by a sense of well-being than by the absence of disease. The World Health Organization (1986) and the South African Department of Health (2000) use the terms 'health' and 'well-being' repeatedly, but not 'wellness'. Wissing (2000:5), on the other hand, says that 'health' and 'wellness' have similar denotations and connotations and can be used interchangeably (although the meanings might differ depending on the context). Van Eeden (1996:9) noted in (Kirsten, van der Walt, & Viljoen, 2009) similarly with respect to 'health', 'well-being' and 'wellness' in a psychological context. Recently, Walsh (2005:955) remarked that well-being has been variously interpreted as 'living and faring well' or 'flourishing', and that the notion of well-being is intricately bound up with our ideas of what constitutes human happiness and the sort of life that is good to lead.

Health and Well-Being in Indian Culture

The most common word for health have its Sanskritic origin, *swastha*, literally meaning 'that which is situated in own-self'. Monster-Williams dictionary (Monier-Williams, 2008) termed *swastha* as 'being in one's self', 'being in one's natural state', 'relying upon one's self' and 'self-sufficient'. Health, thus, means the state of being, located inside the self. It is the inner state not contingent on nutritional physical and material factors but on individual's entire existential conditions.

Combining different conceptual relationship of well-being, health, wellness with the Indian culture perceptions, the conceptualization of the state of well-being is comes closer to the concept of mental health and happiness, life satisfaction and actualization of one's full potential. In this regard, Verma & Verma (1989) have defined 'general well-being' as the subjective feeling of contentment, happiness, satisfaction with life experiences and of one's role in the world of work, sense of achievement, utility, belongingness, and no distress, dissatisfaction or worry.

Further, in Indian tradition health is not related to one's well-being only but co-related and conjoint with the wellness of wider groups. As Sinha (1990) that the state of well-being and happiness is contingent on happiness and health of all others living begins and that no one wishes unhappiness to anyone. This clearly represented in following lines:

Om Sarvey Bhavantu sukhinah sarve santu niramayah,
Sarve bhadrani pashyantu ma kashchid dukhabhag bhavet.
(Om, May All be Happy, May All be Free from Illness,
May All See what is Auspicious, May no one Suffer).

Health and well-being are thus presumed to be contingent not only on the state of one's own self, but also on the state of other's selves, which includes all living creatures. This is clearly gives the notion human and his ecology which consist of both social and biological environment. It is well represented when life-cycle approach used in medical anthropology.

Medical Anthropology

Current approaches in medical anthropology study relationships between cultural and social structures, people's beliefs about cause, course, cure and prevention, and their health behavior. The term `Culture' extends and include many issues like of power, control, resistance and defiance as well, and anthropology seeks to understand the links between social stratification (gender, ethnicity, social class), access to material and immaterial goods (food, water, health services, education), illness representations, cultural constructions of femininity and masculinity, attitudes to health promotion, and health behavior (Krumeich, Weijts, Reddy, & Meijer-Weitz, 2016). The combination of all formed the human behaviour of the community. And the human behaviour -much of which is influenced by social, cultural, economic and political factors- is clearly related to health and wellbeing of particular community. Whether, it is intentional or not, human behaviour affects health-promoting and disease-preventing activities, in some instances increasing risk and in other reducing it (Lobo, 2010).

These elements form a specific cultural system in which tasks, responsibilities and proper conduct have become self-evident (Lock & Scheper-Hughes, 1990; Morsy, 1990; Singer, 1990). Describing the relations between these elements is called a `thick description' (Geertz, 1973). Thick descriptions are based on meticulous fieldwork which may include participant observation, open-ended, unstructured or semi-structured interviews and many other techniques.

Unraveling the way in which a specific culture links notions on the human body with life cycle constructions and perceptions of health and illness provides a fruitful basis for the understanding of that culture. In the next section, author explores the potential of this type of analysis for understanding health and wellbeing among Jats of Western Uttar Pradesh, India. The author will present `thick descriptions' that highlight the role of cultural constructions of the different stages of life-cycle events among the Jats and their relation with body, gender and illness in community.

PART II: MAIN FOCUS OF THE CHAPTER

Ethnographic Dimension

The Jats of Western Uttar Pradesh

The Jat is one of the important community of South Asia constituting over 123 million people together in northwest region of Indian and Pakistan (Mahal & Matsoukas, 2017). The term 'Jat' has several insignia. As per Westphal-Hellbusch & Westphal (1964), the term is an Arabic origin which mean 'men from India'. In South Asia, the term also means as 'bunch of hair'. This also have some deeper meaning for Jats, as they themselves considered that they have descended from the hair of Lord Shiva[1]. While some earlier scholar, such as Ibbetson (1916), positioned them as Indo-Aryan or Indo-Scythian descent. The name so prevalent in Punjab region (both India and Pakistan) that the term jat means an agriculturalist (Ibbetson, 1916). While some other traced them term as more central Asian origin and attempt to meant the term as 'grazer' or 'herder (Bowles, 1977). It is often used together with another equivalent term '*Zutt*'. The term pronounced differently in different region. In Punjab, it is pronounced with special emphasis on 'tt', as '*Zutt*' while in Haryana and western Uttar Pradesh, it has more relaxed pronunciation of 't' sound, hence 'Jat'.

Usually, the migration influences the population of a community. Prior to independence the Jat's population was mixed in term of religion wise in northwestern part of India. However, after partition of India in 1947, Hindu and Sikh Jats have lived primarily in India, and the Muslim Jats have lived primarily in Pakistan. It is important to note that last time caste based census was done in 1931 and India and Pakistan population was taken together and constitute of three main religions. They were 47 per cent, 33 per cent and 20 per cent of Hindus, Muslims and Sikhs respectively (Burdak, 2016). As far contemporary population of the community is concerned, we can have extrapolation through some study to arrive approximate numbers. Chatterji (2012) reported the combined Hindu and Sikh Jat population in India as 82.5 million people.

Like the variety of explanation for their group name, Jat, they have different internal segmentation at various levels. For example, Jats are not monotheistic group. In north-west India, they follow at least three religions- Hindu Jat, Sikh Jat and Muslim Jat- also called as *Mule* Jat. Further, they are distributed over a wide a diverse geographical area- from the hot and humid regions in northwestern India to the hill sand plains in southern Pakistan- setting extensive cultural, linguistic, and religious diversity.

Overview of Culture

Among Jats, a lot of diversity restrict for a sweeping generalization about them. They are different as per geographical locality, speak different language, follow differ religion and sects and have different culture. So instead of presenting a generalized picture, this section is focused on the Jats of western Uttar Pradesh. Uttar Pradesh is a most populous state of the India with inhabited of 16 per cent of total population of the country. Due to large territory it had enough diversity. The state can be divided in different regions based on some key geo-sociological features. Every region is different than other. Western Uttar Pradesh comprises the western districts of Uttar Pradesh state, including the areas of Rohilkhand and Braj. The region has demographic, economic and cultural patterns that are distinct from other parts of the state. The region is more closely resembled with the neighbouring state of Haryana, Punjab and Rajsthan than the other region of the state itself, say Eastern Uttar Pradesh. The region experience great economic growth in a similar way of the neighbouring states, Haryana and Punjab. The Jat comprises in almost 15 percent of the Western UP's population. While in eastern Uttar Pradesh growth is slow and Jat is conspicuously absent. While in Hindu religion, they are not considered as higher socio-cultural status. In fact, there considerable debates about their hierarchy in caste system (Kumar & Mishra, 2017).

Historically there were much conundrum for the Jat in British colonial literature, as they were simultaneously labelled as all, a caste, a race and a tribe. Coming to local perception also the picture was not clear. Several scholars, politicians and activists during the period have used three very different labels for them. Some have identified them as a member of warrior group, Kshatriya (Qanungo, 1982) while other argued that they were more related to the backward castes. At the same time, ethnographers reflected from the field data also have different option. Freed and Freed (Freed, Ruth S. and Freed, 1990; Freed & Freed, 1993) studied the change in Jat's status. As per them, until 1958, they were not considered members of the three twice-born "*dwij*" Varna. The *dwij* are called twice born and wear sacred thread for this. Instead Jat were ranked as "clean menial workers: Shudra status. While some other ethnographer is of the opinion that they were ranked below than Rajputs in the warrior group because of the practice of widow remarriage (Lewis, 1958).

It is important to note that at the advent of the last century several reform had influenced Jat community of Western Uttar Pradesh. One of the main were Arya Samaj movements. The movements, started during 1870s by Dayanand Saraswati, promoted the value and practices based on the belief in prime authority of the Vedas. According to some, Datta (1999), primarily because of the influence of the Arya Samaj, the Jats claimed a Rajput descent and a Kshatriya status. The motto of the Samaji was 'return to the Vedas' (in local language *Lauto Vedon ki Or*). They believe in one god and reject the idol worshipping. Their movement started from Jat region. Hence a large number of the western population, including Jats, is followed Arya Samaj. They are followed more a kind of *Vaishya* status and also achieved empowerment (Datta, 1999b). Through this following, Jats started the wear sacred thread, followed Vedic rituals, etc.

Followed by this, they also influence by British effort to improve the region. Jats have increased their productivity by the help of the various British efforts like Yamuna Canal in western Uttar Pradesh. So, this community get more dominant as compared to others. Now, they act more as pressured group. They are termed as OBC group in state and as well of central list. Fuchs (1974) opines that Jat as a central Asian nomadic group that were immigrated into western India. Several serological ad anthropometrics studies on Jats of north India also suggest their close affinities with the Rajputs (Khanna, 1995).

In spite of their above said diversities, Jats are one of the major landowning agrarian people of the state. Generally, Jats in India primarily engage in agriculture and live in permanent village settlements in rural and urbanizing areas. As agriculturalists, the Jats grow cereals such as wheat, maize, and millet, and cash crops such as sugarcane, fruits, and vegetables. Typically, Jats live in villages in which their community is in numerical majority and dominates the economic and sociopolitical aspects of the village life. In fact, the villager were known by the dominant Jat clan found in the village. Locally, they are referred to as chiefs (*chowdharies*). The title symbolizes their ancestral control over the village land and their socioeconomic dominance in the village (Pradhan, 1965b, 1965a). They characterize by the ancient 'brotherhood', *'biradari' or 'pattadari'* type of land relations which is still present in the village (Kumar, 2018).

Generally, Jat practice clan (*Got*) exogamy in arranging marital alliances. There is ideally four -got rules found in avoiding, father, mother, father's mother and mother's mother (Tiemann, 1970). They followed patrilocal residence and patrilineal system of inheritance. The place of land is primeval important to Jat community. Some scholar observe, because of this, they readily practices the widow remarriage especially with leviratic union (Chowdhry, 1994). The widow remarriage is simple process without any pomp up. It is called as '*Chaddar Odhana*' or '*Chuda Pahnanana*'. It involves man throwing a white sheet (or *chaddar*) over the widow's head, signifying his acceptance of her as his wife. Sometimes levirate alliances are primarily symbolic in order to protect the right over property and to avoid a sexual indiscretion on the part of the widow (Chowdhry, 1994). However, this system have imprint in their kinshp terms. As younger brother called elder's brothers in-laws with the same name as – his in-laws (Kumar, 2018).

Context of Health: Environmental Economic Social and Political Factors

In western Uttar Pradesh, and particularly in Meerut region, health care system is multilevel and multiservice system. As far as the most common health care system concern in the region, it is given by modern medicine system through various channels. The state-sponsored health care delivery program and services combined with the various non-governmental organization efforts have led to significant improvement in health care access to the Jat community. They receive health care from allopathic and non-allopathic medicinal system. Further, the government sponsored maternal child health (MCH) program and the integrated child development schemes (ICDS) have spread and expanded health care in remote rural area of the region. These programs consist of various level health support system. They use village-level workers (*Anganvadi*) and provide them training in prenatal, perinatal, and neonatal care to the village population. These health care workforce serve as crucial links between the community as stakeholder and government trained health care systems.

Most Jat village, in the region, are part of the Maternal Child and Family Welfare (MCFW) target zones of the regional Primary Health Centre (PHC). Scholars have suggested about high level acceptance of family planning methods among the Jats of the region (Khanna, 1995, 1997, 2001). They also immunized timely to their children due to availability and applicability to have good care in private healthcare these also increased their network in the near about towns such as Mawana, Meerut, Daurala etc. Overall, in the studied village, Liloha, increasing awareness of healthcare, close proximity of state sponsored private run health care, have let a lot of overall increase in the utilization of these services and corresponding decrease in family size among the community. Jats are maintaining a low fertility rate by using contraceptives and achieving the desired family composition.

Jat, traditionally, received the health care from diverse ways, what we can call, multi-medical system perspective due to their historical legacy. They received health care from traditional medicine- person (*Vaidyas)* practicing Ayurveda and Greek (*Yunani*) medicine, homeopathic physicians, midwives and local self-trained villager healers who practice popular medicine. Out of these, Vaidya generally have impact of Vedic system or so called traditional medicine system. While, others like Unani, homeopathic systems are influence from western medicine system time to time. In post-colonial India with increase of government support and sponsorship, western medicine become an dominant medical system providing allopathic doctors at local dispensers, PHCs, hospital and private clinics.

Traditionally Jat women folk used to prefer at-home deliveries with the assistance of local village midwives. In Liloha, the village midwife comes from low caste of untouchables, Jatav (Chamar or leather-workers or tanner) community. It is imperative to note that due to increase urbanization and improvement of state sponsor health care delivery, most of the village community have access to biomedical services in near about town and cities, like Mawana and Meerut (Kumar, 2018). This brought a significant change in birth practice among the women. Pregnancies and child birth are increasingly medicalized. In recent times, more assistance from medical health care system are taken. Resultantly, role of midwives from the village decreasing day by day. Now, they do not seek the local Jatav midwife traditional one, but now take care assistance and help of modern midwives and biomedical doctors for prenatal, perinatal and postnatal health care. Role of the anganvadi worker also get more important. Apart from these changes, the health are during prenatal and perinatal period is mainly responsibilities of Jat women. Jat men play little or no role in this area, or we can say it is outside of their purview.

Classification Illness

In spite of increasingly using western medicine and technology for various health care services, Jat still cognize or have a core belief, of the traditional idea of health, illness, healing and wellness. As said these ideas are not generated overnight but yield of a long term associated with the different societies and their influence. Jat people, during their life span, associated health, illness, healing with Ayurvedic, homeopathic, and Unani healing system generally at their core theories of illness. Generally, they use non-biomedical system of healing for non-chronic health conditions through herbal and plant medicine, seasonal do's don'ts and dietary beliefs etc. These changes are associated basically with the two cycles imperative for them. One is seasonal cycle of weather which is associated with the agriculture, which is their basic livelihood pattern, and the second cycle is human life cycle, changes of a human body through different biological and cultural stages. As said earlier, no biological cycle is only important, but it is often associated with the social of cultural attributes. Among them, no biomedical categories hot and cold foods (Freed and Freed, 1993) are generally associated with seasons and physiological effects which often associated with or mixed interpretation of the two cycles.

The Ayurvedic system of medicine adopts a holistic approach through dietary and lifestyle changes, herbal medicine, an exercise to cure chronic diseases and maintain individual health. This medical system is based on the ancient knowledge contained in Atharvaveda[2], the fourth Veda. In fact, Ayurveda is a way of life based on certain emphasis on diet, lifestyle and yoga practices suitable for an individual according to his/her own body constitutions. The body constitutions, in turn is determined on the basis of the predominance of or loss of equilibrium in one or more of the four basic things, the humar, viz Gas (*Vata*), bile (*Pitta*), or phlegm (*Kapha*). Based on the symptoms produced due to excess or deficiency of particular fault (*dosha*), the Ayurvedic practitioner selects remedial measures in the form of herbs, plant medicine, and metal salts.

Apart from the multi-medical system, Jats in western Uttar Pradesh continue to believe in numerous spirituality conditions. As per the local conditions, spirituality is one of the important conditions of health and illness system of behaviour. They believe in numerous male god and mother goddess. A number of the god goddess are associate with the particular medical conditions, especially related to epidemiological conditions related to children. Most of the villagers identify two mother goddess namely Sitala mata and Khasra mata for small pox and skin rashes, respectively. These deities have been propiated with the regular interval, often a cyclic one, of the seasonal calendar for the prevention and cure of the illness.

Further, Jats also believe some other kind of behaviour commonly held for healing or curing illness. In order to protect children and family member form illness, evil eyes and harmful spirits, the villager ties protective amulets made of metals, like iron, gold, silver, copper, bead, cloths and stings (usually black and red) on children wrists, ankles and around their necks (Freed ad freed, 1993). More commonly in Jat villages, diseases like tetanus, diarrhea, and measles are often associated with the spirit possession and evil eyes. Jat women are expected to worship local deities and do charm (*tona- totakas*) in order to ward off evil spirits and cure disease among family members especially children (Chowdhry, 1994). Apart from that there are some health behavior which combine both part spirituality with the using some herbal medicine of the various diseases like for Jaundice. The affected person tied a necklace of thread with having twigs (*Chhoti Lakdi*) of special plant to cure the Jaundice.

Jat Sexuality and Reproduction

Prior to discussing the sexuality and reproductive behaviour of the Jat, few things needed to understand. Jat do not live in isolation. They shared their space with the other community and also influenced rapidly from the ongoing technological transformation in western medicine in the region. Because they are the dominant community, numerically and economically, in the region, they are first to use the westernized health care facilities. In this way, they are experiencing a significantly shifting to their overall social structure; including their health and economical behaviour, their cognition of well-ness, health and illness; and their traditional cultural identity.

As with any other community, Jats sexuality and reproduction are cultural bound. Their basic wellbeing, health and illness concept regarding reproductive and sexual behaviour are associated with the prevailing believe patterns about gender, conception, prenatal period, child birth, postpartum care, childhood, puberty, adulthood and old age. Such believes and related practices are significantly influence their health care practices.

As per Jat peasantry patriarchal system, there is little equality or symmetry between men and women. As compared to men counterpart, Jat women are generally given a little choice especially with regard to marriage, mobility, education and employment. Extensive ethnographic evidences suggests that women faces gender specific neglect (Das Gupta, 1987; Khanna, 1995, Tieman (1970). Earlier, the gender contrast more prevalent as compared to contemporary time. The custom of patriarchal leads to overall neglect of women leading to her overall poor physical health (Jeffery & Jeffery, 1997; Khanna, 1997) more recent one (Kaur and Kochar, 2017). These studies conclusively demonstrate the adverse effect of the culturally prescribed subordination of Jat women on their productive halt and survival. Further, cultural prescribed practices associated the usually based allocation of intra-household resources for health care and food have been argued to be responsible for poor overall health and high morbidity rate among the Jat women (Chaudhry, 2004) and it is more prevalent among the middle aged group (40-59) women (Kaur & Kochar, 2017).

Marriage, among the Jats, is life stage marks the socially accepted initiation of reproductive behaviour. The important life stage can be distinct into two events the actual social events associated with the marriage and the consummation of marriage. As per traditional system, marital alliance are arranged with the help of the village barber, who generally associated with *Jajmani* relation with the family. Barber help parent in finding suitable match for their children and finalizing the timing, exchange and other important details associated with the marriage. Thus, the barber becomes the most important person in marriage, generally worked as the middle man between the two parties, and generally worked with barber with other side (prospective spouse). The barber from both sides meet and discuss the details then their clients (*Jajmans)* will come front to front and alliance is fixed.

Followed by this, an elaborate religious ceremony marks the martial bonds. The consummation of marriage, locally called *gauana*, (some say second marriage), however, takes place usually within one or two years after the marriage. The term *liviayo*, refers to the time of the *gauana*. It also involves the ceremony when bridegroom, along with this other relative comes to take the bride to her affinal village and household. Earlier, these gap of duration used to be long. As early marriage is prevailed combined with the long gap for second marriage. However, recently, there has been considerable decrease in the time gap between the marriage and consummation. Earlier there was also double marriage system prevailed, where marital alliances between sets of sisters and sets of brother were conducted. In those case, siblings or cousin sibling will be seek in the alliances. Such marriages are described by Jats as more realistic and suitable to an agricultural way of life and three generation patrilocal extended family system (Khanna, 2003; Kolenda, 1987). Among jats, earlier endogamy was prevailed, which is not breaching by the several phenomena urbanization, and skewed sex ration to other areas and often long distance cross region marriages (Kukreja, 2018).

Health Through the Life Cycle

The Jats recognize an individual life cycle into the four major stages what locally called as Ashram. This ashram system prescribed the traditional Hindu views of every individual life in mainly four stages. First, in *Bhrahmachara* (student)-ashram, the individual as a student follow a strict code of chastity (*Brahmacharaya*) and learn from his teacher (*Guru*), the things needed for the future life. It is a kind of preparation of future life. In the second stage, called as *Grihastha* (householder)-ashram, the individual is expected to take household responsibilities and fulfill his duties towards his family, household and dharma. The third stage, *Vanaprastha* (retired)- ashram, marks the third state of life in which the individual begins the hermitage phase of life and returns to the contemplation and for guiding household, family and society. The fourth and final stage of *Sannyasa* (renunciation) - ashram, renunciation marks the beginning of the renounce all the outer world and begin learning about the spirituality away from all social and political concerns (Lewis, 1958).

It is important to note that these stages prescribed by traditional view but ground reality may be different. Although general population noted and praised these ashram but rarely conform it verbatim. They have different cognition of lifecycle of the individual in tier society. It is very much on line of at ground level happens to be debate of ideal culture and real culture. Society often prescribed a few standardized set up behaviour which rarely conform present day population. As found in the field data, every villager tell that this four ashram system is perfect and good and should be followed. But when asked how many of the villager followed this pattern. They answered negatively.

Instead they have separate cognition, often specific to Jat community, regarding individuals and their life cycle and its role to wellness and healing behaviour of the individual. Among them, specific ceremonies or events are often associated with the transition of an individual through different stages of life. During each life stage individuals are expected to perform the social roles prescribed for that life stage. It is however, important to note that traditional Hindu view do not separate life stage based on gender. However, among Jats, peasant patriarchal system and the corresponding gender stratification place sever constraints upon the activities and roles of community's women throughout the life cycle. These constraints directly affect Jat women's ability to access health care practices and in total their health behaviour.

Pregnancy and Childbirth

Pregnancy and childbirth, both process, are considered as very auspicious events of a Jat person. Childbearing constitutes an important part of an adult Jat women's life. It was said that a female became women after bearing a child. *"Ma banne par hi asali aurat banti*". During the time of the woman's labour, family members gather in the house and women perform important roles associated with the childbirth. If the newborn is a boy, the relatives bang a metal place (*Thali*) or fire in the air to announce his birth. Because of the strong son preference among the Jats, the birth of the son is considered as auspicious occasion of cheerfulness and jubilation. No such celebration take place on the birth of girl. The happiness on the birth of a son is shared by mother's affinal and natal families together. As the birth of a son improves the social status of the mother not in her household only but in whole affinal patrilineage. Also, this event happily shared by her natal family. The affinal household and family of the mother receives gifts, special food items, and money from her natal family. However, in the case birth of daughter, these contribution are comparatively smaller. That to, this practice is limited to first born child daughter.

Infancy

In Jats, the sex differential in health and mortality during infancy and early childhood. Further, these differences are also based on gender. Culturally prescribed pattern of son preference and neglect of daughter considered an important for gender differentials in morbidity and mortality among the Jats. The mortality patterns among the Jats correspond with the South Asian pattern of sex differentials males. They males generally have equal or slightly higher mortality rates than females during the first month of life and lower mortality rate than female after the first month of life (Khanna, 2004). The field notes suggests that parents tend to show preferential treatments for sons, generally investing more household resources towards ensuring their survival. Infant girls are considered relatively more resistant to disease than an infant boy.

A daughter is often compared and quoted with *kikkar (Acacia Nilotica)* plant- a xerophytics, a thorny bush that grows wild and does not require much nurturing.

Childhood

Gender role is socialized very early in the life of an individual. Often before children are aware of their sexual identity. It is important to note every society gender role is more cultural having a basic of biological facts. The socialization start as per gender role, behaviour what should be done or what should not. This may happen even before the development of an internal motives for conforming to sex role standards. Parents and community play important roles in in reinforcing norms of expected behaviour. Girls, generally socialized under strict patriarchal control, came to understand their limited role, selective option for future life and rigid patterning of these option during their upbringing. For the young girl, discrimination in term of nutrition and health care allocation occur in juxtaposition with the perpetual reinforcement of her gender identity.

It is important to note that, apart from health care, education of female, is second important dimension where gender role has been reinforced differential treatment. Thus, the individual and combining effect cultural and biological factors invariable lead community's differential behaviour of boy and girl. This negatively influence girls overall growth and development patterns, reproductive health and fertility (Khanna, 1997).

Adolescence

Son presence and daughter neglect has not limited to infancy state but continued an along term process. It is also founding among the Jats in spite of increasing urban contact as well as access to utilization education and health care services. In Liloha, few household for which economic and occupation based agriculture to urban jobs based economic means. Means one or few girls or children are doing white collar jobs in nearest big cities, such as Delhi (Kumar, 2018). These households have improvement of education and health care facility still followed the same son preferences patterns. So, it is not the urbanization that will remove this gender differentiation.

It is observed in the field that for a Jat, most important thing after agriculture and his buffalo is his son. He always compare his son and buffalo and takes good care of both. For him, both will repay in the agriculture and future development of household and family. Author often heard saying that ultimately girl will left the household and family and become member of a different family. It is said she is not theirs. As, *'chhori to paraya dhan hai'* (girls are another's wealth), so why invest in another wealth. Means it is destined to married away and all the good things she achieved will go with her. Whereas sons are viewed as economic and political assets addition to strength and prestige of the family. The daughters are perceived as an economic and moral burden. While parents expect their teenage sons to enroll in good school and colleges. Nowadays, they tend to see the 'good' means private school and college. So they readily invest for their teenage son future education. On the other hand for girls, adolescence invariably marks the end of their education experience. However in recent times, people send their girls to educate till the intermediate level as now village have one inter-college of its own.

However, changes are coming in the village. Nowadays, few private schools came up. Earlier, people used to send only son to private English medium schools but now they send their daughter also. Secondly, now girls are studying not only at nearest town and city, Mawana and Meerut, but also few girls are studying in University of Delhi. Moreover, they are now giving competition to the boys for getting government job. Earlier which is used to be only boy's domain. Boys of the village generally get selected for police, CRPF, and military services. These services of boys are limited to state and neighbouring or bordering state, Delhi. But now cities are filled with the village Jat girls enrolled in various sector from teaching to service industries. This is a new things happening. Earlier elders of the family does not allowed the girls to city for education of service purposes. They thing differently of cities. As anthropologists have written about the contempt that the Jats had for city life. They believed people living in the towns were 'gasping, greedy and lacking in dignity', apart from being physically weak, wrote JNU professor Surinder Jodhka, quoting from the research of J Pettigrew published in 1992.

Among the Jats, after development of secondary sexual characteristics and menarche signal several restriction imposed on them. The girls expected to spend more times in the house and take responsibility of the domestic workload. She, expected to help prepare and serve food and take care of their younger siblings. Jat culture mediated the concerns for the parents regarding their daughter's virginity, marriage and workload expectation. This expectation lead the parents to enforce seclusion and strict parental control of mobility, education and occupation of their daughters. The imposition of strict conduct of behaviour enviable leads to agitation, apprehension, and emotional anxiety among the girls. Although, the starting of menstruation is regarded as a natural event, women rarely discuss this issue among themselves. Delay menarche is often considered as indicator of infertility. Irregular menstrual cycles are believed to be associated with the sexual carelessness on the part of girls and a source of great anxiety for parents. Among the parents, one of the major concerns is fear of emerging sexuality of their daughter and possible dishonor which her sexual activity could bring to the family. This brings the anxiety complex among the Jat girls. Coupled with lack of knowledge, this anxiety brings the emotional distress to the psychosocial development of adolescent girl. Health care behaviour among the Jats also indicates a strong bias favoring son over their daughters. Generally Jat sons receive modern health care at an earlier stage of their illness than Jat girls. With comparison to girls, Jat boys are more likely to be taken to biomedical 'specialist' doctors and clinics. An ill son is a matter of great concern and anxiety for the family where as an ill daughter soon become the target of insult and parental frustration. Girl during this stage of their life have little or no control over their health and are dependent on decision of their family elders.

An adolescent girl's life in her natal home is often described as life in a state of transition, the threshold of living in between two worlds. She is considered as someone else's commodity (*paraya dhan*). Life stage puberty and development of secondary sexual characteristics emphasize her temporary existence in her natal home. As compared to daughter, the son always considered more than the permanent member of the family. As he is only who inherit the property directly from parents.

Adulthood

Traditionally Jat prefer early marriage, especially in the case of girls. Among the Liloha Jat, parent observe strict pattern of sub caste or clan (*Got*), village and at times, regional, exogamy while arranging marital alliances for their children. At her affinal home, the adjustment process for the young bride involves meeting conjugal responsibilities, often from a position of complete ignorance, and dealing with the daily demands of the households. She expected to maintain veal from senior men in the family and the community. At the outside the village, *purdhah* observed even from the villager elders, who may belong to other castes.

The also practice patrlineality and patriarchal system among themselves. Expectation to produce a son is very high among them. This also resulted to early marriage and early pregnancy in their married life. Early pregnancy increases the risk of obstructed labour and reproductive morbidity. Easily available of health care practices in most of the rural areas of northwestern India increases the awareness to seek prenatal and perinatal health care from Government sponsored clinics. Women in household are primarily responsible for health care during and after the pregnancy. Among the Jats, sex and gender are contrasting concepts. Jat parent do not think of their children only in terms of child's sex because what concerns them most is whether the child is son (*beta*) or daughter (*beti*). These terms, used to represents two gender, invoke an entire set of cultural values and behavioral norms associated with the sex of the child. While the birth of a son is considered a good sign or an indication of the family's good fortune, that of a daughter is considered as sign of distress and anxiety. Local folklore more clearly reflects these every day realty.

Some of the commonly used proverbs expressing strong son preference among the Jats of Liloha. Like:

jitney ladke utne lath, jitne lath utna kabza
(Number of sons is equal to number of sticks and the number of sticks determine the amount of land controlled by a family)
jisne ghar ka dudh bech diya usne apna poot bech diya
(selling milk is equivalent to selling a son)

On the other hand, common household names for daughter includes like *Rambatheri* (God this one is enough) or *Rambheji* (this daughter belongs to God and he will take care of her). It was observed during the interview that majority of parents expressed desired for a small household size, and considered two sons and a daughter to be the ideal family composition. In fact, during the field work author lived with the parents who have such ideal composition and for that household and their family members have great value in the family and relatives. In this case, the daughter is younger than two sons. But married first, and later on elder brother married. Daughter is married in Daurala (roughly 40 km west) in a different regional marital alliance. While elder son is married near Pilkuha (nearly 35 km east). They rarely go beyond some distance in eastern direction.

The Old Aged

Among Jat, older members command considerable social prestige, respect and authority over other group of population in household, family and village. They prefer to live in joint families with older men as heads of the household. While men enjoy high status and prospection the family primarily by virtue of their gender, Jat women have to contribute male hires to the husbands' patrilineage in order to gain authority and power in the household and family. Often older women's primarily responsibilities include direct supervision of their children's socialization care. Among the Liloha, the elderly women lack physiological knowledge associated with the menopause an experience a wide range of menopausal symptoms such as tension, headaches, swelling and loss of appetite Some informants also reported a feeling resentment and anger. Although the elderly Jats rarely seek health care for minor health problems, the joint family system amount Jats provide financial security and facilities time health care as compared to other communities in the village. Even at this stage in life, men have privileged social status over their female counterpart.

Dying and Death

There are different pattern of the observation of pollution after the death, The Jat generally observe 13 days of pollution after death of Jat men. While when Jat women dies, they observe pollution for 12 days. Jat men are expected show considerable behaviour restraints during the day of pollution while Jat women expected to express their grief in public. The dead are cremated by following the traditional Hindu ritual of cremation in which he eldest son plays an important role. At the death of married women, ritual and practices reinforce the notion that she does not belong to her husband patrlineage. Her sister's and natal women relatives prepare the body for cremation and funeral rites.

CONCLUSION

So, health and well-being is beyond the disease or cure and represented in notions, behaviour and belief patterns which is an integral part of the culture of the social group. It is argued that medical and health care systems are cultural systems consonant with the groups and social realities that produce them. As time is an important factor for every culture, so that it is related to human health and well-being domains. For proper understanding the health, well-being and healing behaviour, that are well drenched in culture system, we need to look into health as a culture system where every aspect of the life has health concept. So we need to look beyond the biomedical model of health and diseases. Here, life-cycle approach, a well-researched approach in anthropology, would fit perfectly to describe the equilibrium homeostatic of the health system in the human body. Human being have different life stages, that are repetitive in nature, as cycle remains, only persons replaced to other persons. Every stages of life be it child, adolescent, adult or any other culture system perfectly have a cultural design of each and every stages. Culture can be defined as a set of elements that mediates and qualifies any physical or mental activity that is not determined by biology and which is shared by different members of a social group. They are elements with which social actors construct meanings for concrete and temporal social interaction, as well as sustain existing social forms, institutions and their operating models. Culture includes values, symbols, norms and practices. Culture is shared and patterned, because it is a human creation shared by specific social groups. Material forms, as well as their symbolic content and attributions, are patterned by concrete social interactions of individuals. That stages more of nature of cultural bound pertaining to particular cultural community. Here, we have shown the Jats have well defined several stages of life cycle which can be explored to understand the health and welling among themselves. The cultural system of health emphasizes the symbolic dimension of the understanding of health and includes the knowledge, perceptions and cognitions used to define, classify, perceive and explain disease. Each and all cultures possess concepts of what it is to be sick or healthy. They also have disease classifications, and these are organized according to criteria of symptoms, severity, etc. Their classification, as well as the concepts of health and illness, are not universal and rarely reflect the biomedical definitions.

ACKNOWLEDGMENT

Author thanks profoundly to Prof. Lancy Lobo, Director, Centre for Culture and Development, Vadodara for providing very conducive environment and constant encouragement. He is also very much grateful of the people of Liloha village, district Meerut, Uttar Pradesh, for their readily co-operation for the providing the insight of their health and belief systems.

REFERENCES

Bowles, G. T. (1977). *The People of Asia*. London: Weidenfeld and Nicolson.

Burdak, L. (2016). *Jat Belt: Distribution of Jat Population*. Academic Press.

Capra, F. (1982). *The Turning Point: Science, Society and the Rising Culture*. London: Fontana Paperbacks.

Chatterji, S. (2012, January). Government Turns focus on Jat Quota. *Hindustan Times*.

Chowdhry, P. (1994). *The Veiled Women: Shifting Gender Equations in Rural Haryana 1880–1990*. New Delhi: Oxfor University Press.

Dalal, A. K. (2016). *Cultural Psychology of Health in India: Well-being, Medicine and Traditional Health Care*. New Delhi: Sage Publication.

Datta, N. (1999a). *Forming an Identity: A Social History of the Jats*. New Delhi: Oxfor University Press.

Datta, N. (1999b). Jats: Trading Caste Status for Empowerment. *Economic and Political Weekly*, *34*(45), 6–12.

Freed, R. S., & Freed, S. A. (1993). Ghost: Life and Death in North India (No. 72). New York: Academic Press.

Freed, R. S., & Freed, S. A. (1990). Ghost Illness in a North Indian village. *Social Science & Medicine, 30*(5), 617–623.

Fuchs, S. (1974). *The Aboriginal Tribes of India*. Delhi: Macmillan.

Geertz, C. (1973). *The Interpretation of Cultures: Selected essays*. New York: Basic Books Inc. Publishers.

Green, J., & Shellenberger, R. (1991). *The Dynamics of Health and Wellness: A Biopsychosocial Approach*. Chicago: Holt, Rinehart & Winston.

Ibbetson, D. (1916). *Punjab Castes*. Lahore: Indian Press.

Jeffery, R., & Jeffery, P. (1997). *Population, Gender and Politics: Demographic change in rural North India*. Cambridge, UK: Cambridge University Press. doi:10.1017/CBO9780511621550

Kaur, M., & Kochar, G. K. (2017). Impact of Anaemia on Morpho-physiological Variables of Rural Jat Women. *Journal of Life Science*, *2*(1), 17–20. doi:10.1080/09751270.2010.11885148

Khanna, S. K. (1995). *Gender Discrimination, Maternal Health, and Pregnancy Outcomes in North India*. Syracuse University.

Khanna, S. K. (1997). Traditions and Reproductive Technology in an Urbanizing North Indian Village. *Social Science & Medicine*, *44*(2), 171–180. doi:10.1016/S0277-9536(96)00144-X PMID:9015870

Khanna, S. K. (2001). Shahri Jat and dehati Jatni: The Indian peasant community in transition. *Contemporary South Asia*, *10*(1), 37–53. doi:10.1080/09584930120062029

Khanna, S. K. (2003). Jat. In Encyclopedia of Medical Anthropology: Health and Illness in the World's Cultures Topics - Volume 1; Cultures (pp. 777–783). Springer International Publishing.

Kirsten, T. G. J. C., van der Walt, H. J. L., & Viljoen, C. T. (2009). Health, Well-being and Wellness: An Anthropological Eco-systemic Approach. *Health SA Gesondheid*, *14*(1), 1–7. doi:10.4102/hsag.v14i1.407

Kolenda, P. (1987). *Regional Differences in Family Structure in India*. Jaipur: Rawat Publications.

Krumeich, A., Weijts, W., Reddy, P., & Meijer-Weitz, A. (2016). The Benefits of Anthropological Approaches for Health Promotion Research and Practice. *Health Education Research*, *16*(2), 121–130. doi:10.1093/her/16.2.121 PMID:11345657

Kukreja, R. (2018). Caste and Cross-region Marriages in Haryana, India: Experience of Dalit cross-region brides in Jat households. *Modern Asian Studies, 52*(2), 492–531. doi:10.1017/S0026749X16000391

Kumar, D. (2018). Changing Agricultural Practices and their Impact on Rural Social Institutions in Uttar Pradesh, India. National Institute of Technology, Rourkela.

Kumar, D., & Mishra, N. R. (2017). Caste Hierarchy and New Agro-technological Practices : Some Anthropological thoughts on Western Uttar Pradesh. *Man in India, 97*(11), 285–300.

Lewis, O. (1958). *Village Life in Northern India: Studies in a Delhi Village*. New York: Vintage Books.

Lobo, L. (2010). *Malaria in the Social Context: A study in western India*. New Delhi: Routledge.

Lock, M., & Scheper-Hughes, N. (1990). A Critical Interpretive Approach in Medical Anthropology: Rituals and Routines of Discipline and Dissent. In T. M. Johnson & C. F. Sargent (Eds.), *Medical Anthropology. Contemporary Theory and Method* (pp. 47–72). New York: Praeger Publishers.

Mahal, D. G., & Matsoukas, I. G. (2017). Y-STR Haplogroup Diversity in the Jat Population Reveals Several Different Ancient Origins. *Frontiers in Genetics, 8*, 121. doi:10.3389/fgene.2017.00121 PMID:28979290

Meyer, W., Moore, C., & Viljoen, H. (2002). *Personology: From Individual to Ecosystem*. Johannesburg: Heinemann.

Monier-Williams, M. (2008). *A Sanskrit-English Dictionary (revised)*. Delhi: Motilal Banarsidas Publication.

Morsy, S. (1990). Political Economy and Medical Anthropology. In T. M. Johnson & C. F. Sargent (Eds.), *Medical Anthropology. Contemporary Theory and Method* (pp. 26–46). New York: Praeger Publishers.

Myers, J. E., Sweeney, T. J., & Witmer, J. M. (2000). The Wheel of Wellness Counselling for Wellness: A Holistic Model For Treatment Planning. *Journal of Counseling and Development, 78*(3), 251–266. doi:10.1002/j.1556-6676.2000.tb01906.x

Pradhan, M. C. (1965, Dec. 11). The Jats of Northern India: Their Traditional Political System-II. *The Economic Weekly*, 1821–1824.

Procter, P. (Ed.). (2002). *Cambridge International Dictionary of English*. Cambridge, UK: Cambridge University Press.

Qanungo, K. (1982). *History of the Jats: Contribution to the history of northern India*. New Delhi: Surajmal Memorial Education Society.

Sinclair, J. M. (Ed.). (1998). *Collins Concise Dictionary*. Glasgow, UK: Collins.

Singer, M. (1990). Postmodernism and Medical Anthropology: Words of Caution. *Medical Anthropology*, *12*(3), 289–304. doi:10.1080/01459740.1990.9966027 PMID:2233174

Sinha, D. (1990). Concept of Psychological Well-being: Western and Indian Perspective. *Nimhans Journal*, *8*, 1–11.

The New Oxford Dictionary of English. (1998). London: Oxford University Press.

Tiemann, G. (1970). The Four-got-Rule among the Jat of Haryana in Northern India. *Anthropos*, *65*(1/2), 166–177.

Van, H. V., & Neves, D. (2004). Activity Theory as a Framework for Psychological Research and Practice Developing Societies. In *Self, Community and Psychology* (pp. 9–20). Lansdowne: UCT Press.

Verma, S. K., & Verma, A. (1989). *Manual for PGI General Wellbeing Measure*. Lucknow: Ankur Psychological Agency.

Walsh, P. (2005). Well-being. In T. Honderich (Ed.), *The Oxford Companion to Philosophy* (pp. 955–956). Oxford: Oxford University Press.

Wass, A. (2000). *Promoting Health-The Primary Health Care Approach*. Marruckville: Harcourt Australia.

Wehmeier, S. (Ed.). (2002). *Oxford Advanced Learner's Dictionary*. Oxford, UK: Oxford University Press.

Westphal-Hellbusch, S., & Westphal, H. (1964). *The Jat of Pakistan*. Berlin: Duncker & Humbolt.

Wissing, M. P. (2000). Wellness: Construct clarification and a framework for future research and practice. *First South African National Wellness Conference*.

World Health Organization. (1978). *Alma-Ata Declaration*. Geneva: WHO.

World Health Organization. (1986). *Young People's Health – A Challenge for Society. Technical Report Series 731*. Geneva: WHO.

KEY TERMS AND DEFINITIONS

Health: A state of complete physical, mental, and social well-being and not merely the absence of disease or infirmity.

Jats: Traditional agriculturalist people residing western part of India.

Life-Cycle: The life cycles refers to maturational and generational processes in natural population. In human being, it starts from conception and ends with death through travelling from different stages (e.g., infancy, childhood, adolescence, and adulthood).

Medical Anthropology: A subfield of Anthropology that draws upon social, cultural, biological, and linguistic anthropology to better understand those factors which influence health and well-being.

Thick Description: It is a term used to characterize the process of paying attention to contextual detail in observing and interpreting social meaning when conducting qualitative research

Village Ethnography: A branch of ethnography that focus on the systematic study of people and culture of the village.

Village Studies: The studies focus on village and its people. It may done through different perspective. Started by seminal works of famous anthropologist, M. N. Srinivas. The 1950s and late 1960s witnessed the publication of a large number of village studies by Indian and other anthropologists; more village studies have been made by anthropologists in India.

Well-Being: Well-being is the experience of health, happiness, and prosperity. It includes having good mental health, high life satisfaction, and a sense of meaning or purpose. More generally, well-being is just feeling well.

Wellness: The state of being in good health, especially as an actively pursued goal. Wellness is an active process of becoming aware of and making choices toward a healthy and fulfilling life.

ENDNOTES

[1] Lord Shiva, also known as Mahadeva or Maheshvra (Deity of Deity), is one of the three primary deities of the Hindu trinity and is worshiped as the destroyer and transformer of the world.

[2] Literally means knowledge storehouse of Atharvanas, the procedures for everyday life. The knowledge gained and needed for everyday life. The fourth Veda, though added later to the Vedic scriptures of Hinduism.

Chapter 8
The Impact of Assistive Technologies on Quality of Life and Psychosocial Well-Being

Michael R. Schwartz
WEAR Lab, USA

Paul Oppold
University of Central Florida, USA

ABSTRACT

Health-related quality of life is a comprehensive term to describe a person's experiences of health and illness. Quality of life (QOL) is a dynamic psychological construct encompassing interacting subjective and objective dimensions; thus, it is not directly observable. There is no gold standard for measuring quality of life due to the differing interests of doctors, caregivers, patients, and researchers. This chapter examines the research needs in the area of improving QoL through the proper implementation of AT. The authors also make recommendations for incorporating the needs of users and caregivers in the design, deployment, and use of AT to reduce device abandonment.

INTRODUCTION

Quality of life (QoL) is a comprehensive term to describe a person's experiences of health and illness; it is a personal, dynamic and amorphous concept. There are multiple ways to assess QoL: measuring physical health and functional ability, emotional assessment, measuring psychological well-being, and assessing social

DOI: 10.4018/978-1-7998-1185-5.ch008

well-being. While some QoL factors can be measured objectively, there is evidence to support the utility of measuring subjective well-being (Mroczek & Kolarz, 1998). The multidimensionality of QoL presents a challenge to researchers: causal factors are interrelated and affect overall well-being. A person's subjective well-being will also change over the lifespan due to health status and life events; therefore, any QoL assessment must be considered a snapshot of well-being at that point in time and at least occasional reassessment is necessary. Quality of life is personal because needs, desires and priorities are different from person to person. Quality of life assessment is used to supplement objective, or clinical, measures of medical conditions. The increasing usage arises from a shift in contemporary healthcare organizations from a medical care model to a person-centered, social care model (Walsh & O'Shea, 2008). In a social care model, importance is placed on disease outcomes, satisfaction with treatment, and how patients feel. Assessing treatment, services, assistance, and outcomes is especially important for people who have a chronic medical condition, such as a disability, and is understudied. A disability occurs when a person, in an environment, cannot complete a task. For example, a wheelchair user (person) would have difficulty ascending (task) a flight of stairs (environment). Elevators and wheelchair ramps are examples of assistive devices that enable a wheelchair user to navigate not just the environment, but tasks within environments. An additional area of QoL research that needs to be further developed is the impact of assistive devices on a person's life (i.e., how a person's life is changed because of using or not using a device or service that accommodates a disability). The Technology Related Assistance for Individuals with Disabilities Act of 1988 (the United States Tech Act) defines an assistive device as "any item, piece of equipment, product, or system, whether acquired commercially off the shelf, modified or customized, that is used to increase, maintain or improve functional capabilities of individuals with disabilities". This broad definition is by design and highlights the unique needs of individuals and classifies a device as assistive whether it was originally developed to accommodate for a disability. AbleData, an online database of assistive technology resources and information, contains information on over 35,000 assistive technology devices and products. For the purposes of this chapter the terms "assistive device", "assistive technology" and "assistive technological device", all common terms in the industry and scientific literature, are referred to synonymously as "assistive technology (AT)". As important as the devices themselves is the procurement process. People cannot be satisfied or dissatisfied with a product if they cannot obtain it; therefore, researchers are also examining the QoL impact of AT services (Jutai, Fuhrer, Demers, Scherer, & DeRuyter, 2005).

BACKGROUND

Quality of life measurement is a broad field and one challenge for researchers is the lack of a scientific consensus on what constitutes quality of life. There are hundreds of QoL measures and many are manifestations of researchers' and clinicians' interests (Bowling, 2003). Patient-centered measures have been developed to investigate the gaps not addressed by questionnaires developed through the medical care model and the disparities between doctors' assessments and those of patients (Addington-Hall, & Kalra, 2001; Slevin, Plant, Lynch, Drinkwater, & Gregory, 1988). New QoL measures are frequently added to the many that already exist and choosing the correct measure for a specific clinical or research situation can be a difficult and laborious process. Validity, reliability and practicality are important; however, the choice of instrument will vary depending on the purpose and population for which it is used. Measures used as part of a population-based survey must be efficient, concise, and broadly applicable. An instrument used to detect the impact of treatment for a particular disease or condition must be responsive to the specific functional and social consequences of the condition and associated treatments. A useful measure for one situation may not be appropriate for another. For studying the impact of ATs on a person's QoL, the wide range of disabilities, devices and research purposes makes selecting an appropriate QoL measure a time-consuming process.

MAIN FOCUS OF THE CHAPTER

Quality of life instruments can be used for a variety of purposes: to assess the effectiveness of treatments, evaluate quality of care, quantify a population's QoL, and investigate the impact of disease. The choice of QOL questionnaire is a result of three factors: 1) what is the purpose of measuring quality of life, 2) whose quality of life is being measured and 3) how and at what level will data be analyzed? Measures are either generic or condition-specific (Patrick & Deyo, 1989). Generic measures are broad and examine general health-related QoL across different diseases or populations. The content covers most aspects of QoL that are important to most people, such as freedom from pain or discomfort and physical and social functioning. The broad applicability allows for comparison between people or groups with different conditions, such as comparative studies of the impact of different conditions. Examples of generic QoL measures include EuroQoL-5D (EQ-5D), the Nottingham Health Profile and the World Health Organization Quality of Life (WHOQoL) measure. Generic QoL measures may ignore some aspects of a condition that are important to specific groups, such as adults in a certain age range or with a more severe medical case. By excluding certain domains, generic measures can lack the necessary precision to distinguish between groups of people or respond to treatment-induced changes, thus limiting their usefulness in research trials and clinical practices. Condition-specific QoL instruments address the limitations of generic measures by focusing on specific diseases, anatomical systems, or aspects of a medical condition; therefore, they are more responsive to changes within patient groups and are more appropriate for use in clinical research trials. The Voice-Related Quality of Life (V-RQoL) scale and the Pulmonary Embolism Quality of Life (PEmb-QoL) scale are examples of disease-specific QoL measures (Kahn et al., 2017; Roy, Tanner, Merrill, Wright, Miller, & Kendall, 2016). The narrow focus of condition-specific instruments prevents their use in population studies or cross-condition comparisons and could mean that some consequences of a medical condition remain undetected. The choice of generic or specific measure will involve compromising between the advantages and disadvantages of both. Valid and reliable generic instruments can perform as well as specific tests, in some situations (Parkerson, Connis, Broadhead, Patrick, Taylor, & Tse, 1993). Researchers can use both generic and specific measures to address the limitations of each and obtain a more holistic view of a person's QoL (Scott & Garrood, 2000; Wacker et al., 2016). Comprehensive assessment is ideal; however, researchers must use caution when asking patients and clients to complete more complex and demanding questionnaires. Greater complexity can result in more errors, lower completion rates, and higher burdens for both participants and researchers. A suitable compromise between adequacy of data and participant burden must be reached before assessment begins. Questionnaire length, ease of completion, and whether participants are limited in their ability to complete a survey on their own must be considered. Some measures may be too complex for people with dementia to complete. For people with visual impairments, a written survey would be inappropriate; alternate formats, such as interviewer-administered or audio-based, are needed. Some specialties have a large selection of QoL instruments, while others are lacking in measure development (Bowling et al., 2015; Heinl et al., 2016; Schwartz & Oppold, in press). Even well-developed research areas often lack the necessary validation studies of the QoL instruments being used (Heinl et al., 2017). More research is needed to validate new and existing measures to ensure proper interpretation, applicability of results, and sound implementation when put into practice.

Healthcare practitioners have started examining the psychosocial impact that assistive technological devices (ATDs) have on the QoL of people who use them. Patients, practitioners, and providers operate with limited time and funding; finding and using resources that are efficient and cost-effective is important. There is a need for more research in this area because healthcare providers do not want to spend time and money on products and services that do not work or for which the evidence is inconclusive. Assistive technology can help overcome the negative impact disability has on a person's QoL (Tabrizi & Radfar, 2015). The effect AT can have on a person's QoL is multidimensional: QoL is a combination of physical, emotional, mental, and social functioning. Examples of assistive technology include white canes, wheelchairs, computers, ramps, and aids for activities of daily living such as tactile overlay buttons. The goal for assistive devices is to reduce or eliminate problems faced by people with disabilities and allow for full participation in society. For example, a wheelchair helps someone physically move around; however, the ability to be mobile affects how often, where and in what manner a person socializes. Thus, a wheelchair affects physical, psychological, and social aspects of a person's life. If not properly designed, accessed or used, AT can decrease QoL and the AT is abandoned (i.e., no longer used). The motivation for studying the impact of assistive devices arose from the realization that abandonment of AT occurs up to 75% of the time (Phillips & Zhao, 1993; Seale & Turner-Smith, 2003; Tewey, Barnicle, & Perr, 1994). Researchers began to ask why someone would stop using technology that improved functioning (an objective, quantifiable metric). Factors other than functioning and presence of symptoms influence AT use. Mental and emotional factors cannot be directly observed; however, assessment is still necessary. Rehabilitation professionals have expressed dissatisfaction adapting medically-oriented, generic QoL measures to assess the impact of AT on QoL (Oldridge, 1996; Seale & Turner-Smith, 2003). Kemp (1999) highlighted that more emphasis needs to be given to the impact of social activities on a person's life.

The assessment of participation in social activities is not easily accomplished. Participation is complex, consisting of behavioral patterns across time and context. There are several dimensions: individual interests and preferences, what is done, where, with whom, and how much satisfaction is achieved. Participation, like disability, is a phenomenon involving the person, the environment, and the tasks; measurement occurs at the intersection of these domains. Across all age groups, disability has a prolonged and substantial effect on participation; social isolation is significantly associated with disability severity (Law, 2002). A person living with a disability is more likely to have fewer social relationships, engage in less active recreational activities, be unemployed, and be confined to home more. Less participation is associated with decreased mobility and experiencing difficulties in performing activities of daily living (ADLs). ATs are meant to help someone overcome a disability, thereby increasing participation in ADLs and social activities; however, to do so ATs must be effective, usable, and accessible to increase QoL. Therefore, investigating the psychosocial impact of ATs on QoL is a worthwhile endeavor that seeks to increase benefits to people who use AT and decrease the abandonment of devices. Measures for assessing impact, however, are few and many still require validation.

The LIFE-H scale examines the quality of individual social participation by operationalizing life habit as a construct of social participation. Life habits are sorted into twelve categories, six for ADLs and six for social roles, and defined as activities or social roles valued by a person in a specific socio-cultural context. People complete the scale by indicating the degree of difficulty and types of assistance required (human assistance or technical aid) to perform a task. Noreau, Fougeyrollas and Vincent (2002) argue that when someone is unable to perform ADLs social participation is restricted and, thus, a handicap occurs. While the LIFE-H was not developed for assessing ATs, it can be used to examine the impact of AT on social participation. The LIFE-H has not been used extensively to test the impact of AT; however, the scale has been tested with a variety of populations including traumatic brain injury (TBI), spinal cord injury (SCI), myotonic dystrophy, and cerebral palsy (Noreau, Fougeyrollas, Labbé, & Laramée, 1998). Also, the LIFE-H is not specific to one profession and the theoretical development of the scale is grounded in an internationally accepted understanding of disability, the World Health Organization's International Classification of Functioning, Disability and Health (ICF). However, the LIFE-H is not without limitations; the short version of the scale contains 69 items and may place a large burden on participants, the scale was not developed to examine AT, and more validation studies are needed before extensive use is warranted.

The Psychosocial Impact of Assistive Devices Scale (PIADS) was developed to assess feelings of adaptability, competence, and self-esteem (Jutai, 1999). The PIADS is useful for comparing populations of people who use specific ATs. People with some disabilities may require more than one AT and the PIADS can be completed to assess the psychosocial impact of each device. Originally used to measure the impact of eyeglasses and contact lenses on people who use them, the measure has also been used to examine the impact of continence pads, wheelchairs, and more (Day, Jutai, Woolrich, & Strong, 2001; Ding et al., 2008; Long, Southall, Fowler, Cotterill, Van Den Heuvel, & Jutai, 2014). The variety of disabilities that a person can have is a complicating factor for research in the area of psychosocial health and wellbeing. It is not unusual for a person to have multiple medical conditions at once as a result of underlying genetic and disease-related factors. To validate a measure, such as the PIADS, researchers must find people with a specific type and level of disability, without confounding comorbid diseases or conditions, within a confined geographic area, and of a similar age or functional ability. Recent years have seen progress in validating the PIADS with people who speak different languages, people who speak the same language but live in a different culture, and people who use ATs or have medical conditions that have not been studied before (Long et al., 2014; Orellano & Jutai, 2013). However, more research is needed to validate the PIADS in specific contexts, such as languages, cultures, age groups and medical conditions.

Identifying the changes of AT in the lives of assistive technology users requires generating sufficient evidence that AT interventions are the cause of the measured outcomes. While the examples of AT interventions in this chapter come from the domain of mobility research, the themes are applicable to AT interventions across domains. AT interventions are a combination of the devices themselves and the associated services (e.g., obtaining devices, receiving AT training); however, this chapter focuses on assessing the impact of devices and not AT services. Some ATs are ubiquitous and have a long history: canes, wheelchairs and eyeglasses, for example; it is difficult to doubt the benefit of these devices. The impact of other ATs is unclear and there is some evidence to indicate ATs can decrease QoL, such as by increasing stigma, for some conditions (Southall, Tuazon, Djokhdem, van den Heuvel, Wittich, & Jutai, 2017). Obtaining research funding is difficult as outcome studies are often expensive and participants with some medical conditions can be difficult to find and gain access to. While companies that manufacture and sell diagnostic and therapeutic devices are required by United States federal regulatory agencies (e.g., FDA) to produce evidence confirming the benefits of the technologies, ATs are not held to the same standard. The suggestion to consumers is that sales revenue is proof of the benefits conferred by devices despite a lack of research-based evidence that establishes value.

Physical therapy and occupational therapy are two health professions that rely on evidence-based practices (EBPs) and frequently use ATs to provide services to clients (Holm, 2000; Manns & Darrah, 2006). AT providers who rely on EBPs to support clinical decision making will have difficulty finding sufficient evidence to make definitive claims. It is worth noting that the Institute of Medicine's definition of EBPs is "…the integration of best research evidence with clinical expertise and patient values", which emphasizes the role of individual psychological and emotional differences between people (Baker, 2001; Straus, Glasziou, Richardson, & Haynes, 2018). Programs such as Medicare, the largest third-party provider of mobility ATs in the United States, increasingly rely on evidence-based outcomes to justify payment decisions about which ATs are covered (Carlson & Ehrlich, 2006). Advancements in AT research and development may not be held back by a lack of innovation, but by a lack of scientific evidence confirming the value of new devices. There is also uncertainty about which alternatives among device types are best for people with a specific set of medical conditions (e.g., between manual and powered wheelchairs). Further complicating the study of psychosocial impact, ATs influence the psychosocial well-being of family and caregivers of AT users. For example, there is evidence to indicate that ATs diminish the physical and emotional burden of caregivers when supporting someone who has a disability; however, the weak study designs used in prior research undermine researchers' ability to make causal connections (Mortenson, Demers, Fuhrer, Jutai, Lenker, & DeRuyter, 2012). There is also a need to investigate how even ATs with widespread usage fail to meet users' requirements. AT outcomes are the aggregate of many factors—the device, use of the device, caregiver benefit, services associated with the device—all of which mediate the outcomes of interest (e.g., user satisfaction, contributions to QoL, functional improvements, increased social participation).

Novel ATs need to undergo outcome studies as well, especially those which have two characteristics. First, the devices should have the ability to enhance users' functioning, satisfaction and psychological well-being beyond what is available with current ATs. Second, the ATs should incorporate novel design and engineering concepts, which may lead to the next generation of AT devices. For example, a white cane used by people with visual impairments is useful; however, a haptic cane may serve all the functions of a white cane with the added benefit of alerting the user about obstacles above waist height, such as a tree branch or sign post (Wang & Kuchenbecker, 2012). A haptic cane could save someone from head injury, thereby increasing physical functioning, and could reduce incidences of social stigma, thereby encouraging someone with a disability to engage in more social participation. The sensor technology could also lead to additional innovative devices being produced and further aiding AT users. However, each new device has multifaceted research questions that require investigation: usability studies assessing efficiency and effectiveness, the incidences of secondary conditions that may result from use (e.g., does using a heavier cane lead to wrist-joint deterioration?), and psychosocial factors on users and caregivers (e.g., does a haptic cane allow users to walk with increased self-confidence and safety from head injury?) all need to be studied. Until such investigations are performed, the likelihood of third-party payers paying for ATs is unlikely as the added benefit has not been shown to justify the higher cost. Rigorous outcome studies that demonstrate the psychosocial benefits of ATs increase the likelihood that the technologies will be provided to the people who can benefit from their use.

No single study can address all the issues involved in AT outcomes research. First, the study must employ a representative population. The AT and associated services must be causally responsible for the observed changes. Finally, the research conditions should approximate the real-world scenarios in which users obtain their devices. All three conditions are necessary to ensure internal and external validity of research findings and a body of research is required to address the tradeoffs between the two. Ideally, at least one efficacy study which prioritizes internal validity and one effectiveness study prioritizing external validity would be performed. The approximate number of studies required will be determined by user populations, service settings, and the requirements of the scientific community and third-party payers. Concerns about cost-effectiveness affect AT innovation, similar to the concerns about advanced health technologies, namely, increases in healthcare costs. Knowledge about the benefits of AT can help to overcome those concerns by demonstrating the value of AT interventions to patients, practitioners and third-party payers. Assistive technology that helps someone regain lost abilities (e.g., when recovering from a stroke), live more independently (i.e., require less caregiver intervention) or return to work and not require welfare payments benefits the AT user, his or her family and society at large. For example, in frail elderly patients, rate of functional decline can be slowed, and institutional and in-home caregiver costs can be reduced through AT use (Mann, Ottenbacher, Fraas, Tomita, & Granger, 1999). However, there are costs to AT interventions beyond the initial purchase price: service-related expenditures such as provision and maintenance, ordering devices, assessing potential users, customizing devices to fit individual needs and providing training. These costs are paid by AT users, caregivers, providers, third-party payers, government agencies, and taxpayers. Andrich and Caracciolo (2007) demonstrate how estimating the complete economic cost of an AT intervention upfront does not have to be an additional barrier to implementing AT; reducing the assistance burden by successfully providing and using AT leads to a significant cost savings over time. This cost savings is in addition to the social benefits users gain from having an AT device available.

Issues, Controversies, Problems

Several challenges exist in AT research and development. Using undergraduate students as participants, as is common in university settings, is suitable for initial prototyping; however, for the results of academic studies to be externally valid, a representative sample must be employed. AT outcomes research is a multidisciplinary field and includes researchers from academia and industry in disciplines such as occupational therapy, medicine, mechanical and electrical engineering, psychology, computer science and education. Assembling and coordinating a diverse group of professionals to form a project team has challenges of its own, especially if the team members have not worked together before.

There is a need to study psychosocial wellbeing and QoL as both relate to the abandonment, or discontinuance, of assistive technologies. If ATs can enhance QoL for people with disabilities, then why would someone cease using their assistive device? Failing to improve a person's quality of life has been identified as a primary reason for ceasing AT use (Day, Jutai, Woolrich & Strong, 2001). Well-designed studies and rigorous research methodologies will not benefit AT users if devices are not used! Phillips and Zhao (1993) examined the factors that predict abandonment of ATs and found that, on average, people discontinue use of their devices 29.3% of the time. Mobility aids were the most likely category of device to be abandoned and were highest in the first twelve months after receiving the device and after five years of use. Four factors were predictive of discontinued use: poor performance of the device, changes in personal needs and priorities, effortless AT procurement and AT designers, manufacturers and providers failing to consider user preferences in device selection. Participants in Tewey, Barnicle and Perr's (1994) study reported abandoning their devices up to 75% of the time. In a follow-up study, the two factors that were significantly associated with abandonment were relative advantage (i.e., device performance) and user involvement (Riemer-Reiss & Wacker, 2000). Relative advantage is not as simple of a concept as it first appears. There are many costs associated with using a device beyond an initial financial investment (e.g., time, mental workload, frustration). The advantages conferred through use of a device must be greater than the costs of use or the person will abandon the device (Schwartz and Oppold, 2019). Thus, it is important to note that while AT can increase psychosocial well-being, using AT that performs poorly can cause feelings of frustration, embarrassment, hopelessness and, eventually, rejection of the device. Discontinued use of AT results in the needs of people living with disabilities being unmet and less funding and resources available for providing AT devices to others who need them. One study found that employing an interdisciplinary approach to the evaluation of a user's needs reduced rates of AT device abandonment from 37.3% to 9.5% (Verza, Carvalho, Battaglia, & Uccelli, 2006). While using an interdisciplinary approach to AT user need evaluation did not eliminate the issue of discontinued use, this method greatly reduces abandonment rates and increases the likelihood that ATs are continuing to benefit those who need them most (Scherer, 1996). Copley and Ziviani (2004) indicate that for ATs to benefit school-age children in achieving desired functional and educational goals, a team model for AT planning and assessment is needed that incorporates children, parents and school employees. Across contexts, a collaborative approach that incorporates AT designers, manufacturers, providers, caregivers and users in the device selection process and usage settings is beneficial for reducing AT abandonment and increasing the likelihood that devices are helping to improve a person's quality of life.

SOLUTIONS AND RECOMMENDATIONS

More research is needed to assess the effect of social interaction on AT use. A cycle exists between psychosocial well-being and AT usage. Assistive devices can convey to the world that the device user has a disability. Shinohara and Wobbrock (2011) indicate that two misperceptions are commonly held about AT use: (1) ATs eliminate a functional disability, and (2) a person is helpless without their AT device. The authors suggest three solutions to making AT more socially acceptable. The first proposed solution is that accessibility be considered from the start and built into mainstream environments and technologies. Second, AT should include emerging and innovative technologies. Finally, designing for social acceptability is proposed as a way to avoid discouraging people from abandoning their AT because of social pressures.

FUTURE RESEARCH

The issue of changing personal needs and preferences is an area of AT research that requires more investigation. People's needs change over time. As we age, our mental and physical abilities may decline and specific types of AT may be required to overcome the process of aging into or with a disability. On the other hand, AT may only be needed temporarily (e.g., using a wheelchair while recovering from a broken leg, using a text-to-speech device while recovering from a stroke). In these cases, discontinued use of AT is desirable as the person may have recovered their previous abilities. It should be noted, however, that some individuals may cease rehabilitative therapy and use of AT before rehabilitation is complete and it cannot be assumed that AT abandonment in a rehabilitation setting is always desirable. More research is needed to determine the nature of AT abandonment as a result of age, gender, condition, prognosis and device type. The issue of AT abandonment has been addressed by occupational therapists by focusing on providing additional training on AT devices; however, this approach assumes that the user's skill level and confidence of one's own ability to use AT are the root cause of discontinued use. Hocking (1999) demonstrates that AT abandonment may be due to someone's perception of themselves as disabled and relates to issues of identity and self.

CONCLUSION

Current demographic trends indicate that, worldwide, more people are living longer and there will be an increased demand for AT devices in the future as more people age into or with a disability. Consequently, AT designers, manufacturers, providers and healthcare professionals will need to ensure that resources and funding are being used effectively. As part of this effort, it is imperative that the evidentiary body of research indicates how AT can be deployed and used to provide the most benefit to the most people. More research is needed to indicate how this can be accomplished. Further, the needs of AT users and caregivers should be incorporated in the device design, selection and use process in order to reduce abandonment of AT. The prevalence of some ATs (e.g., wheelchairs, eyeglasses) indicates the ability of these technologies to improve the lives of people who use them. However, some

ATs can emphasize the stigma surrounding disability and care should be taken in the design, deployment and use of AT to reduce social pressure toward people living with a disability.

REFERENCES

Addington-Hall, J., & Kalra, L. (2001). Who should measure quality of life? *BMJ (Clinical Research Ed.)*, *322*(7299), 1417–1420. doi:10.1136/bmj.322.7299.1417 PMID:11397754

Andrich, R., & Caracciolo, A. (2007). Analysing the cost of individual assistive technology programmes. *Disability and Rehabilitation. Assistive Technology*, *2*(4), 207–234. doi:10.1080/17483100701325035 PMID:19263539

Baker, A. (2001). Crossing the quality chasm: A new health system for the 21st century. *BMJ (Clinical Research Ed.)*, *323*(7322), 1192. doi:10.1136/bmj.323.7322.1192

Bowling, A. (2003). Current state of the art in quality of life measurement. *Quality of Life, 2003*, 1-8.

Bowling, A., Rowe, G., Adams, S., Sands, P., Samsi, K., Crane, M., ... Manthorpe, J. (2015). Quality of life in dementia: A systematically conducted narrative review of dementia-specific measurement scales. *Aging & Mental Health*, *19*(1), 13–31. doi:10.1080/13607863.2014.915923 PMID:24881888

Carlson, D., & Ehrlich, N. (2006). Sources of payment for assistive technology: Findings from a national survey of persons with disabilities. *Assistive Technology*, *18*(1), 77–86. doi:10.1080/10400435.2006.10131908 PMID:16796243

Copley, J., & Ziviani, J. (2004). Barriers to the use of assistive technology for children with multiple disabilities. *Occupational Therapy International*, *11*(4), 229–243. doi:10.1002/oti.213 PMID:15771212

Day, J., Woolrich, W., & Strong, H. (2001). The stability of impact of assistive devices. *Disability and Rehabilitation*, *23*(9), 400–404. doi:10.1080/09638280010008906 PMID:11394591

Fitzpatrick, R. B. (2010). AbleData: A resource of assistive technology information. *Medical Reference Services Quarterly*, *29*(3), 260–268. doi:10.1080/02763869.2010.494510 PMID:20677066

Heinl, D., Prinsen, C. A. C., Deckert, S., Chalmers, J. R., Drucker, A. M., Ofenloch, R., ... Apfelbacher, C. (2016). Measurement properties of adult quality-of-life measurement instruments for eczema: A systematic review. *Allergy*, *71*(3), 358–370. doi:10.1111/all.12806 PMID:26564008

Heinl, D., Prinsen, C. A. C., Sach, T., Drucker, A. M., Ofenloch, R., Flohr, C., & Apfelbacher, C. (2017). Measurement properties of quality-of-life measurement instruments for infants, children and adolescents with eczema: A systematic review. *British Journal of Dermatology*, *176*(4), 878–889. doi:10.1111/bjd.14966 PMID:27543747

Hocking, C. (1999). Function or feelings: factors in abandonment of assistive devices. *Technology and Disability, 11*(1, 2), 3-11.

Holm, M. B. (2000). Our mandate for the new millennium: Evidence-based practice. *The American Journal of Occupational Therapy*, *54*(6), 575–585. doi:10.5014/ajot.54.6.575 PMID:11100239

Jutai, J. W., Fuhrer, M. J., Demers, L., Scherer, M. J., & DeRuyter, F. (2005). Toward a taxonomy of assistive technology device outcomes. *American Journal of Physical Medicine & Rehabilitation*, *84*(4), 294–302. doi:10.1097/01.PHM.0000157313.88732.DC PMID:15785265

Kahn, S. R., Akaberi, A., Granton, J. T., Anderson, D. R., Wells, P. S., Rodger, M. A., ... Dennie, C. (2017). Quality of life, dyspnea, and functional exercise capacity following a first episode of pulmonary embolism: Results of the ELOPE cohort study. *The American Journal of Medicine*, *130*(8), 990–e9. doi:10.1016/j.amjmed.2017.03.033 PMID:28400247

Kemp, B. J. (1999). Quality of life while aging with a disability. *Assistive Technology*, *11*(2), 158–163. doi:10.1080/10400435.1999.10131999 PMID:11010065

Law, M. (2002). Participation in the occupations of everyday life. *The American Journal of Occupational Therapy*, *56*(6), 640–649. doi:10.5014/ajot.56.6.640 PMID:12458856

Mann, W. C., Ottenbacher, K. J., Fraas, L., Tomita, M., & Granger, C. V. (1999). Effectiveness of assistive technology and environmental interventions in maintaining independence and reducing home care costs for the frail elderly: A randomized controlled trial. *Archives of Family Medicine*, *8*(3), 210–217. doi:10.1001/archfami.8.3.210 PMID:10333815

Manns, P. J., & Darrah, J. (2006). Linking research and clinical practice in physical therapy: Strategies for integration. *Physiotherapy*, *92*(2), 88–94. doi:10.1016/j.physio.2005.09.006

Mortenson, W. B., Demers, L., Fuhrer, M. J., Jutai, J. W., Lenker, J., & DeRuyter, F. (2012). How assistive technology use by individuals with disabilities impacts their caregivers: A systematic review of the research evidence. *American Journal of Physical Medicine & Rehabilitation*, *91*(11), 984–998. doi:10.1097/PHM.0b013e318269eceb PMID:22955027

Mroczek, D. K., & Kolarz, C. M. (1998). The effect of age on positive and negative affect: A developmental perspective on happiness. *Journal of Personality and Social Psychology*, *75*(5), 1333–1349. doi:10.1037/0022-3514.75.5.1333 PMID:9866191

Noreau, L., Fougeyrollas, P., Labbé, A., & Laramée, M. T. (1998). Comparison of 2 measurement tools addressing the concept of handicap: CHART and LIFE-H. *The Journal of Spinal Cord Medicine*, *21*(2), 192.

Noreau, L., Fougeyrollas, P., & Vincent, C. (2002). The LIFE-H: Assessment of the quality of social participation. *Technology and Disability*, *14*(3), 113–118. doi:10.3233/TAD-2002-14306

Oldridge, N. B. (1996). Outcomes measurement: Health-related quality of life. *Assistive Technology*, *8*(2), 82–93. doi:10.1080/10400435.1996.10132278 PMID:10163932

Orellano, E. M., & Jutai, J. W. (2013). Cross-cultural adaptation of the psychosocial impact of assistive device scale (PIADS) for Puerto Rican assistive technology users. *Assistive Technology*, *25*(4), 194–203. doi:10.1080/10400435.2012.761292 PMID:24620702

Parkerson, G. R. Jr, Connis, R. T., Broadhead, W. E., Patrick, D. L., Taylor, T. R., & Tse, C. K. J. (1993). Disease-specific versus generic measurement of health-related quality of life in insulin-dependent diabetic patients. *Medical Care*, *31*(7), 629–639. doi:10.1097/00005650-199307000-00005 PMID:8326776

Patrick, D. L., & Deyo, R. A. (1989). Generic and disease-specific measures in assessing health status and quality of life. *Medical Care*, *27*(Supplement), S217–S232. doi:10.1097/00005650-198903001-00018 PMID:2646490

Phillips, B., & Zhao, H. (1993). Predictors of assistive technology abandonment. *Assistive Technology*, *5*(1), 36–45. doi:10.1080/10400435.1993.10132205 PMID:10171664

Riemer-Reiss, M. L., & Wacker, R. R. (2000). Factors associated with assistive technology discontinuance among individuals with disabilities. *Journal of Rehabilitation*, *66*(3).

Roy, N., Tanner, K., Merrill, R. M., Wright, C., Miller, K. L., & Kendall, K. A. (2016). Descriptive epidemiology of voice disorders in rheumatoid arthritis: Prevalence, risk factors, and quality of life burden. *Journal of Voice*, *30*(1), 74–87. doi:10.1016/j.jvoice.2015.02.011 PMID:25888079

Scherer, M. J. (1996). Outcomes of assistive technology use on quality of life. *Disability and Rehabilitation*, *18*(9), 439–448. doi:10.3109/09638289609165907 PMID:8877302

Schwartz, M., & Oppold, P. (in press). Cross-cultural Adaptation of the Psychosocial Impact of Assistive Devices Scale (PIADS) for South African Exoskeleton Users. *Human Factors*. doi:10.4018/978-1-5225-7949-6.ch007

Schwartz, M., Oppold, P., & Hancock, P. A. (2019). Wearables and Workload. In Critical Issues Impacting Science, Technology, Society (STS), and Our Future (pp. 145-170). IGI Global.

Scott, D. L., & Garrood, T. (2000). Quality of life measures: Use and abuse. *Best Practice & Research. Clinical Rheumatology*, *14*(4), 663–687. doi:10.1053/berh.2000.0106 PMID:11092795

Seale, J., & Turner-Smith, A. (2003). 8: Measuring the impact of assistive technologies on quality of life: can rehabilitation professionals rise to the challenge? *Alison J Carr*, 79.

Slevin, M. L., Plant, H., Lynch, D. A., Drinkwater, J., & Gregory, W. M. (1988). Who should measure quality of life, the doctor or the patient? *British Journal of Cancer*, *57*(1), 109–112. doi:10.1038/bjc.1988.20 PMID:3348942

Southall, K., Tuazon, J. R., Djokhdem, A. H., van den Heuvel, E. A., Wittich, W., & Jutai, J. W. (2017). Assessing the stigma content of urinary incontinence intervention outcome measures. *Journal of Rehabilitation and Assistive Technologies Engineering, 4*.

Straus, S. E., Glasziou, P., Richardson, W. S., & Haynes, R. B. (2018). *Evidence-Based Medicine E-Book: How to Practice and Teach EBM*. Elsevier Health Sciences.

Tabrizi, F. M., & Radfar, M. (2015). Fatigue, sleep quality, and disability in relation to quality of life in multiple sclerosis. *International Journal of MS Care*, *17*(6), 268–274. doi:10.7224/1537-2073.2014-046 PMID:26664332

Tewey, B. P., Barnicle, K., & Perr, A. (1994). The wrong stuff. *Mainstream*, *19*(2), 19–23.

Verza, R., Carvalho, M. L., Battaglia, M. A., & Uccelli, M. M. (2006). An interdisciplinary approach to evaluating the need for assistive technology reduces equipment abandonment. *Multiple Sclerosis Journal*, *12*(1), 88–93. doi:10.1191/1352458506ms1233oa PMID:16459724

Wacker, M. E., Jörres, R. A., Karch, A., Wilke, S., Heinrich, J., Karrasch, S., ... Vogelmeier, C. (2016). Assessing health-related quality of life in COPD: Comparing generic and disease-specific instruments with focus on comorbidities. *BMC Pulmonary Medicine*, *16*(1), 70. doi:10.118612890-016-0238-9 PMID:27160582

Walsh, K., & O'shea, E. (2008). Responding to rural social care needs: Older people empowering themselves, others and their community. *Health & Place*, *14*(4), 795–805. doi:10.1016/j.healthplace.2007.12.006 PMID:18289914

Wang, Y., & Kuchenbecker, K. J. (2012, March). HALO: Haptic alerts for low-hanging obstacles in white cane navigation. In *2012 IEEE Haptics Symposium (HAPTICS)* (pp. 527-532). IEEE. 10.1109/HAPTIC.2012.6183842

KEY TERMS AND DEFINITIONS

ADL: Activity of daily living.
AT: Assistive technology.
ATD: Assistive technological device.
EBP: Evidence-based practice.
Pemb-QoL: Pulmonary embolism quality of life scale.
PIADS: Psychosocial impact of assistive devices questionnaire.
QoL: Quality of life.
SCI: Spinal cord injury.
TBI: Traumatic brain injury.
V-RQoL: Voice-related quality of life scale.
WHOQoL: World Health Organization quality of life measure.

Chapter 9
Emotional Intelligence as a Moderator in Reducing Academic Stress Among School Students

Elavarasi Dhanakotti
Central University of Tamil Nadu, India

Poornima Rajendran
Central University of Tamil Nadu, India

ABSTRACT

In this chapter, the authors reviewed the dimensions/subscales of emotional intelligence and deliberated its significance associated in enhancing emotional competencies, thereby overcoming academic stress in students. The present review makes the reader understand and rationalize the significance of emotional intelligence for students to develop their emotional competencies to empower themselves and combat academic stress and enhance their academic performance.

INTRODUCTION

The common insight of our current education system is to give more significance to the cognitive domain that ignores the other major domain including the emotional domain (affective domain). Majority of the parent community are unaware of their children ability and thus not giving enough importance to their desires and so pressures are building on children to learn to attain intense goals in their life (Deb, Strod &

DOI: 10.4018/978-1-7998-1185-5.ch009

Sun, 2015). All this problems may leads to suicidal tendency, drug habits, low test grades, poor performance in their academics and illegal activities (Utting, 2007).

Maladaptive students can generate reactive behaviours such as fear, stress, confusion, overwhelm, lack inspiration, anxious, affection, affairs and passion among the parents. According to Sylva (1994 & 2000) teachers will play as a role model for their students and some teachers will share the student's criticism with other teachers, whereas friends' only acts as a determining factor of student's nature and characters. Students spend most of the day with friends and sometimes they will get spoil by irregular and bad activities like smoking, alcoholism, teasing, skipping class, which creates some excitement and nervousness among them. All these behaviours adversely affect their academic achievement of the students. Jordan and his colleagues (2010) stated, that the attention towards emotion, stress and social skills are required to make many changes from the students in the primary to secondary school level.

Some of the emotions like anger, envy, jealousy, anxiety, fright, guilt, shame and sadness were usually arise during stressful situations, which refers to harmful, threatening or challenging conditions (Lazarus, 1990). Both emotion and stress are the motivational related factors which plays an important role in students learning and achievement (Zhan and Hu Mei, 2013). Emotions has a major concern in one's adjustment to self and the surrounding environment. When an individual is emotionally balanced, then that person can be able to express their emotions in a proper way in every situations. So, the student should have to understand the need of emotional intelligence and related factors to manage the situations and these factors can affect a person in different aspects. Academic performance and achievement is one of the chief aspect in students that will be affected by emotional intelligence. By considering all the previous study, some strategies to overcome the Academic stress among school students are discussed in detail below.

STRATEGIES TO OVERCOME ACADEMIC STRESS AMONG SCHOOL STUDENTS

Academic stress is the common burden faced by all the students in their school life. Sarita (2015) states that academic stress among students can be elevated due to parents and other students' intervention. In this context, academic stress is creating both personal and social relationship problems to the students. Nowadays, students use many techniques to cope up with stress, either in a positive or negative way. Some students alleviate their stress in a negative way by consuming alcohol, drug, refusal and behavioural changes (Sarita, 2015). On one hand researcher like Claeys-Jackson (2017) states that there are many techniques to manage stress, those are managing time, exercise, get some fresh air, stay positive, spend time with friends, free mind, and cognitive behavioural therapy.

On another hand emotional intelligence will help to manage stress with actions such as handling problems, active dealing and positive thought for acceptance (Al-Dubai, Al-Naggar, Al-Shagga & Rampal, 2011). Stress management can have a positive impact while poorly managed or neglected stress leads to major issues in life (Ardic & Ozturk, 2018). In this context, emotional intelligence is an essential aspect for school students to overcome academic stress. Meanwhile, Gujral (2013) pointed that students are capable to overcome academic stress with improving emotional intelligence. Emotional intelligence focuses on balancing the negative emotions such as anger, stress, depression, anxiety. And it also focuses on positive emotions such as patience, hope and empathy. According to Garg & Rastogi (2009), the components of emotional intelligence are self-motivation, emotional stability and self-development. Even from childhood years every students requires training to improve their emotional intelligence that help them to cope up with any situation in their life.

SIGNIFICANCE OF EMOTIONAL INTELLIGENCE IN SCHOOL STUDENTS

Youth suicide rate were found highest in south part of India across the globe. The researchers like Aaron, Joseph, Abraham, Muliyil, George, Prasad, Minz, Abraham & Bose (2005) and Das (2017) have found that academic failure is one of the major contributing factors for suicide. This problem is getting increased not only in India but all over the globe. Kundi (2016) highlighted that

India has one of the highest rates of suicides among people aged between 15 and 29. Although the reasons are myriad but failure in examination, unemployment, and depression are some the reasons why people put their life at risk.

IQ alone is not an absolute measure for success, it only counts about 20%, and the rest are emotional and social intelligence and luck (Goleman, 1995). But in Tamil Nadu, most of the schools include the scholastic component in their curriculum which are considered vital for student's success. The academic success of students is based on different aspects rather than a single concept. The student's expectation with regard to their academics are overwhelming even at the entry level itself. Also, stressors are standing as a great obstacle to perform academically high among secondary grade students apart from the adolescent age factor.

The academic stress in students creates a sort of negative emotions. It was also observed that student's mental health is dependent on their appropriate behaviour with their society. It is also evident from researches (Gupta and Kumar, 2010; Kaur, 2018; Al –Nawasrah, 2019) that mental health of students are influenced by their emotional intelligence. The students who are well adapted to their environment possess better mental health and stay away from negative emotions.

The researchers, like Kauts (2016), Rowniyar (2016), Arslan (2017) and; Subramanyam (2016) stated that emotional intelligence is involved in reliving any kind of stress in an individual. Goleman (1998) also referred that emotional intelligence includes the ability to solve emotional problems, flexibility and ability to regulate and alter the effective reactions to reduce stress in different emotional crisis.

Freedman & Jensen (2008) noted that the components of emotional intelligence are believed to increase student attention and it strengthen relationship between teachers and students. Emotional Intelligence improves students learning experience, a positive verbal statements, enhanced collaboration and cooperation and decreases *put-downs*. Similar views were also expressed by Trinidad & Johnson (2002) where students with high Emotional intelligence can read better than others, find the pressure of unwanted peers and manage their own emotions and therefore can be concentrated in their studies. Bar-On (1997) reported that emotional intelligence levels from early adolescents have been significantly increased, than the adults (as cited by Parker, Summerfeldt, Hogan & Majeski, 2004). Emotional intelligence and its dimensions are essential for school students for their advance career.

EMOTIONAL INTELLIGENCE FOR SCHOOL STUDENTS

According to Goleman (1995), emotional Intelligence is 'the ability to know and manage one's own emotions, recognize them in others and handle relationships'. Emotional intelligence skills help to identify a person's emotions, which make it easy for self-reliance and others to deal with all feelings and use them efficiently. Emotional intelligence is an ability to make sense of emotions and their relationships with each other can find a solutions to their problems occurred in their life (Mayer et al., 1999). The variety of dimension attained by emotional intelligence are having ability to express emotions, appraise and perceive accurately. Besides that, it had ability to access and create feelings and facilitate thought. Furthermore, the ability to understand emotions and emotional knowledge, regulating emotions to promote emotional and intellectual maturity are some part of emotional intelligence (Mayer and Salovey, 1997).

In this chapter, the investigator refers 'emotional intelligence' as defined by Bar-On (1997). Bar-On's Mixed Model of Emotional intelligence is a cross-section of interconnected emotional and social capabilities and abilities. Bar-On (1997) defines emotional intelligence as "an array of non-cognitive capabilities, competencies and skills that influence one's ability to succeed in coping with environmental demands and pressures". He states that Emotional Intelligence is essential to be successful in dealing with environmental demands such as, relating well to people, adapting and coping with immediate environment for a better understanding. Bar-On Model divided into two basic parts, in which first part is theory/construct and the second part is psychometric aspect which is significant to measure the emotional-social intelligence. According to Bar-On (2006), Emotional Quotient Inventory Youth Version (EQi-YV) for student from age of 7 to 18 years divided into 6 dimensions such as Interpersonal, Intrapersonal, Stress Management, Adaptability, General Mood and Positive Impression each of these consist of 15 sub-factors. The dimensions are explained in the next section of this chapter.

Authors refer stress as defined by Selye (1983) that identifies stress as the body's nonspecific response to some demand placed upon it. Other potential sources of stress for students include excessive homework, unclear assignments, and uncomfortable classrooms (Kohn & Frazer, 1986) and refer academic stress as defined by Banerjee (2011). He refers that academic stress as a type of stress that arises due to academic factors such as heavy school schedule, unrealistic expectation and demands of parents and teachers, low academic performance, poor study habits and not having enough time to deal with school's multiple responsibility.

EMOTIONAL COMPETENCIES AS MODERATOR OF ACADEMIC STRESS IN SCHOOL STUDENTS

Intrapersonal

According to Bar-On (2007) Intrapersonal relationship is an ability to understand emotion as well as to express one's feelings and themselves. In common, it is called as 'Inner self in an individual' which indicates the inner feelings related to the individuals. According to Armstrong (2009) multiple intelligences defines intrapersonal as a self-knowledge and the ability to act adaptively based on the knowledge. Intrapersonal includes one's strength, awareness, attitudes, intention, motivation, limitation, desires, capacity, self-discipline, self-understanding and self-esteem (as cited in Gleason, 2011). Intrapersonal is an ability to understand about ourselves and manage the situations of individual.

In other words, Intrapersonal are highly innate as it helps individual to be emotionally self-confident in expressing their feelings and strong in expressing their ideas and beliefs (Esmaeili & Jamkhaneh, 2013). Students need intrapersonal competencies to be: effective, ethical, self-regulate and administer meta-cognitive skills both in personal and classroom environment. So, Intrapersonal is essential for students to identify themselves thereby reduce stresses that arises due to personal factors. This in turn will help to promote self-confidence in students. According to Bar-On (2006), intrapersonal component consists of five sub-factors such as Self-regard, Emotional Self-Awareness, Assertiveness, Independence and Self-Actualization.

Self-Regard

Self-regard is also known as Self-esteem, which refers to accurately perceive, understand and accept oneself. It is an ability to recognize and feel their strength and weakness. According to Bar-On (2007) self-regard is an ability to accept positive and negative characteristics, strength and weakness. Self-regard is the way to regard oneself to think about themselves and to view own self as capable, assertive, worthy and acceptable (Cory, 2015; Jorfi, Jorfi, Yaccob & Shah, 2010).

Possessing high levels of self-regard decreases negative stress by increasing their sense of being in control the situations they face in life. Self-regard is essential for students to learn better and it enhance good communication skills to achieve personal goals that will make them feel superior about themselves and leads to improve academic achievements. In other words, Roosevelt (2017) explained, that self-regard has a capacity to honour, accept, know the individuals strengths and weaknesses. A student with high level self-regards tends to be associated with feelings of self-worth, self-confidence, inner strength, believes in own self, stress less and capabilities. The essential component of self-regard is to image the inner self (Levus, 2012). The inner-self can be determined by the self-assessment. Students can create a self-assessment by assessing it more sufficiently evaluates themselves in various manner such as performing essays, reports, performances, projects, dissertations and exams. The self-regard will get boosted, if the students will work hard to meet the demand and succeed with the help of self-esteem. However, the demand seems beyond their abilities, so students are likely to feel distress. Hence, Self-regard will help the students to understand themselves to analyse inward, perfectly perceive and accept their inabilities and set the goals within their scope and abilities.

Emotional Self-Awareness

One's ability to be attentive, recognise and understand their own emotions is called emotional self-awareness. Emotional Self-awareness is a strong predictability of work or performance, know the inner strength, priorities, resources and instincts (Igbinovia, 2016). Once Crompton (2010) documented that individuals with high emotional self-awareness identify the sources and recognize how others could feel. Self-awareness refers to a complex variety of events which involve various self-respect, self-realization and discipline for students. It helps the students to aware, identify, understand, and cope up with those problems.

Bar-On (2007) perceived that emotional self-awareness is an ability to distinguish between their various emotions and able to identify those feelings. For instance, when students face angry or fear, they should know the difference between both and should be able to identify the situation or the reason causing those emotions. Stein & Book (2011) defined that emotional self-awareness as a skill to recognize the feelings and to identify the impact of those feelings on others. And also to understand how it happened. In short, students with emotional self-awareness can recognise their own feelings that will influence their actions. Igbinovia (2016) highlighted that emotional self-awareness precedes all phases of emotional intelligence. Emotional self-awareness leads the students to understand their own feelings in each situation and regulates thinking accordingly. For instance, students should understand their strengths and weaknesses for to complete a work. They can identify what they have to do, find mistakes or make changes in studies, recognize their needs and also they thinks how their behaviour affects others.

Assertiveness

Assertiveness plays a key role of a person to manage his or her own emotions (Stein and Book, 2011). Confident and forceful behaviour are referred as assertiveness. A person with assertiveness have their ability to express thoughts and feelings clearly. It is otherwise called as Emotional Self-expression. According to Bar-On (2007) assertiveness is a capability for effective and constructive way to express their feeling themselves in general.

Stein and Book (2011) states that assertiveness includes three basic components: the ability to express (1) feelings (2) beliefs and thoughts openly and (3) to stand up for personal rights respectively. Assertive students are controlled by their feelings since, they are able to express their opinion and feelings without being aggressive. Assertive behaviour promotes to turn into their own interests to stand up for themselves without worries and show the real joyful feeling. It also help the individual to fight for their personal rights without rejecting the rights of others. According to Bar-On (2007) assertive students are not much restricted to express their feelings more often, without destruction. Individuals those who score low on assertiveness were normally calm; individuals with high assertiveness show more interest in talking with accuracy in every aspect (Norton & Warnick, 1976). In addition, assertive students are often guided by their strategy, courage, polite and positive behaviour of themselves which involves a process to develop a skill and behaviour. So assertive students will develop their academic qualities and attain success in their life.

Independence

One's ability to make decisions, not depending on others and doing things without being rely others is independence. However, they may consider the opinions of others before reaching any conclusion. In other words, independent students have the capacity to think, act and play like self-directed, self-ruling and self-control (Stein and Book, 2011).

Bar-On (2007) states that independent individual try to achieve individual goals and often controls stress which affects circumstances. In short, it is called one's ability to take care of themselves. Genc, Kulusakli, Aydin (2016) stated that individual with high level of independence will get high level experience with self-confidence and better to do risky actions. In this context, students with emotional ability to be self-independent will be able to take own responsibility, feelings, emotions, thoughts and actions. So, students can face any sort of problem, and they can solve it independently without depending on parents or elders.

Self-Actualization

Self-actualization means to understand or completion of individual's talents and potentialities especially considered as a drive or need of an individual. Self-actualization is a chance to feel their capacity and comfortable from students. Furthermore, Panda (2015) stated that self-actualization is meant to understand one's ability to make everything with good manner. Self-actualization in students are associated with good well-being, higher emotional intelligence, competent to do better outcomes, healthy and interpersonal adjustment. Pajouhandeh (2013) documented that self-actualization refers to the desire for self-fulfilment which has the tendency to acquire the inherent potential. According to Maslow opinion, that if an individual achieving self-actualization will be able to satisfy their social or personal needs.

Self-actualization students shows their ability to set goals and drive to attain them in order to realize their prospective. According to Bar-On (2007), that self-actualized person have desire to work towards personal goals with self-fulfilment that includes realization in general, as well as a sense of direction of life. Self-actualization is more relevant which often leads to self-satisfaction. Students can motivate themselves and finish their work according to their desire and fulfil the parents and teacher's needs.

Interpersonal

It is the ability to communicate with the people and understand the feelings of others. It is a skill that everyone required, but it will turn into a quality for them, if they are a students, teacher, doctor, seller or politician. The classroom is a social environment for students to understand about the teachers and peer group. Students having interpersonal abilities can better understand teachers mainly their teaching, way of handling class which processes their challenges and assumption. Behaviors of teachers or peers in school will have varying effects on those students, depending on their behavioral individuality. The teacher's instructional style and the syllabus, the students' feelings about themselves and their academic abilities, and the nature of the interpersonal relations in the classroom are major influences on this teaching-learning process (Schmuck, & Schmuck, 1975). According to Bar-On (2006) interpersonal component consists of three scales: Empathy, Social Responsibility and Interpersonal Relationship.

Empathy

Empathy is capacity to share and understand the 'mind or mood or emotions of others' (Ioannidou & Konstantikaki, 2008). It has the ability to understand, what others can feel, think, and appreciate the thoughts and feelings of others. Empathy is an attribute to understanding others that depends on their priority and by this attribution we can understand ourselves (Bar-On, 2007). According to Badea & Pana (2010) opinion empathy is based on the emotions, interaction, gestures and movement of others. For example, a person with stress would speak with hesitating tone, low strength, irritations and anxiety. By all these previous statement, "Empathy is having the capability to share, understand and respond with care to the experiences of others. Being empathic involves cognitive and emotional reactions, such as actively listening, identifying, understanding the concerns and emotions of others".

The researchers like Abe, Niwa, Fujisaki and Suzuki (2018) explained, that empathy is found to be associated with intelligence and emotions. Sharing stories is a great way to create empathy will make the students to read many story books from the school library. If they like any particular story books, they will start portray the same character in which they got attracted from the book. Empathy connects them towards the particular character of the story books. Like empathy helps the student to understand their parents or teachers or friends at a certain situation (Jones, 2017). Empathy is an essential part in student's life. Students acquire knowledge about empathy during the learning stage itself, after that they can understand about the perspective of others. Empathy helps the students in getting high score in assignment, academic achievement, creating a flexible classroom community with strong communication abilities. Moreover, their behaviour will change with reduced emotional complaints and they will not involve in destructive performance and lesser opportunities for harassment and also have more positive interactions (Ashoka, undated).

Social Responsibility

Social responsibility is an ability to prove as a cooperative, contributing, constructive member of a social group (family, friends and at work place) (Al-Faouri, 2011) and also exhibit co-operation, community and unity in the social environment. An individual can obey, cooperate and understand others in a social group. Bar-On (2007) defines the social responsibility is related to the most cooperative which indicates that, they share similar well-suited ideas to the society. Social responsibility has a capacity to be in support to the contributing members of a social group in the society (Stein & Book, 2011).

Social responsibility helps to behave, collaborate, benefit and influence on others. To improve the social responsibility of children they should involve in various extracurricular activities like National cadet corps (NCC), National service scheme (NSS), Red Cross, Scouts and Guides, etc., that are being conducted in schools. Other activities like attending health education and anti-violence program including visiting the homeless shelter clinics. Student's social responsibilities are essential for taking their own actions and responsibility. It also initiates social, cultural and environmental responsibilities in every student. Moral control of these responsibilities on each student will try to reduce the harmful effects on their surroundings. Some other social responsibilities such as to be a volunteer and accountable to one self with respecting elders and follow the ethics, traffic rules, value diversity and working together.

Interpersonal Relationship

Some researchers consider that interpersonal relationships include a behaviour of sense of humour and intimate friendship and involves interaction between the social, family, friends and peer groups (Yang & Mossholder, 2002). Student's well-being remains on positive interpersonal relationships with all elders, family and teachers. Previous research study (Dolev & Leshem, 2016) indicates that interpersonal relationship will develop the importance of social emotional skills and academic success of students at their learning stage. They often contribute to a positive work environment everywhere. Moreover, interpersonal relationship is dependent only on the relationship of families, school and society. It is an ability to understand emotions and feelings in those relationships of students (Hsieh, Wang, Fan & Huang, 2014).

Interpersonal relationship establish mutual satisfying relationships and relate well with others. School stimulates as a forum for the life of each student that will develop peer relationships and helps to acquire several experiences.

Interpersonal relationship helps the student to interconnect with others and to establish a balanced satisfying relationships (Dolev & Leshem, 2016). Weaker students are often shy, less motivated, unwillingness to read and become a target of others. Their character may change to avoid social contact with each other. Interpersonal relationship is having efficiency to maintain a purposeful relationship and help each other. It is ability to establish a good bond between the teacher and the student. If the teacher is a compassionate with students based on their interpersonal relationship behaviour, it will automatically improve the learning, gestures, non-verbal communication between teachers and students (Opic, 2016). So, it is a basic necessary for the flick of life.

Stress Management

It is the ability to manage and control their stress behaviour. It is concerned about the ability of someone who has to endure stress without fatigue, falling down, losing control or going down. Some strategies like listening music, watching videos and planning games can help the students to perform better on whatever they do, furthermore they will turn out to be less tense without stress and silent (Rizzolo, Zipp, Stiskal & Simpkins, 2009). High trait emotional intelligence individuals exhibit a good stress management skills having capability to appraise, express and manage their emotions with others.

The stress management realm concerns the capacity to be flexible, tolerate stress and control impulses (Stein and Book, 2011). Stress is being experienced by everyone in this world. Managing stress is an ability which is found essential for all the individuals in this society. Stress among students can be a significant for the welfare of the family. Many factors cause stress and can change the relationship dynamics in the family, especially adolescents. Stress management is an ability to understand and analyse the significant impact of life will help the students by reducing the stress. According to Bar-On (2006) stress management dimension consists of two scales: Stress tolerance and Impulse Control.

Stress tolerance

Stress tolerance is an ability to withstand during stressful situations, adverse events and strong emotions without falling apart but actively coping with stress (Sunil & Rooprai (2009). Stress tolerance is a skill to remain calm and focused. Moreover, Stein and Book (2011) refers that stress tolerance is a capacity to develop physical or emotional symptoms by active and positively coping with stress. Bar-On (2007) mentioned that stress tolerance is ability for leadership, challenging position of individuals in pressure situation. It is very important skill for the leader to manage with complexity, effort and worrying situation. In short, stress tolerance is the ability to be effective and constructively handle the emotions for a successful life. It is the capability to stay calm and pressure to constructive fight against negative events and contradictory feelings. Students with pressure will have less academic achievements compared to those who are not having it.

Stress tolerance is the key to live without stress, minimise damage of health, relationships, performance and intelligence of individuals. In addition, such individual can develop their emotional intelligence and stress tolerance for their health and success. There are six approaches to enhance stress tolerance like, a step away from the place, get enough sleep, daily exercises, focus on a balanced diet, improve happiness and flexibility, build mind against stress (Sunil & Rooprai, 2009). Stress tolerance will also enable students to get motivated and persist, despite frustrations and become more resilient to stress and enhance their IQ and EQ. Some variables can decrease the bearing of stress on watching television, counselling, doing exercise, playing, watching comedy, physical and mental health of students. Such variables are social support, hardness, trust, emotion holding, and auto-reaction which helps the students to tolerate stress. Creating programs, innovative classes, counselling by health educators or psychiatric can teach students for best and most practical ways to handle stress (Welle & Graf, 2011).

Impulse Control

According to Bar-On (2007), impulse control is the capability to resist or delay an impulse or test to act. Impulse controls are an ability to accept aggressive stimuli during unfavourable condition and ineffective careless behaviour. It is also capable of maintaining strength, controlling challenges, and seeking a sense of situations. Impulse control is necessary for students, if students can control their emotions and it will make beneficial and successful relationship with the surroundings.

Stein and Book (2011) identifies that impulse control entails avoiding the rash behaviours, it is also a tendency for decision making, spontaneous or restricted happiness of being composed students. One must have enough impulse to control and not to express the disapproval feeling, anger without letting it to increase, aggressive and unwanted behaviour. Therefore, impulse control enable students to find out solutions to incapacities, interpret the chances that will promote learning hopefulness, high self-esteem and self-efficacy. In fact, if students can develop emotional intelligence, impulse control will expand the strength of self-control and it leads into the holistic development of students. Students learn some strategies to increase their impulse control to maintain smooth surroundings. Impulse control training is a type of intellectual-behavioural intervention to improve attention and decrease the problem of students.

Adaptability

It is an ability to manage the changes and resolve interpersonal and intrapersonal issues. According to Kalanjiam & Manoharan (2016), stress plays an important role in affecting the adaptability of a person that leads to various negative effects in daily life. Adaptive learning is broadly concerned with academic work and stresses, while adaptation focuses particularly on changing, new and uncertain circumstances and situations. It is a specific type of emotional regulation that involves plans that are intended to control feelings in originality, variety and uncertain situations (Collie & Martin, 2017). For example, students will adapt to their new syllabus, adjust with friends, parents and teachers, etc.

Some researchers like Leary & De Rosier (2012) stated that, the transition from one school to another can be a source of thrilling, stressful due to leaving their friends and family and adapt a new situation, environment, academic features and society for adjusting to a new life in an unfamiliar environment. Moreover, Collie & Martin (2017) demonstrated that students' self-reports of adaptability had the strong association with academic achievement. In this context, students are using an ability to manage surrounding to solve the internal and external problems. Adaptability refers the student capacity to employ a new plan to regulate their response to innovation, change or ambiguity. Students adaptability in examination parameters that embrace the students' education system, change their group team, stimulus, communication, cognition, and regulatory problems. For instance, NEET (National Eligibility cum Entrance Test) has been introduced by the Govt., of India for students who wish to study any graduate medical course, dental course or postgraduate course in govt., or private medical colleges in recent times. This made the students to develop stress owing to preparations and new syllabus. In this regard, student's adaptability is expected to the new exam patterns by accepting the reality and being flexible to solve the problem. Bar-On (2006) opined that adaptability consists of three scales: Reality-Testing, Flexibility, and Problem Solving.

Reality Testing

Reality testing involves identifying and understanding the reality happening around their surroundings and to change the current situations accordingly. According to Stein & Book (2011), the reality testing is the capacity to see a things exactly and act upon the real situation. It is also a skill to stay attentive when trying to assess and survive with the emotions associated with things happening. An individual needs objective evidence to settle emotions, perceptions and thoughts. Reality Testing helps to remain disconnected, so it can accurately identify emotions and deal with them. It is an ability to assess the correspondence between what's experienced and objectively exists. It also involves on 'tuning in' to the immediate situation.

Arnott (2015) refers that reality testing is a capability to remain detached from seeing things as they really needed. It is interesting to note, that reality testing is part of a complex of emotional intelligence skills that includes decision making, impulse control and problem solving. Reality testing refers to validate the individuals feelings and thinking with external reality. The concept above gives an idea of accuracy and recognition of thoughts. In this context, students has to show their ability to evaluate different feelings and thinking objectively with unambiguous reality. Reality testing searches for confirmation, justification, support for feelings, spirits and ideas. The strategy of reality testing that can help the realistic test are: objectiveness, thinking, reacting, controlling, deliberate, searching for the perspectives of others and looking for a successful trainer. Students decide their career with decision making with emotional intelligence skills. This also in turn helps them to reduce their stress in about the future.

Flexibility

It is to adapt and adjust an individual feelings, thoughts, actions, changes which are challenging during unfamiliar conditions and thinking to a new situations refers as flexibility. According to Bar-On (2007), flexible student is capable of changing the reactions without awareness of inactivity, integrated and inefficient. The component of flexibility of students with a high feeling of self-efficacy have shown more flexibility. Foster (2016) refers that both emotional intelligence and psychological flexibility are concerned with encouraging positive outcomes in examination within this context of flexibility.

Yazdi, Farahi, Farahi & Hosseini (2018) states that students with low flexibility are affected with low attention, performance, cognitive flexibility, less activity, low performance and low cognitive flexibility. Flexibility helps the students to be attentive, active and perform the cognitive well than others. According to Kashdan & Rottenberg (2010) shows that flexibility is included as a fundamental aspect of health and by, adjusting with the social environment and abilities to face any difficulties (as cited in Hochmair, 2013). Emotional intelligence has an ability to contribute positive thought and work-related psychological flexibility through emotional self-efficacy training. Flexibility involves in being able to train our self for unexpected situations that may at inspire first towards inspire mental depression due, because to adjust the others emotions, thoughts, condition and behaviour in certain situations (Stein & Book, 2011).

Students who were less satisfied with their performance are well-known by their flexibility and if students were high in flexibility then they can be able to get high in grasping and well- adjusted with all. Rye (2008) describes flexibility as the steady component of occurrence that will assure its continuing reality in a continuous process. Student's flexibility is determined by teachers, syllabus, time, surroundings, assessment, objects like books, computers, notes, etc. In flexible learning there is a no stress for interactive and collaborative nature of learning offered by the environment and surroundings (Nagy & McDonald, 2007). The students' flexibility is associated with cognitive, self-regulation, attention and mindfulness.

Problem Solving

Problem solving is an organized process focusing on difficult situations and acts as a part of decision making. Problem solving is a step focus on the internal problems in decision making, and analysing the cause of problem and how to solve it, what it is and what it should be to solve the problem (Hosseini, 2007). Researchers like Moattari, Soltani, Mousavinasab, Aiattollahi, (2005) concluded that students had problem solving skill, when the emotional intelligence are in high level. Problem solving is a base of the training process as it is very essential for an effective interventions. Emotional intelligence of students in all activities are directed towards a high level of thinking to problem solving. Emotional skill is a vital part of achievement, where problem solving skills in individuals depend on their cognitive and behavioural abilities. The higher ability of problem solving is due to knowing and analyzing the situation better (as cited by Shewchuk, Johnson, Elliot, 2000). The level of emotional intelligence affects to solve the individuals' problem, if individuals are high in emotional intelligence also increases the problem solving ability (Esmaeily, Ahady, Delavar, Shafiabady, 2007).

Khona, Kima & Aidossovaa (2016) refers that emotional intelligence dimension like self- concept and self-management can be improved through the problem solving training approach. Emotional intelligence training is a design for solving problems and the evidence shows that it is useful for self-understanding and emotional regulation. Furthermore, Deniz (2013) states that some student will take the different problem solving ability like confidence, challenge, belief, time, effort, determination and pledge to solve the problem and tackle every situation. All these are the main characteristics of positive problem orientation and appraisal.

Salovey and Mayer (1990) proposed that individuals differ greatly in their ability to organize their emotions to solve problems. Both emotions and moods have a subtle influence over the strategies involved in problem solving. Emotional intelligence is designated as efficient processing of emotional sensation (Barzegar, Afzal, Maleki & Koochakyazdi, 2013). Emotional intelligence factor can identify, define, create and implement potentially effective solutions for the problem. Students share all their problem with well-wishers, friends, family members, parents or teachers to solve academic and personal problems.

General Mood

Mood is generating ability to cognitive process of attention, expectation and, behaviour. Mood is stimulated from the situation, so it is a great consequence for regulation of mood (DeSteno & Salovey, 1997). It is concerned about individual's personality and ability to feel about sharing the whole feeling with the others, sometimes it will be satisfying and dissatisfying from their performance. Stein and Book (2014) states that the general mood is a strong predictor of resilience. Positive mood has shown an enabling impact on remembrance, learning and behaviour; whereas negative mood effect has a depressing impact. A positive mood has been found to improve the performance of behaviour that leads to more positive effects like increasing energy and freedom to act by their wish. But the negative mood decreases the accessible goal (Febrilia & Warokka, 2014, Fishbach & Labroo, 2007). Also, moods decides the individual ability to reach their goals and further it is decided by one's happiness, stress and interprets in social behaviour. If student win in a team play match will leads to their elevation of enthusiastic mood and have a positive impact on their outcomes. According to Bar-On (2006) General mood consists of two scales: Optimism and Happiness.

Optimism

As per Stein and Book (2011) optimism approach is to be positive and always look at the brighter side of life (It is an ability to maintain a realistic positive approach). Bar-On (2007) states that optimism (also called as enthusiasm) plays a key role in self-motivation which represents a very important aspect to reduce depression and achieve goals, and attribute a valuable and desirable leadership. Also, Stein and Book (2011) noted that generally, optimistic individuals can stay with confidence in each difficult situation in general and not worried about themselves in most of the situations. Moreover, they can stay confidently in each difficult situation and also motivate themselves and others during difficult situations and never compromised. So, optimistic students can easily face challenges.

Moreover, Mo (2010) documented optimistic students can focus on the positive qualities on their study. By having these qualities, students can improve their achievement by generating and maintaining excitement, enthusiasm, confidence, and optimism (as cited in George, 2000). Optimism indicates an effective use to help with stress reduction and maintain a positive attitude. Student community is very dynamic one and that needed more attention to grow. So, during on this period optimism is an important thing for the students to become more efficient and to cope up in every situation in future. Optimistic students have a better connection with surroundings, because they work hard with, have good confidence level and so they will be ready to do work anywhere (Carver & Scheier, 2014). The same author explained that student with optimism are more persistence in academics, manage stress, increase goals and make professional efforts. Optimistic students have the characteristics of positive thinking, problem-solving, strengths, good content, mental health, well-being, faces obstacles and decreases suicidal ideation.

Happiness

Happiness is an ability to feel content with oneself and others and life in general (Bar-On, 2013). It is one's capability to feel satisfied in their life, and enjoying with other activities. Furnham & Petrides (2003) said that happiness is the response which indicates a person who feels generally satisfied with life. Students with happiness probably have a happy and pleasant disposition that will help to maintain positive

Figure 1.
Source: Mohanadasan, (2014). Emotional intelligence and managerial skills: A comparative study on the managers of selected public sector and private sector banks in Kerala.

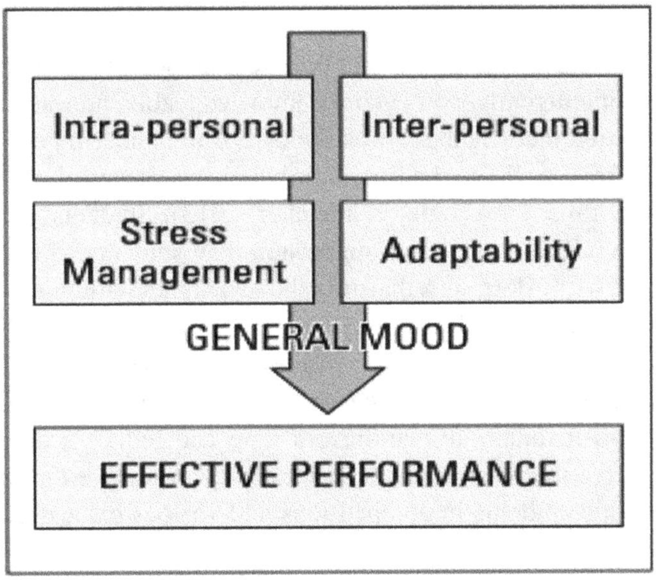

feelings. Positive atmosphere can make more energetic to do things and it lifts the overall performance. It is evident that cheerful people often feel better and easier in their work and use every moment for entertainment.

The essential components of happiness are positive emotions, life satisfaction, lack of negative emotions and positive relations with others, purposeful life, personal growth and love on others (Sasanpour, Khodabakhshi & Kh, 2012). According to the principle of pleasure-seeking state, happiness is maximising pleasure and minimising pain to attain life fulfilment (Khosla & Dokania, 2010). On the other hand, happy life is one which enhances good feelings (pleasure) and illuminate the bad feelings (pain). Hence happiness is the sum total of the lifetime of all these specific feelings (Kahneman, 1999). The happiness among students may help to change their whole life pattern, definitely they will show the difference on their achievement in academics. The increase of happiness in a student is vital, it makes to live healthy both physically and psychologically; it shows success in academics, social life and professional life.

Positive Impression

Impression is defined as the initial awareness and creation of feelings about others. Impression on others is very truthful during first sight. As such, first impressions can facilitate our survival and interaction with the environment. First impressions are formulated in each occasion like we observe a new, unfamiliar, individual or phenomenon. Collon (1987) opined that the purpose of the first impression is to help to learn about existing strengths and weaknesses as seen through the eyes of the first time visitor.

Kwon (1994) described some people believe that well-dressed person can communicate very intelligently, competently, knowledgeable, honest and reliable. This raises the question that whether a weak body posture undermines the positive impression created by a well-fitted garment or whether a powerful pose enhances the effect (Howlett, Pine, Orakçoglu, & Fletcher, 2013). Students with a higher grade point average (GPA) make good impression than students with lower GPA. Gender is associated with effort, such that girls shows a higher willingness to manage desired impressions in the school environment. The positive impression on oneself makes them to see themselves as always positive and others too. Even though they were ready to take effort for change the negative vibrations to positive. This positive attitude is helping to maintain an equilibrium state and reduce academic stress. On one hand, positive impression in students help them to face the people with confidence. It also aid students in competitions and various exams. On the other hand, it develops positive outlook in them.

DISCUSSION

Bharti & Sidana (2012) pointed Emotional intelligence is necessary for the success path in present life. Students with average academic stress were more emotionally stable as compared to the students having high academic stress (Bharti & Sidana, 2012). Schutte, Malouff, Thorsteinsson, Bhullar & Rooke, (2007) opined that Emotional intelligence (EI) is associated with good health and it effectively contributes to one's benefit (as cited in Por, Barriball, Fitzpatrick, & Roberts, (2011). Bharti & Sidana, (2012) illustrates that emotional intelligence should be well-known not only for academic interest but also for success in life. Emotional Intelligence also need to be self-reliant (intrapersonal) and decisive (Independence), in making realistic (Reality-Testing) and effective solutions to problems as they arise (Problem-solving). This often requires having the ability to work well under pressure (Stress Tolerance), happiness, emotional self-awareness, and maintain a positive approach (Optimism). Especially, five specific components of Emotional Intelligence namely empathy, stress tolerance, independence, optimism and interpersonal relationships were found to relate to transformational leadership. Hence the dimension of Emotional intelligence is very helpful for the effective performance of students.

De Villiers (2010) classified Emotional Intelligence into five main categories of general skills like 1) Communication skills, 2) Problem solving skills and critical thinking, 3) Leadership and work, 4) Moral and spiritual values and 5) Self-management.

CONCLUDING REMARKS

Based on the above review and discussions, one can conclude that the sub-competencies of emotional intelligence will help the students to cope with the stressors arising from parents, teachers, academic and from peers and manage their academic stress. Once the students mastered over these emotional competencies they can easily face the challenges that are arising in this complex and dynamic environment. These emotional competencies determine how the student can grow, how to win in the school, how to succeed in their life and how to maintain purposeful relationships with others. Therefore, emotional intelligence is significant in everyone's life for their betterment in each stage. No doubt that emotional intelligence will play a significant role in moderating the academic stress and increasing individual resilience. This in-turn enhances student's mental health and wellbeing. The student with better mental health perform well in any tasks with involvement and also exhibit appropriate desired behaviour both in the school and the community. It is possible to enhance mental health of students through emotional intelligence training, and will act as an extra power to succeed in their life both personally and professionally. Assessing student's emotional intelligence will be of prime use as it help the teachers to plan their teaching accordingly and help them to enhance emotional intelligence among students.

REFERENCES

Aaron, R., Joseph, A., Abraham, S., Muliyil, J., George, K., Prasad, J., ... Bose, A. (2005). Suicides in young people in rural southern India. *Lancet, 363*(9415), 1117–1118. doi:10.1016/S0140-6736(04)15896-0 PMID:15064031

Abe, K., Niwa, M., Fujisaki, K., & Suzuki, Y. (2018). EI and empathy have been found to be associated. Empathy is viewed as an ability to understand and share the feelings of another. It is a multi-dimensional construct which includes both cognitive and affective elements. *Bio medical centre*, 2 -9.

Al-Dubai, S. A. R., Al-Naggar, R. A., AlShagga, M. A., & Rampal, K. G. (2011). Stress and coping strategies of students in a medical faculty in Malaysia. *The Malaysian Journal of Medical Sciences: MJMS, 18*(3), 57. PMID:22135602

Al-Faouri, A. H. A. (2011). Investigating the impact of emotional intelligence on technology learning. *IACSIT International Journal of Engineering and Technology, 11*(3), 58–78.

Al-Nawasrah, F. A. (2019). The Relationship between the Mental Health and the Emotional and Social Intelligence among Talented Students in Ajlun Schools. *Brock Journal of Education, 7*(1), 77–93.

Ardic, C., & Ozturk, G. Z. (2018). The role of stress management and interpersonal communication in preventing violence against family physicians. *International Journal of Research in Medical Sciences, 6*(4), 1094–1100. doi:10.18203/2320-6012.ijrms20181262

Armstrong, T. (2009). *Multiple intelligences in the classroom*. Ascd.

Arnott, S. (2015). *Reality testing*. The Emotional Intelligence Training Company Inc. Retrieved from https://www.eitrainingcompany.com/2015/12/show-notes-episode-11-reality-testing/

Arslan, N. (2017). Investigating the relationship between educational stress and emotional self-efficacy. *Universal Journal of Educational Research, 5*(10), 1736–1740. doi:10.13189/ujer.2017.051010

Ashoka. (n.d.). *Be fearless be kind, empathy toolkit from rules of kindness*. Retrieved from https://befearlessbekind.hasbro.com/wp-content/uploads/pdf/Ashoka_empathytoolkitfromRules ofKindness.pdf

Badea, L., & Pană, N. A. (2010). The Role of Empathy in Developing the Leader's Emotional Intelligence. *Theoretical & Applied Economics, 17*(2).

Bar-On, R. (1997). *Bar-On Emotional Quotient Inventory: A Measure of Emotional Intelligence: User's Manualcby Reuven Bar-On*. MHS.

Bar-On, R. (2006). The Bar-On model of emotional social intelligence (ESI). *Psicothema, 18*, 13–25. PMID:17295953

Bar-On, R. (2007). *Description of the EQ-i, EQ-360 and EQ-i: YV*. Retrieved November.

Bar-On, R. (2013). *The 15 factors of the Bar-On model*. Retrieved from http://www.reuvenbaron.org/wp/the-5-meta-factors-and-15-sub-factors-of-the-bar-on-model

Barzegar, M., Afzal, E., Maleki, M., & Koochakyazdi, S. (2013). The relationship between Emotional Intelligence and Decision-making Quality in Hospital Managers. *International Journal of Hospital Research, 2*(2), 64–69.

Bharti, R., & Sidana, J. J. (2012). A study of emotional intelligence in relation to academic achievement and academic stress of student-teachers. *Indian Streams Research Journal., 2*(9), 1–6.

Collie, R. J., & Martin, A. J. (2017). Students' adaptability in mathematics: Examining self-reports and teachers' reports and links with engagement and achievement outcomes. *Contemporary Educational Psychology, 49*, 355–366. doi:10.1016/j.cedpsych.2017.04.001

Collon, D. (1987). *First impressions: cylinder seals in the ancient Near East*. London: British Museum Publications.

Cory, D. (2015). *Healthy self-regard in effective leaders*. The Emotional Intelligence Training Company Inc. retrieved from https://www.eitrainingcompany.com/2015/02/healthy-self-regard-in-effective-leaders/

Crompton, M. (2010). *Improving self-awareness increases your emotional intelligence. inter business issues*. Retrieved from https://peoriamagazines.com/ibi/2010/apr/improving-self-awareness-increases-your-emotional-intelligence

Das, S. (2017). Suicide among the elderly: A psychological perspective. *International Journal of Social Work and Human Services Practice, 5*(1), 35–42.

De Villiers, R. (2010). The incorporation of soft skills into accounting curricula: Preparing accounting graduates for their unpredictable futures. *Meditari Accountancy Research*, *18*(2), 1–22. doi:10.1108/10222529201000007

Deniz, S. (2013). The relationship between emotional intelligence and problem solving skills in prospective teachers. *Educational Research Review*, *8*(24), 2339–2345.

DeSteno, D. A., & Salovey, P. (1997). The effects of mood on the structure of the self-concept. *Cognition and Emotion*, *11*(4), 351–372. doi:10.1080/026999397379836

Dominic Claeys-Jackson. (2017). *5 ways to manage student stress*. Retrieved from https://www.prospects.ac.uk/applying-for-university/university-life/5-ways-to-manage-student-stress

Esmaeili, N., & Jamkhaneh, E. B. (2013). The relationship between emotional intelligence and mental health in humanism college students at IAU, Qaemshahr Branch, Iran. *Journal of Basic and Applied Scientific Research*, *3*(2), 68–76.

Esmaeily, M., Ahadi, H., Delavar, A., & Shafiabadi, A. (2007). Effects of emotional intelligence training on enhancing mental health. *Majallah-i Ravanpizishki va Ravanshinasi-i Balini-i Iran*, *13*, 158–165.

Febrilia, I., & Warokka, A. (2014). *The effects of positive and negative mood on university students' learning and academic performance: Evidence from Indonesia*. Academic Press.

Fishbach, A., & Labroo, A. A. (2007). Be better or be merry: How mood affects self-control. *Journal of Personality and Social Psychology*, *93*(2), 158–173. doi:10.1037/0022-3514.93.2.158 PMID:17645393

Foster, R. M. P. (2016). *The power of emotional intelligence for facilitating psychologically flexible thinking: a contextual perspective in decision making and workplace flourishing*. Academic Press.

Freedman, J., & Jensen, A. (2008). A case for emotional intelligence in our schools. *Six seconds: The Emotional Intelligence Network.*

Furnham, A., & Petrides, K. V. (2003). Trait emotional intelligence and happiness. *Social Behavior and Personality*, *31*(8), 815–823. doi:10.2224bp.2003.31.8.815

Garg, P., & Rastogi, R. (2009). Emotional intelligence and stress resiliency: A relationship study. *International Journal of Educational Advancement*, *1*(1), 1–16.

George, J. M. (2000). Emotions and leadership: The role of emotional intelligence. *Human Relations*, *53*(8), 1027–1055. doi:10.1177/0018726700538001

Gleason, M. E. (2011). Intrapersonal intelligence strategies in the developmental writing classroom. *Inquiry*, *16*(1), 95–105.

Goleman, D. (1995). *Emotional intelligence: why it can matter more than IQ?* New York: Bantam.

Goleman, D. (1998). *Working with Emotional Intelligence*. New York: Bantam Books.

Gujral, D. H. K. (2013). Emotional intelligence buffers stress: A study on emotional intelligence and coping styles. *EXCEL International Journal of Multidisciplinary Management Studies*, *3*(11), 76–82.

Gupta, G., & Kumar, S. (2010). Mental health in relation to emotional intelligence and self-efficacy among college students. *Journal of the Indian Academy of Applied Psychology*, *36*(1), 61–67.

Hochmair, I. (2013). The importance of being flexible. *Nature Medicine*, *19*(10), 1240–1244. doi:10.1038/nm.3341 PMID:24100995

Hosseini, H. S. (2007, September). *Problem solving by intelligent water drops. In 2007 IEEE congress on evolutionary computation* (pp. 3226–3231). IEEE. doi:10.1109/CEC.2007.4424885

Howlett, N., Pine, K., Orakçıoğlu, I., & Fletcher, B. (2013). The influence of clothing on first impressions: Rapid and positive responses to minor changes in male attire. *Journal of Fashion Marketing and Management: An International Journal*, *17*(1), 38–48. doi:10.1108/13612021311305128

Hsieh, M. C., Wang, T. S., Fan, C. P., & Huang, C. I. (2014). A study of the emotional intelligence and interpersonal relationships of college students in Southern Taiwan. *Universal Journal of Management*, *2*(8), 133–138.

Igbinovia, M. O. (2016). *Emotional Self Awareness and Information Literacy Competence as Correlates of Task Performance of Academic Library Personnel.* Academic Press.

Ioannidou & Konstantikaki. (2008). Empathy and emotional intelligence: What is it really about? *International. Journal of Caring Sciences*, *1*(3), 118.

Johnson, K. K., Schofield, N. A., & Yurchisin, J. (2002). Appearance and dress as a source of information: A qualitative approach to data collection. *Clothing & Textiles Research Journal*, *20*(3), 125–137. doi:10.1177/0887302X0202000301

Jones, N. B. (2017). An Ethological Study of Some Aspects of Social Behaviour of Children in. *Primate Ethology*, 347.

Jordan, J. A., McRorie, M., & Ewing, C. (2010). Gender differences in the role of emotional intelligence during the primary–secondary school transition. *Emotional & Behavioural Difficulties, 15*(1), 37–47. doi:10.1080/13632750903512415

Jorfi, H., Jorfi, S., Yaccob, H. F. B., & Shah, I. M. (2010). Emotional intelligence: The relationship between self-regard and communication effectiveness. *World Academy of Science, Engineering and Technology, International Journal of Social, Behavioral, Educational, Economic. Business and Industrial Engineering, 4*(9), 1989–1995.

Kahneman, D. (1999). Objective happiness. *Well-Being: The Foundations of Hedonic Psychology, 3*(25), 1-23.

Kalanjiam, V., & Manoharan, M. G. (2016). A study of the relationship between stress, adaptability and temporomandibular disordersy. *International Journal of Current Research and Review, 8*(4), 1.

Kashdan, T. B., & Rottenberg, J. (2010). Psychological flexibility as a fundamental aspect of health. *Clinical Psychology Review, 30*(7), 865–878. doi:10.1016/j.cpr.2010.03.001 PMID:21151705

Kaur, S. (2018). Emotional intelligence in relation to mental health and adjustment among students. *International Journal of Advanced Research and Development., 3*(1), 304–308.

Kauts, D. S. (2016). Emotional Intelligence and Academic Stress among College Students. *Educational Quest, 7*(3), 149.

Khona, N., Kima, A., & Aidossovaa, Z. (2016). *Problem Solving Design for Emotional Intelligence Training of Middle Managers*. Academic Press.

Khosla, M., & Dokania, V. (2010). Does happiness promote emotional intelligence. *Journal of the Indian Academy of Applied Psychology, 36*(1), 45–54.

Kundi, G. (2016). *Why Indian Students are more stressed than ever?* Retrieved October 18, 2016, from http://www.studyin-uk.in/blog/why-indianstudents-are-more-stressed-than-ever/

Kwon, Y.-H. (1994). Feeling toward one's clothing and self-perception of emotion, sociability, and work competency. *Journal of Social Behavior and Personality, 9*(1), 129–139.

Lazarus, R. S. (1999). *Stress and emotion: A new synthesis*. New York: Springer.

Leary, K. A., & DeRosier, M. E. (2012). Factors promoting positive adaptation and resilience during the transition to college. *Psychology (Irvine, Calif.)*, *3*(12), 1215–1222. doi:10.4236/psych.2012.312A180

Levus, N. (2012). Self-regard in the structure of personality behavioural manifestations. *Journal of Education Culture and Society*, (2).

Mayer, J. D., Caruso, D. R., & Salovey, P. (1999). Emotional intelligence meets traditional standards for an intelligence. *Intelligence*, *27*(4), 267–298. doi:10.1016/S0160-2896(99)00016-1

Mayer, J. D., & Salovey, P. (1997). What is emotional intelligence? *Emotional development and emotional intelligence: Educational implications, 3*, 31.

Mo, Y. Y. (2010). *Measuring and enhancing the emotional intelligence of built environment students* (Doctoral dissertation).

Moattari, M., Soltani, A., Mousavinasab, M., & Aiattollahi, A. (2005). The effect of problem solving skill training on self-concept of nursing students of the Shiraz faculty of nursing & midwifery. *Iran J Educ Med Sci., 5*(14), 147-55. (in Persian)

Mohanadasan, T. (2014). *Emotional intelligence and managerial skills: A comparative study on the managers of selected public sector and private sector banks in Kerala*. Academic Press.

Nagy, J., & McDonald, J. (2007). New models for learning flexibility: Negotiated choices for both academics and students. In *Proceedings ASCILITE 2007: 24th Annual Conference of the Australasian Society for Computers in Learning in Tertiary Education: ICT: Providing Choices for Learners and Learning* (pp. 737-746). Nanyang Technological University, Centre for Educational Development.

Norton, R., & Warnick, B. (1976). Assertiveness as communication construct. *Human Communication Research*, *3*(1), 62–66. doi:10.1111/j.1468-2958.1976.tb00504.x

Opic, S. (2016). Interpersonal relations in school. *International Journal of Cognitive Research in Science, Engineering and Education, 4*(2), 9-21.

Pajouhandeh, E. (2013). Personal Development and Self-Actualization of Students in the New Environment. *International Journal (Toronto, Ont.)*, *2*(1), 2307–227X.

Panda, M. (2015). Emotional intelligence as a correlate of self-actualization among teachers at secondary teachers training college. *International Journal of Multidisciplinary Research and Development.*, *2*(12), 158–168.

Parker, J. D., Summerfeldt, L. J., Hogan, M. J., & Majeski, S. A. (2004). Emotional intelligence and academic success: Examining the transition from high school to university. *Personality and Individual Differences*, *36*(1), 163–172. doi:10.1016/S0191-8869(03)00076-X

Por, J., Barriball, L., Fitzpatrick, J., & Roberts, J. (2011). Emotional intelligence: Its relationship to stress, coping, well-being and professional performance in nursing students. *Nurse Education Today*, *31*(8), 855–860. doi:10.1016/j.nedt.2010.12.023 PMID:21292360

Rizzolo, D., Zipp, G. P., Stiskal, D., & Simpkins, S. (2009). Stress management strategies for students: The immediate effects of yoga, humor, and reading on stress. *Journal of College Teaching and Learning*, *6*(8), 79–88.

Roosevelt, E. (2017). Emotional Intelligence Skills – Self-Regard. *Apex Leadership Mastery*. Retrieved from https://www.apexmastery.com/emotional-intelligence-skills-self-regard-1/

Rowniyar, P. (2016). Emotional intelligence as a key to reduce academic stress among adolescence student. *The Signage*, *4*(1), 2455–0051.

Rye, S. A. (2008). Dimensions of flexibility-students, communication technology and distributed education. Seminar.net, 4(1), 1-18.

Salehi, M., Zadeh, M. A., Ghaderi, A., & Tabasi, A. Z. (2016). Study of the Effect of Education and Academic Environment on Emotional Intelligence on Accounting Students in Iran. *International Education Studies*, *9*(1), 182–188. doi:10.5539/ies.v9n1p182

Salovey, P., & Mayer, J.D. (1990). Emotional Intelligence. *Imagination, Cognition and Personality, 9*, 185-211.

Salovey, P., & Mayer, J. D. (1990). Emotional intelligence. *Imagination, Cognition and Personality*, *9*(3), 185–211. doi:10.2190/DUGG-P24E-52WK-6CDG

Sarita, S. (2015). Academic stress among students: Role and responsibilities of parents. *International Journal of Applied Research*, *1*(10), 385–388.

Sasanpour, M., Khodabakhshi, M., & Kh, N. (2012). The relationship between emotional intelligence, happiness and mental health in students of medical sciences of Isfahan University. *International Journal of Collaborative Research on Internal Medicine & Public Health*, *4*(9), 1614–1620.

Schmuck, R. A., & Schmuck, P. A. (1975). *Group processes in the classroom.* Academic Press.

Schutte, N. S., Malouff, J. M., Thorsteinsson, E., Bhullar, N., & Rooke, S. (2007). A meta investigation of the relationship between emotional intelligence and health. *Personality and Individual Differences*, *42*(6), 921–933. doi:10.1016/j.paid.2006.09.003

Shewchuk, R. M., Johnson, M. O., & Elliott, T. R. (2000). Self-appraised social problem solving abilities, emotional reactions and actual problem solving performance. *Behaviour Research and Therapy*, *38*(7), 727–740. doi:10.1016/S0005-7967(99)00122-9 PMID:10875194

Stein, S. J., & Book, H. E. (2011). *The EQ edge: Emotional intelligence and you success*. John Wiley.

Subramanyam, K. (2016). Impact of emotional intelligence, nature of course and gender on academic stress among college students. *The International Journal of Indian Psychology, Volume 3, Issue 4, No. 60*, 120.

Sunil, K., & Rooprai, K. Y. (2009). Role of emotional intelligence in managing stress and anxiety at workplace. *Proceedings of ASBBS*, *16*(1), 163–172.

Sylva, K. (2000). School influences on children's development. *Psychology of Education: Schools. Teachers and Parents*, *1*, 51.

Trinidad, D. R., & Johnson, C. A. (2002). The association between emotional intelligence and early adolescent tobacco and alcohol use. *Personality and Individual Differences*, *32*(1), 95–105. doi:10.1016/S0191-8869(01)00008-3

Utting, D. (2007). *Parenting and the different ways it can affect children's lives: research evidence*. Joseph Rowntree Foundation.

Welle, P. D., & Graf, H. M. (2011). Effective lifestyle habits and coping strategies for stress tolerance among college students. *American Journal of Health Education*, *42*(2), 96–105. doi:10.1080/19325037.2011.10599177

Yang, J., & Mossholder, K. W. (2004). Decoupling task and relationship conflict: The role of intragroup emotional processing. *Journal of Organizational Behavior*, *25*(5), 589–605. doi:10.1002/job.258

Yazdi, S. A. A., Farahi, S. M. M., Farahi, S. M. M. M., & Hosseini, J. (2018). Emotional Intelligence and its role in Cognitive Flexibility of Children with and without Attention Deficit Hyperactivity Disorder. *Anales de Psicología/Annals of Psychology, 34*(2), 299-304.

Zhan, Z., & Mei, H. (2013). Academic self-concept and social presence in face-to-face and online learning: Perceptions and effects on students' learning achievement and satisfaction across environments. *Computers & Education*, *69*, 131–138. doi:10.1016/j.compedu.2013.07.002

Chapter 10
Technological Issues in Emotional and Mental Health

Suresh K.
https://orcid.org/0000-0003-1328-7576
Central University of Tamil Nadu, India

Manimozhi G.
Central University of Tamil Nadu, India

Elango M.
Central University of Tamil Nadu, India

ABSTRACT

In the 21st century, people are connecting with technology, and most of the people are spending time in social networks for sharing information. For the most part, spending time on social media is linked with an increased risk of loneliness and depression. Negative effects of social media and social network are affecting the person's mental, emotional, and physical health. The World Health Organization (WHO) reported that 8,000,000 people are dying due to suicide every year, and especially, every 40 seconds teenagers are dying. Generally, most of the teenagers are emotionally imbalanced; most of the suicide is committed on high depression. Depression is the foremost cause of emotional and mental illness. Emotional health is a state of emotional wellbeing, and it's a hidden and invisible factor as well as a factor for good mental health; mental health is a deep-seated problem for most humans. With this background, this chapter discusses the emotional and mental health with respect to technological issues.

DOI: 10.4018/978-1-7998-1185-5.ch010

INTRODUCTION

Emotional health is so important of every human's life because no humans can live without emotions such as smile, enjoy, angry and so on. Emotions are innate characteristics, and exposing and realizing of emotions are depends on individuality. Emotions play a crucial role in human life for their happiness and mutual understanding with the society. Emotionally healthy persons can control their emotions, feelings, thoughts, overall behaviour and realize the potential of them. Generally, emotional outburst created by destructive emotions suffers other seriously. An emotionally unstapled administrator always getting angry easily and scolds his/her subordinate is an example for emotional outburst. Emotions cannot be controllable but manageable. Some peoples are not compromise with their negative/destructive emotions that directly suffers others and themselves also. Suicidal activities are the result of uncontrollable destructive emotions. Everyone take care about

World Health Organization (WHO) reported that 8, 00,000 people are dying due to suicide every year and every 40 seconds 15-29 years old people are dying is deployable news. Roving the blue whale game also is one of the best examples of illness of emotional health problems. American Association of Suicidology (AAS), 'Blue Whale Challenge' is a social media game and the teenage people addicted to this game. It purposefully encourages the activity of hold in self-harm and suicidal behaviour to the young people. AAS also insisted that the teenage people directed by the game to do suicidal activities and ending their lives. Because of teenage people are not known to how rightly deal with their own emotions.

Emotionally Healthy person is an individual who knows how can aware of negative emotions, how to manage their negative feelings and they can handle the emotional problems. Maintaining emotional health is one of the skills to improve our lifestyles and travel our life path in positive manner. Emotional healthy persons always manage the destructive emotions and he/she follow some management strategies. They always prefer constructive emotions for maintaining the mental and emotional health. Emotional health is linked with one's mental health and physical health and so on.

Meaning of Mental Health

WHO (2004), Mental Health is a "state of well-being in which the individual realizes his or her own abilities, can cope with the normal stresses of life, can work productively and fruitfully, and is able to make a contribution to his or her community".

Medical dictionary (2012), mental health is "emotional, behavioural, and social maturity or normality; the absence of a mental or behavioural disorder; a state of psychological well-being in which one has achieved a satisfactory integration of one's

Figure 1. 15-29 years ages causes of suicides (WHO, 2017)

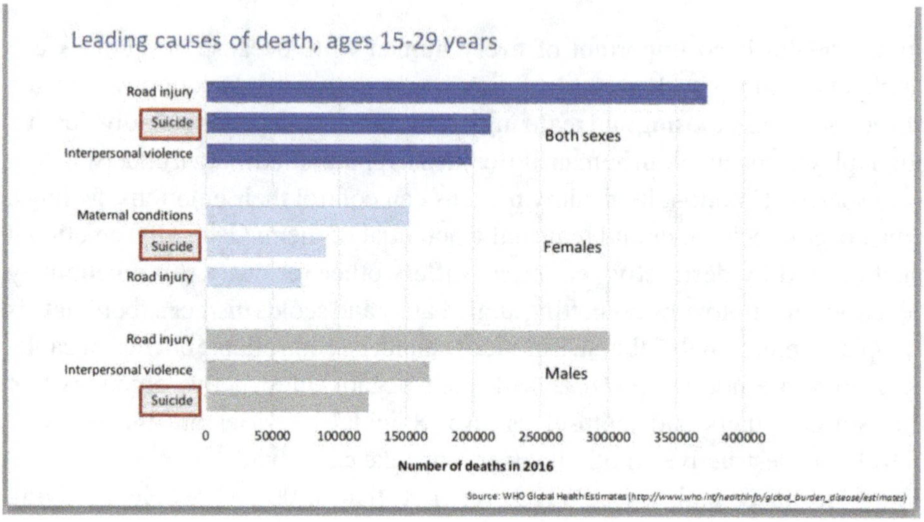

instinctual drives acceptable to both oneself and one's social milieu; an appropriate balance of love, work, and leisure pursuits"

Public Health Agency of Canada (PHAC, 2006) states that ——mental health is the capacity of each and all of us to feel, think, and act in ways that enhance our ability to enjoy life and deal with the challenges we face. It is a positive sense of emotional and spiritual well-being that respects the importance of culture, equity, social justice, interconnections and personal dignity.

With the help of above definitions, some of the common things are listed below and they are representing the mentally healthy person.

- One can easily solve the emotional problem and manages the challenges of their stresses.
- Mental health persons comprise the psychological well-being such as oneself and surrounding of others also accepting social integration behaviour.
- Mentally Healthy person having a positive sense of emotions and give respect to the values and the honesty of the rules.
- Mental Health persons also be emotionally healthy, psychologically healthy and socially well-beings.

Factors Affecting Mental Health

Mental health disturbed with internal or external. Internal factors like emotions, feeling and external factors like fevers, different type of aches and diseases may decide the status of one's mental health. Every individual should care with these factors to maintain their mental health and they are briefly explained below,

- *Internal factors:* The factors that relevant to the individual that are also called as psychological factors. The internal factors like self-esteem, emotions, feelings, stress and depression are involving the increase or decrease the level of mental health.
- *External factors:* Other than the internal factors which are not relevant to the psychological factors of an individual and they are indicates the outside of the individual. Physical conditions, different aches, diseases, fever, abuse, ill-health, family breakup, loneliness, bereavement, homelessness and environment are the external factors.

On the other side, mental health may be affected by the environment in which the persons belong. Generally, the learners' mental health affects in two environments, they are briefly explained below,

- *Home environment:* Home is an innate environment to the learners, because the learners were born in a home where they remain in the company their mothers in the formative years of infancy. The home is the first community and school to the learners and it is a first place to engage the character and personality development. The parents of the learners always care about their future. Of course, the parents control the learner over to childhood for discipline. The first important requisite condition for learners is affection should feel secure and loved in their home. But, Parents meet the legitimate needs of their child. This legitimate atmosphere cannot be accepted by the learners. The learners always want to be free. But, the home atmosphere made these opportunities ever. Thus, the home environment turned to make metal illness of learners and it affects mental health. The ideal home atmosphere provides proper and conductive environment up to early childhood. Pleasant and satisfaction giving experiences should be provided for harmonious development of the personality of the child. The parents should keep the following things into consideration.
    - Provide proper affection and love to the child.
    - Provide conductive environment in home.
    - Do not criticize the child.
    - Do not compare the child with other children.

- Don't ask irritable questions to the child
- Be a friend in time
- Don't use harsh words to the child while they did wrong
- Do not reject or overprotect the child.
- Do not quarrel in present of the child.
- Do not be over anxious about the future of the child.
- Try to be democratic in your dealings.
- Meet legitimate needs of your child.
- Provide guidance where necessary and build self-confidence in the child.

These points will assist the parents to create mental healthy individuals. Otherwise the learners become mental illness which affects the academic performance and other outcomes on the child.

- *School environment:* Schools are the second community or social place. In India, most of the parents are illiterate and ill informed who cannot be charged with the responsibility of providing proper guidance for mental health. The school has the great responsibility in harmonious development of personality of the learners. Normally, the learners spend six to seven hours in schools. Schools are in position to help in the development of children potentialities by catering their needs. In schools, the teacher should maintain the students' mental health when they are learning. The atmosphere of the schools is in the hands of the teachers. The teacher is a second parent of the students. It is one of the responsibility of the teacher who providing proper guidance for developing mental health. Because of the school are in a position to help in the developing of children's potentialities. The following school factors may affects the students' mental health.
    - Bad environment of school leads to make fear tension and frustration of the students.
    - The teacher autocratic style leads the authoritative environment in schools.
    - The undesirable participation of teacher to forget makes the positive attitude.
    - Some time the school rejects proper human relations.
    - Less facility of schools.
    - Irrespective activities of teachers and the head.

Qualities of a Mentally Healthy Person

Like a proverb 'Face is the index of the mind', the face is also the index of the mentally healthy persons. Emotionally disturbed persons never behave with the qualities of a normal person and their qualities are generally different from a normal person. The following qualities are identified and it's mostly fit for the mentally healthy persons. Jha and Bhatt (2010) quoted the following qualities are possessed by the mentally health persons and they are;

- *Adaptability and resilient mind:* The individual, who is adaptable to the changing conditions of his environment receptive and not rigid in his behaviour, can be said mentally healthy.
- *Social adaptable:* A mentally healthy person is socially awakened. He participates in social activities and his personality functions properly under strain ad stress of emotional disturbances.
- *Emotionally satisfied:* The emotions of mentally healthy persons are well trained and controlled. He is free from persistent emotional tensions in his life.
- *Desires are in harmony with socially approved goals:* The mentally healthy person does not indulge in anti social activities. The goals of the person of life are in accordance with social norms. The person's objectives are harmony with other people.
- *Insight into his own conduct:* The mentally healthy person has insight into his own conduct He self evaluates his behaviour. He improves his behaviour on the basic of his self-examination.
- *Enthusiastic and reasonable:* He has enthusiasm in life. He works with curiosity and is devoted to his profession. He is responsible in his actions. He accepts criticism sportingly.
- *Good Habits:* The healthy person has good habits. He is balanced and is not easily annoyed.
- *Philosophy of Life:* The healthy person has his own philosophy of life. He develops definite attributes towards values of life.
- *Provision for sex and moral education:* Most of the problems of adolescents are concerned with sex and moral conflicts which cause mental disturbances. It will be great use if sex and moral education are made an integral part of regular curriculum.
- *Art and craft:* Writing for understanding and release of emotional tensions can also be used in mental hygiene programme.

- *Guidance:* School students should be given guidance through guidance services for their benefit. This is of three types: personal, educational and vocational.

Meaning of Emotional Health

Mental health and emotional health are interrelated but both are slightly different. Ones lack mental health; those persons can be affected mental illness such as depression/ mood disorder, anxiety, personality disorder. National Alliance on Mental Illness quoted in their report that one in five adults in the United State suffers mental illness each year.

According to Peterson (2015), Emotional health is a psychological functioning and it's based on a positive manner. Emotional health is the extension of mental health and its function the inner and outer worlds of human to build one's thoughts, feelings and behaviours.

According to mental health foundation, "Emotional health is a positive sense of well being enables an individual to be able to function in society and meet the demands of everyday life."

From the above definitions, Emotional Health comes from several common points that common points are,

- To build up the thoughts, feelings, and behaviour from the ones psychological functioning.
- Emotional health is fully depending on the positive manner and engages with society in optimistically.

Factors Affecting Emotional Health

There are many factors contribute increase or decrease the level of emotional health and it is a key factor in promoting or de-promoting the mental health. So, the before said factors in the topic 'factors affecting mental health' also affects the emotional health. In addition to that the following factor also affects the emotional health and they are;

- *Level of anxiety:* It is a basic emotion that assists an individual from the dangers. Fluctuation in anxiety causes emotional imbalance and it directs less emotional health. Anxiety is a manageable emotion by the interventions and strategies like relaxation and mindfulness.
- *Level of self-confidence:* It is a belief of one's to reach the goal or the task assigned to the individual. Self-confidence makes the person to face

the challenging, difficult and complex situations. The poor self-confident individual easily getting fear and anxiety which pushes the imbalance in emotions.

- *Physical illness:* It is also changes the level of emotions. Diabetic persons always feel about the activity of injecting artificial insulin in their body and kept medicine with themselves as well as their eating styles. This may repress the emotions in negative directions. On the other side, fever, diseases may make emotional instability.
- *Undesired events:* Pleasant events makes the desired emotions and opposite are vise versa. An individual getting happy for pleasant events and upsets if the person facing an unpleasant event.
- *Capacity to manage emotions:* Escaping from the emotional issues, the person may have managing capacity or coping capability (Emotional Intelligence) in outburst of destructive emotions. Some persons having balanced emotions that are they maintain the emotions in average level. These types of persons not excited too for pleasant events and vice versa.

Qualities of Emotional Healthy Person

An emotionally healthy person is having high tolerance because those people are easily adopted in a new situation. They are always feeling free with others. The television Programme titled 'Big Boss" has been organized by Star Vijay Television is showing the emotions of the participants. This programme is normally telecasting for 100 days and the participants are insisted to stay with a group in a closed home. There is no mobile phone, entertainment for the participants and they are requested to cook the food themselves with the limitation of vegetables. Their activities are watching through a camera and high emotional participants are

Emotionally healthy people,

- Try to grow up their self-awareness and self-esteem,
- Known their boundaries of characteristics,
- End a bad relationship for good things,
- Easily adopt any emotional situation,
- Chooses the best approach to others and them following their passion

Barriers of Mental Health Services

Raguram, Weiss, Channabasavanna and Devins (1996) stated that the most important barriers in looking for mental health is unavailability of professional services, low literacy, socio-cultural barriers, traditional and religious beliefs, and shame.

Table 1. Mental Health Atlas. (WHO, 2018)

	Psychiatrists	Psychiatric Nurses	Psychologists	Social Workers
2001	0.4	0.04	0.02	0.02
2005	0.2	0.05	0.03	0.03
2017	1.3	3.5	0.9	0.3

According to WHO (2017), the median number of mental health beds per 100 000 population ranges below 7 in low and lower-middle-income countries to over 50 in high-income countries; from 100,000 people just 0.4 psychiatrists and 0.02 psychologists. Mental disorders are disgustingly underestimated by the community and health system in India and across the world. In the year 2000 estimation of the mental disorder, 12.3% of disability-adjusted life years and 31% of years lived with disability. Projection proposes that the health trouble owed to mental disorders will increase to 15% of disability-adjusted life years by 2020 (Murray and Lopez, 1996).

According to the National Commission on Macroeconomics and Health (2005) shows that at least 6.5% of the Indian population has some form of serious mental disorders. Mental health workforce breakdown per 100,000 populations by WHO region such as noted in the table given below.

Technological Issues and Remedies for Mental and Emotional Health Problems

In the older time, people often used typewriters, cycling, dancing, did puzzle, played board games and played in the ground for entertainment. Nowadays the boom of technology, computers, tablets, and mobile phones has replaced all those things and become very popular. Gaming technology in mobile phones, laptops, tablets and video games like a PUBG and Blue whale, have been as entertainment and hobby of the young students. Many years ago there were not very many forms of technology that stay alive. If an individual is not using technology for some form of entertainment, they are most likely using it for something along the lines of school or work. Technology has gone from being a suitable tool for being a bad impact on society. Not only is it slighting the brainpower and mental health of many people, but it is also taking away from one's social behaviour.

During the past years, the rapid development of technology in human mental health is based on social media such as facebook, twitter, Skype, whatsapp and my space was used to interact and communicate to others.

American Association of Suicidology stated that social media is a significant impact on mental health towards young people. An exception of vague booking, social media usage may be misplaced (Berryman, Ferguson & Negy). Sometimes technology can also offer new ways to treat mental health disorders. More than mental health apps also available for alternative treatments the apps also available in Smartphone such as,

- What's up: Cognitive Behavioural Therapy (CBT) and Acceptance Commitment Therapy (ACT) Method
- Mood kit: Cognitive Behavioural Therapy and Mood improvement activity
- Twenty-Four Hours a Day: Meditation book for people in recovery from addiction. Companion and Focus on moderation of addiction behaviour
- Quit that: strike their habits or addiction, perfect recovery tool and monitoring the progress.
- Mind shift: It is an anxiety app, this app trying to avoid anxious feelings and changing the negative thing about anxiety
- Self-help for anxiety management: Social Cloud" feature to confidentially connect with other users in an online community for additional support
- Bipolar Disorder Connect: Identify the struggles of people and monitor the people moods
- IMoodJournal: Analyze the daily feelings through the summary charts such as noted the stress level based on rising and falling.
- Talk space Online Therapy: This app is used to support one's through the ones own depression
- Happify: This app is fast-track to a good mood. Try various gratitude prompts, activity suggestions, engaging games and more to train your brain as if it were a muscle, to overcome negative thoughts.
- Recovery Record: Recovering from an eating disorder and inadequate to build up a more optimistic body image and used to stick the meal plan.
- nOCD: nOCD giving mainly two treatments such as mindfulness and Exposure Response Prevention Treatment.
- PTSD Coach: to find and giving an opportunity for Post-Traumatic Stress Disorder from a self-assessment
- UCSF PRIME: This app is used for schizophrenia groups. It also lets people track "challenge goals," belongings they'd like to accomplish or improve about them.
- Headspace: This app is used to make meditation in a simple way, that meditation on the lot from stress and anxiety to sleep and focus.
- Calm: Calm provides people experiencing anxiety and stress with guided meditations, breathing programs, sleep stories and relaxing music.
- MY 3: This app is suicidal prevention app and used to recognize ones warning signs through one's safety plan and listed warning plans.

The above apps are using the people to develop mental health in positive manner, technology impact the humans in both way. Technology can impact society in positive and negative. So human only choose the correct way and tools to grow up the living style, personality and so on.

CONCLUSION

In this chapter, the authors discussed various opportunities for all people for maintaining mental health and emotional development. Our focus is that the individuals growing up with good emotional and mental health. For that, the authors briefly discussed technological issues regards to mental and emotional health. Everyone knows that emotions are innate, cannot be controlled but manageable and it is a hidden factor for developing good mental health. Generally, destructive emotions affect an individual's mental health and high on that emotions may throw the individual as a murderer or committing suicide. Constructive emotions ensure stress-free and peace of living, which develops good mental and emotional health. So, emotions play a vital role in maintaining emotional health which is a factor for developing mental health. Notwithstanding this, some technologies also fluctuate emotions and direct emotional and mental health issues. Hence this chapter discussed with technological issues regards to mental and emotional health and providing remedies for emotionally and mentally healthy life.

REFERENCES

All About iMood Journal. (n.d.). Retrieved from https://www.imoodjournal.com/

Berryman, C., Ferguson, C. J., & Negy, C. (2018). Social media use and mental health among young adults. *The Psychiatric Quarterly*, *89*(2), 307–314. doi:10.100711126-017-9535-6 PMID:29090428

Bipolar Disorder Connect - Mobile App. (n.d.). Retrieved from http://ibpf.org/resource/bipolar-disorder-connect-mobile-app

Cale, L. (2018). Young people, social media, physical activity, and health. *Young People, Social Media and Health,* 212-224. doi:10.4324/9781351026987-17

CalmE. (n.d.). Retrieved from https://www.calm.com/

Cozy Apps, L. (2014, August 27). *Quit That! - Habit Tracker*. Retrieved from https://apps.apple.com/us/app/quit-that-habit-tracker/id909400800

Creighton, C. (2018, March 22). *Validity of the Blue Whale Challenge is Disputed, but Social Media's Impact on Young People's Mental Health is Real.* Retrieved from https://www.einpresswire.com/article/393609296/validity-of-the-blue-whale-challenge-is-disputed-but-social-media-s-impact-on-young-people-s-mental-health-is-real

Data Blog. (2018, June 19). Retrieved from https://health-infobase.canada.ca/datalab/blog.html

Everyday Health. (2018, October 25). *Trusted Medical Information, Expert Health Advice, News, Tools, and Resources.* Retrieved from https://www.everydayhealth.com/

Galderisi, S., Heinz, A., Kastrup, M., Beezhold, J., & Sartorius, N. (2015, June). *Toward a new definition of mental health.* Retrieved from https://www.ncbi.nlm.nih.gov/pmc/articles/PMC4471980/

Get the Headspace App. (n.d.). Retrieved from https://www.headspace.com/headspace-meditation-app

Home. (n.d.). Retrieved from https://www.mentalhealth.org.uk/

Home. (n.d.). Retrieved from https://www.mind.org.uk/

Home Page. (n.d.). Retrieved from https://www.treatmyocd.com/

Kumar, A. (2011). Mental health services in rural India: Challenges and prospects. *Health, 3*(12), 757–761. doi:10.4236/health.2011.312126

Mental Health. (2019, June 20). Retrieved from https://www.who.int/mental_health/en/

Mobile, B. (2010, August 30). *Twenty-Four Hours a Day.* Retrieved from https://apps.apple.com/us/app/twenty-four-hours-a-day/id389029534

Mood kit app. (n.d.). Retrieved from http://www.thriveport.com/products/moodkit/

Murray, C. J. L., & Lopez, A. D. (1996). *The Global Burden of Disease.* Cambridge, MA: Harvard School of Public Health.

National Alliance on Mental Illness. (n.d.). Retrieved from https://www.nami.org/

New MindShift™ CBT App Gives Canadians Free Anxiety Relief. (n.d.). Retrieved from https://anxietycanada.com/articles/new-mindshift-cbt-app-gives-canadians-free-anxiety-relief/

Overcome stress and negative thoughts. Build resilience. (n.d.). Retrieved from https://www.happify.com/

Peterson, T. (2015, October 13). What is Emotional Health? And How to improve it. *Healthy Place.* Retrieved on 2019, July 2 from https://www.healthyplace.com/other-info/mental-illness-overview/what-is-emotional-health-and-how-to-improve-it

Raguram, R., Weiss, M. G., Channabasavanna, S. M., & Devins, G. M. (1996). Stigma, depression, and somatization in South India. *The American Journal of Psychiatry*, *153*(8), 1043–1049. doi:10.1176/ajp.153.8.1043 PMID:8678173

SolutionsV. W. (n.d.). *PTSD Coach.* Retrieved from https://mobile.va.gov/app/ptsd-coach

Suicide data. (2018, November 5). Retrieved from https://www.who.int/mental_health/prevention/suicide/suicideprevent/en/

Suicide Prevention App for Android and iPhone - MY3. (n.d.). Retrieved from https://my3app.org/

Talkspace. (n.d.). *Online Therapy: Counseling Online: Marriage Counseling.* Retrieved from https://www.talkspace.com/

Technology enabled best practice for eating disorder treatment. (n.d.). Retrieved from https://www.recoveryrecord.com/

UCSF. (2016, July 13). *UCSF PRIME.* Retrieved from https://apps.apple.com/us/app/ucsf-prime/id1031402495

University of the West of England. (2013, July 4). *Self-help for Anxiety Management.* Retrieved from https://apps.apple.com/us/app/self-help-for-anxiety-management/id666767947

What is Emotional Health? And How to Improve it? (n.d.). Retrieved from https://www.healthyplace.com/other-info/mental-illness-overview/what-is-emotional-health-and-how-to-improve-it

What's Up? - Mental Health App – Apps on Google Play. (n.d.). Retrieved from https://play.google.com/store/apps/details?id=com.jacksontempra.apps.whatsup&hl=en_GB

World Health Organization. (2004). *Promoting mental health: Concepts, emerging evidence, practice: Summary report*. Author.

Chapter 11
Who Lives Healthier in a University?
Faculty, Students, or Administrative Staff

Ahu Ergen
https://orcid.org/0000-0002-2575-9262
Bahcesehir University, Turkey

Aybike Elif Bolcan
https://orcid.org/0000-0003-3947-4070
Bahcesehir University, Turkey

ABSTRACT

Being healthy is an important aspect in life satisfaction. The factors that affect the health status of an individual are environmental, economic, socio-cultural and genetic factors, access to health services, and lifestyle. Since it can be controlled by the individual, lifestyle is a topic with great importance. Understanding the healthy lifestyle behaviors of individuals is important for health and education institutions, companies, and governments to define their strategies accordingly. This quantitative study involves 205 respondents from a university in Istanbul. Data were obtained from self-administered questionnaires with 27 questions. The chapter examines the characteristics of the respondents regarding demographics and healthy lifestyle behaviors. Differences in the sample's healthy lifestyle dimensions were determined according to demographic variables after T-test and ANOVA analysis. This research presents the opportunity for further qualitative research in healthy lifestyle habits especially among university students.

DOI: 10.4018/978-1-7998-1185-5.ch011

INTRODUCTION

The concept of health has always existed for people; because health is the human life itself. The understanding of health has shown changes between individuals and societies from time to time. Until recently, health and illness have been considered together; health has been defined as an absence of illness and illness has been defined as not being healthy.

Healthy lifestyle behaviors are healthy eating, stress management, regular exercise, spiritual wellbeing, high quality interpersonal relations and taking the health responsibility. In many countries, number of people who are adopting healthy lifestyle is increasing. In Turkey this is mostly due to the promotion of healthy lifestyle by media, the awareness campaigns held by governments and the global trend of LOHAS. LOHAS (Lifestyle of Health and Sustainability), is one of the latest approaches about lifestyle bringing a consumer segment who cares about health, environment, social justice and sustainable living (Cohen, 2010).

The objective of the study is to explore the healthy lifestyle behaviors of different groups at a university. In this study the healthy lifestyle behaviors of three different groups (student, faculty, administrative staff) at a university in Istanbul are researched.

Health and Well Being

World Health Organization (WHO) defines health as a state of complete physical, mental and social well-being and not merely the absence of disease or infirmity (www.who.int). This definition is the first modern definition to be described as multi-dimensional. On the other hand, well-being reflects how one feels about life, as well as one's ability to function effectively (Corbin, Welk, Corbin, & Welk, 2008). Like health, wellbeing is a multidimensional concept and is a dynamic balance of physical, psychological, social, and spiritual aspects of an individual's life. Egbert (1980) summarized the central areas of wellness as "being a combination of having a strong sense of identity; a reality oriented perspective; a clear purpose in life; the recognition of a unifying force in one's life; the ability to manage one's affairs creatively and maintain a hopeful view; and, the capability of inspired, open relationships" (as cited in Miller & Foster, 2010). It is often emphasized that well-being is a choice, a process, a way of life; it is multidimensional but has a holistic structure; it is about balance; it is subjective, perceptual, relative and is based on the characteristics of healthy people (Korkut-Owen & Owen, 2012). Health and well-being concepts are often used interchangeably. In fact, these two concepts complement each other. While wellbeing is the positive component of health, health has a positive component led to the use of the term wellbeing (Corbin & Pangrazi, 2001). Health and wellbeing consist of physical, social, emotional, intellectual and

Figure 1. Five dimensions of health and well-being
Source: Corbin, Welk, Corbin, and Welk (2008, p.6).

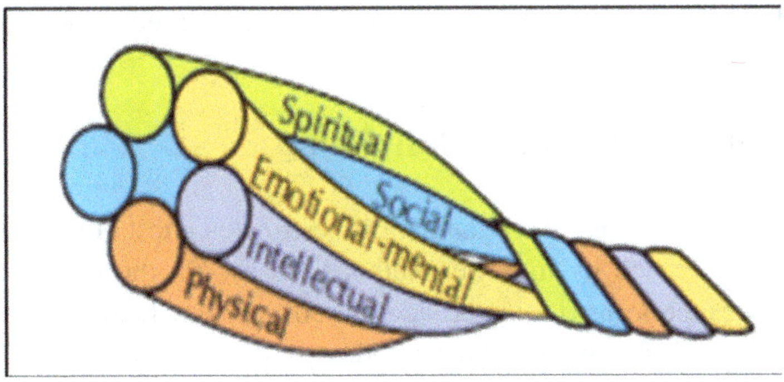

spiritual dimensions. It is thought that these dimensions are in relation to each other and can influence a person's identity.

Physical health is being free from illnesses that affect the physiological systems of the body, such as the heart and the nervous system. Physical well-being is a person's ability to function effectively in meeting the demands of the day's work and to use free time effectively. A physically well person is the one who eats properly and healthily, who is regularly engaged in physical activities (Korkut-Owen & Owen, 2012). Social health is being free from illnesses or conditions that severely limit functioning in society, including antisocial pathologies. Social wellbeing is a person's ability to interact with others successfully and to establish meaningful relationships that enhance the quality of life for all people involved in the interaction (including self) (Corbin, Welk, Corbin, & Welk, 2008). A person with emotional health is free from emotional/mental illnesses such as clinical depression, and possesses emotional wellness. Emotional wellbeing is a person's ability to cope with daily circumstances and to deal with personal feelings in a positive, optimistic, and constructive manner (i.e. being happy instead of depressed) (Corbin, Welk, Corbin, & Welk, 2008). A person with intellectual health is free from illnesses that invade the brain and other systems that allow learning. Intellectual wellbeing is a person's ability to learn and to use information to enhance the quality of daily living and optimal functioning (Corbin, Welk, Corbin, & Welk, 2008). According to Westgate (1996); spiritual wellness, which is synonymous with spiritual health, represents the openness to the spiritual dimension that permits the integration of one's spirituality with the other dimensions of life, thus maximizing the potential for growth and self-actualization and it has four dimensions: meaning and purpose in life, intrinsic values, transcendence and community of shared values and support.

Furthermore, two other dimensions can be added to wellness: occupational wellness, which is the ability to get personal fulfillment from our jobs or our chosen career fields while still maintaining balance in our lives and environmental wellness, which is the ability to recognize our own responsibility for the quality of the air, the water and the land that surrounds us (https://wellness.ucr.edu/seven_dimensions.html).

Determinants of Health and Well Being

According to the World Health Organization's estimates, most of the human deaths in the world are caused by lifestyle-related diseases. On the other hand, health expenditures are increasing day by day and this constitutes a heavy burden on health systems. For this reason, in many countries today, policies are implemented to improve public health and change the lifestyle and social marketing campaigns are carried out in many areas such as balanced nutrition, exercise, smoking cessation, reduction of alcohol use and benefiting from preventive health services (Bozkurt, 2015, p.4).

The factors affecting the health status of an individual are named as the environmental factors, economical factors, socio-cultural factors, genetic factors, access to health services and life style. In other words; where you live, genetics, income, nutrition, education, relationships with friends and family, gender, culture, social status, and personal behaviors can affect our health. In this context, as a person's individual behaviors can be regarded as his/her lifestyle and since it can be controlled by the individual, it can be said that healthy lifestyle has a very important role in healthy living. In other words, health and wellness begins with a conscious decision to shape a healthy lifestyle (Ardell, 2002).

The model in Figure 2 developed by Göran Dahlgren and Margaret Whitehead in 1991, maps the relationship between the individual, their environment and health. Individuals are placed at the center, and surrounding them are the various layers of influences on health – such as individual lifestyle factors, community influences, living and working conditions, and more general social conditions (http://www.esrc.ac.uk). It is observed that people who are poor, have low levels of education, or are socially isolated are more likely to engage in a wide array of risk-related behaviors and less likely to engage in health-promoting ones (www.ncbi.nlm.nih.gov/books/NBK43743/doi: 10.17226/9838).

Furthermore Kickbusch (2012) claims that many of the health challenges we deal with are related to unsustainable lifestyles and unsustainable production and consumption patterns and urbanization, modern media, new forms of work, women's entry into the employment market – all have contributed to time pressure and increased stress, anxiety and depression.

Figure 2. Dahlgren and Whitehead Model of the Determinants of Health
Source: Eikemo, Bambra, Huijts, and Fitzgerald (2016).

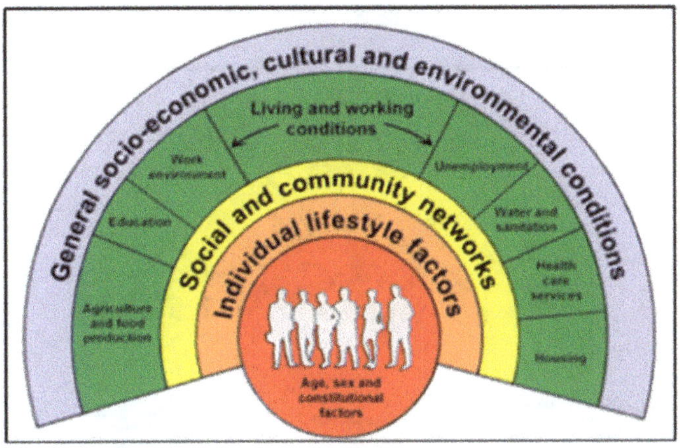

Healthy Lifestyle and Life Satisfaction

Lifestyle can simply be defined as how one lives. In this context, how people spend their time; what interests they have and what importance they place on their immediate surroundings; and their views of themselves and the world around them show their lifestyles (Küçükemiroğlu, 1997). The lifestyle relates to the economic level at which people live, how they spend their money, and how they allocate their time (Anderson & Golden, 1984). In the context of health, lifestyle has been defined as all those behaviors over which an individual has control, including actions that affect a person's health risks (Ardell, 1979) or as discretionary activities with significant impact on health status that are a regular part of one's daily pattern of living (Wiley & Camacho, 1980). The related theories and models reveal that healthy life is a lifestyle, covers different areas of human life, requires a continuous and lifelong effort, is a choice, requires stability, is a proactive approach and covers different dimensions. However, it is noteworthy in the literature that there is no agreement on the dimensions of healthy life (Bozkurt, 2015, p.19).

Myers, Sweeney, & Witmer (2000) define the concept as "a way of life, oriented toward optimal health and well-being in which body, mind and spirit are integrated by the individual to live more fully within the human and natural community".

Corbin, et.al. (2008) developed a model for describing the factors that contribute to health, wellness, and fitness. According to the model shown in Figure 3; heredity, age, and disability are the factors over which an individual has the least control; environmental factors and health-care system are factors over which an individual has some control but less ability to change; however the factors healthy lifestyles

Figure 3. Relationship Between Health and Lifestyle
Source: Corbin, Welk, Corbin, and Welk (2008, p.10).

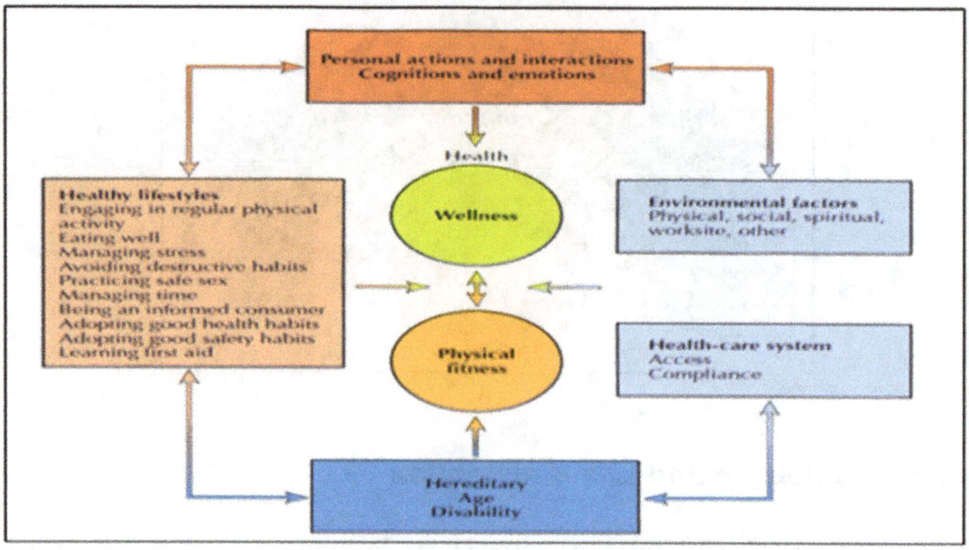

and personal actions and interactions, cognitions and emotions are the ones an individual has greater control.

The basic reasoning behind healthy lifestyle is that people may have health consciousness and may be ready to do something good for their health, or may have favorable environmental attitudes (Chen, 2009). Healthy lifestyle has two components: Health-protecting behavior which aims to decrease the individual's probability of encountering illness and health-promoting behavior which is directed toward sustaining or increasing the individual's level of well-being, self-actualization and personal fulfilment; thus a healthy lifestyle is seen satisfying and enjoyable, not because of a wish to avoid disease (Walker, Noble, Sechrist, & Pender, 1987).

According to Reeves and Rafferty (2000), in the United States and worldwide, chronic diseases account for the greatest overall population disease burden in terms of mortality, morbidity, and decreased quality of life and most people with major chronic diseases share multiple common lifestyle characteristics or behaviors, particularly smoking, poor diet, physical inactivity, and obesity. Moreover according to Cobin et.al., (2008) healthy lifestyles can reduce the effects of aging on health, wellness, and fitness, and extend life and have a positive effect on quality of life. Reeves and

Rafferty (2005) conducted a research with 153,805 U.S adults and estimated the prevalence of 4 healthy lifestyle characteristics (nonsmoking, healthy weight, fruit and vegetable consumption, and leisure time physical activity). The results showed that only 3.0% of US adults followed a combination of these 4 lifestyle characteristics. The Interheart study, which covered 30.000 men and women in 52 countries showed that, factors such as smoking, cholesterol level, high blood temperature, diabetes, obesity, diet, level of physical activity, alcohol consumption, emotional stress and depression are related to various lifestyle factors (Yusuf et.al, 2004). According to the estimations of World Health Organization, 70-80% of deaths in developed countries and 40-50% of deaths in less developed countries result from lifestyle related diseases (Pirinççi, Rahman, Durmus, & Erdem, 2008). One of the most effective approaches to promote healthy lifestyle is using social marketing campaigns which aim to improve health related habits of individuals to the optimal level possible within their environment (Bozkurt & Ergen, 2015).

Healthy lifestyle is also an important indicator of life quality and an important aspect in life satisfaction. Life satisfaction is defined as a judgmental process in which individuals assess the quality of their lives on the basis of their own unique set of criteria (Shin & Johnson, 1978). Therefore, life satisfaction is a conscious cognitive judgment of one's life in which the criteria for judgment are made by the person (Pavot & Diener, 1993) and explains the difference which emerged after the comparison of individual's expectations with the real situation (Naz, 2015). However, Diener et.al. (1985) claim that judgments of satisfaction are dependent upon a comparison of one's circumstances with what is thought to be an appropriate standard and it is important to point out that the judgment of how people are with their present state of affairs is based on a comparison with a standard which each individual sets for him or herself; it is not externally imposed. According to Frijns (2010), life satisfaction is affected by numerous aspects of life which can be classified into two categories: micro-social life domains (or individual living conditions) including features such as work related conditions, subjective health conditions, marital status, financial household status, and macro-social life domains (or societal conditions) including aspects such as governmental performance, political democracy, welfare growth and economic equality.

Researches show that friendship and family relationships, taking part in social activities, and the feeling of being free are important elements to make sense of life, and that these factors can increase life satisfaction (Tambağ & Öz, 2013). In an analysis of health, activity, social-psychological, and socio-economic variables thought to influence life satisfaction in middle age, it was found that self-rated health was the predominant variable (Palmore & Luikart, 1972). According to the research conducted by Strine et.al. (2008), increased life satisfaction is inversely related to mean number of days in the past 30 days of poor mental health, depressive symptoms, and anxiety symptoms, as well as with somatic complaints including poor physical health, sleep insufficiency, pain, and activity limitations.

MAIN FOCUS OF THE ARTICLE

Issues, Controversies, Problems

Nowadays, while the concept of health is being defined, importance is given also to life style, cultural accumulation, beliefs and values, economic and psycho-social situation. Bozkurt and Ergen (2015) state that especially lifestyle is increasingly evaluated as one of the most important factors influencing health status. As increasing health expenditure is an important problem for sustainable development, it is essential to examine the society in terms of their health related habits and promote healthy lifestyle.

Understanding the healthy lifestyle behaviors of individuals is important for health and education institutions, companies and governments to define their strategies accordingly. This study examines the characteristics of the respondents regarding demographics and healthy lifestyle behaviors.

The aim of the study is to explore the healthy lifestyle behaviors of different groups at a university. This exploratory study involves 205 respondents (students, faculty and administrative staff) from a foundation university in Istanbul. Convenience sampling was used and 230 surveys were collected from the respondents in the campus. After eliminating incorrect and incomplete forms, 205 surveys remained for the analysis. Data were obtained from self-administered questionnaires with 27 questions. Healthy lifestyle questions were adapted from Gil et.al. (2000) surveys. After receiving expert opinions, additional questions were added to the healthy lifestyle scale by the authors. Healthy lifestyle dimensions were measured with 21 questions by 5-point Likert scale. The demographic characteristics of the respondents were measured by nominal scale with 6 questions.

SOLUTIONS AND RECOMMENDATIONS

The sample consists of 52,8% female and 47,2% male subjects. 76,5% of the respondents are single and 33,5% are married. 68,3% of the respondents are students, 16,6% are administrative staff and 15,1% are academic staff. 69,3% of the respondents' age is between 18 and 25, 16,1% between 26 and 35, 12,7% between 36 and 49 and 2% is over 50. 48,3% of the respondents have income between 1000 and 4000 TL. 28,7% of them have income between 4000 and 7000 TL. 10,7% of

Figure 4. Frequency of healthy lifestyle behaviors

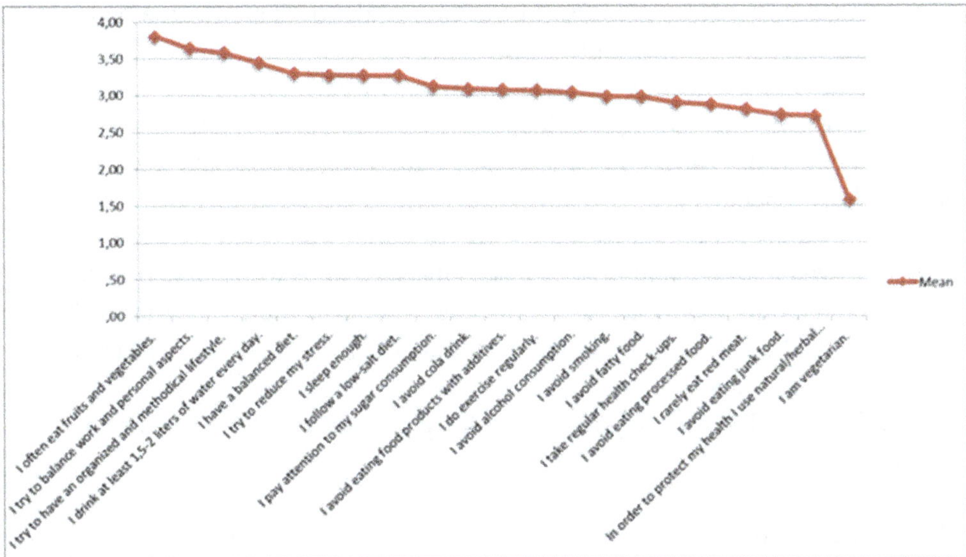

*Table 1. Factor analysis for healthy lifestyle**

Healthy lifestyle	Factor load	Eigenvalue	%Variance	Cronbach's alpha
Avoidance from unhealthy food		3,91	27,97	0,729
I avoid eating processed food.	0,767			
I avoid eating food products with additives.	0,711			
I avoid eating junk food.	0,680			
Mental health		1,78	12,74	0,740
I try to have an organized and methodical lifestyle.	0,805			
I try to reduce my stress.	0,786			
I try to balance work and personal aspects.	0,746			
Avoidance from addictive substances		1,03	7,38	0,699
I avoid alcoholic drinks.	0,827			
I avoid smoking.	0,821			

*KMO=0,779; Bartlett's p<0,005

them have income between 7000 and 10000 TL and 12,2% over 10,000 TL. 12,7% have graduate and master degrees, 14,6% have undergraduate degree and 72,8% have primary, secondary and high school degrees.

The frequency of healthy lifestyle behaviors is given in Figure 4. Fruit and vegetable consumption, having a balance between work and private life are the two most frequent healthy lifestyle behaviors. Being vegetarian is the least frequent healthy lifestyle behavior.

Factor analysis is conducted for healthy lifestyle (Table 1). The first factor is named as "avoidance from unhealthy food"; the second factor is named as "mental health" and the third one is named as "avoidance from addictive substances". The Cronbach's Alpha values of these factors are; 0,729 for Factor 1, 0,740 for Factor two and 0,699 for Factor 3.

After factor analysis, the hypothesis are designed parallel to the research objective accordingly;

H1: Avoidance from unhealthy food varies according to gender
H2: Avoidance from unhealthy food varies according to age
H3: Avoidance from unhealthy food varies according to education level
H4: Avoidance from unhealthy food varies according to marital status
H5: Avoidance from unhealthy food varies according to income
H6: Avoidance from unhealthy food varies according to occupation
H7: Mental health varies according to gender
H8: Mental health varies according to age
H9: Mental health varies according to education level
H10: Mental health varies according to marital status
H11: Mental health varies according to income
H12: Mental health varies according to occupation
H13: Avoidance from addictive substances varies according to gender
H14: Avoidance from addictive substances varies according to age
H15: Avoidance from addictive substances varies according to education level
H16: Avoidance from addictive substances varies according to marital status
H17: Avoidance from addictive substances varies according to income
H18: Avoidance from addictive substances varies according to occupation

The results of the t-tests show that married respondents' avoidance from unhealthy food (mean=3,32) is significantly higher than single respondents' (mean=2,78). So, H4 is supported. Married respondents' avoidance from addictive substances (mean=3,56) is significantly higher than single respondents' (mean=2,84). So, H16 is supported.

The results of the ANOVA tests show that there are significant differences between avoidance from unhealthy food of 18-25 age group (mean=3,36), 26-35 age group (mean=3,36), 36-49 age group (mean=3,52) and over 50 age group (mean=4,19). So, H2 is supported. There are significant differences between avoidance from unhealthy food of high school graduates (mean=2,71) and graduate degree respondents (mean=3,36). So, H3 is supported. There are significant differences between avoidance from unhealthy food of students (mean=2,71) and academic staff (3,28); students (2,71) and administrative staff (mean=3,36). So, H6 is supported. There are significant differences between avoidance from addictive substances of 18-25 age group (mean=2,73) and 26-35 age group (mean=3,76). So, H14 is supported. There are significant differences between avoidance from addictive substances of students (mean=2,80) and administrative staff (mean=3,60). So, H18 is supported. H1, H5, H7-13, H15, H17 were not found statistically significant.

FUTURE RESEARCH DIRECTIONS

For further studies, it is recommended to segment university students according to their lifestyle and motivations for healthy living. The motives for avoidance from unhealthy food and addictive substances of administrative staff can be researched and shared with students.

This research presents the opportunity for further qualitative research in healthy lifestyle habits among university students, academic and administrative staff.

CONCLUSION

A healthy lifestyle emphasizes activities such as healthy nutrition, stress management, regular exercise, spiritual wellbeing, high quality interpersonal relations and taking health responsibility. It also covers physical health-related activities such as natural food consumption, health care, and life equilibrium. (Korkut-Owen & Çelik, 2018). By selecting a healthy lifestyle, an individual tries to maintain and promote his/her health and avoid diseases through having a proper diet, rest/activity, exercising, controlling body weight, not smoking and drinking alcohol and immunizing body against diseases; this set of activities constitutes the lifestyle (Yasobant, 2016, p. 330). Also, inappropriate lifestyle is one of the influential factors for the emergence of chronic diseases like colon cancers, hypertension, chronic obstructive pulmonary diseases, liver cirrhosis, peptic ulcers, AIDS and cardiovascular diseases.

The findings of the study show that married respondents avoid more from unhealthy food. This may be due to having regular life style with family meals. It is also seen that students' eating habits are not healthy. Promoting healthy food in campuses is recommended. Also, using humor in the communication may be effective for this segment. Campus activities can be organized for healthy eating. Carefully chosen influencers may have positive affect on students to have positive attitudes towards healthy eating. For mental health, the results of the research showed no statistically significant difference according to the variables.

Another finding is the increase of avoidance from unhealthy food by high ages. This may be due to seeing the negative results of unhealthy eating such as chronic diseases. Before it becomes too late, young generations must be educated about healthy eating. Government must see this as an important topic since it creates a heavy load for health economy, effects the quality of life and also labor productivity. Increasing the health status is an important factor for sustainable development. Education is an indicator for avoidance from unhealthy food. Highly educated people may have the knowledge and vision to search for healthy products that will support healthy living.

The findings also show that students avoid less from addictive substances. Awareness campaigns and workshops for the dangers of addictive substances and also social media addiction must be organized more. On the other hand, according to the results; it is found that income is not an indicator for healthy lifestyle behaviors. It is worthy to note that, the result is against the general judgment that the higher income, a better lifestyle. Furthermore, it is found in the study that for healthy lifestyle behaviors gender is also not an indicator.

Social and psychological factors must be considered to encourage healthy lifestyle behaviors. Especially, among young people "what do others think about me?" question is very important. For all dimensions of healthy living, a positive and encouraging social environment in the schools and society must be established. Competitions, games, case studies, inviting influencers with healthy lifestyles to the campuses can be good ways to influence the young people in schools and universities.

It is also a good news that income is not an indicator for healthy lifestyle behaviors. There are cheap ways to be healthy such as eating less, drinking more water instead of beverages, walking instead of driving, meditating or doing yoga at home or maybe only praying for mental health. Being aware and conscious about these facts don't always motivate people to directly change their behaviours towards a healthy lifestyle. The challenge is changing the behaviours of people. Models from sociology and psychology such as Theory of Planned Behavior and Social Normalisation may be adapted to healthy living studies to close the gaps between attitude and behaviour towards healthy living. Even neuroscience technics can be helpful for healthy living studies. What part of the brain activates when the person sees the vegetable and what part for the hamburger? Which emotions are stimulated? These questions can be answered by neuroscientists today. By interdisciplinary research and projects, healthy lifestyle can be encouraged among young people. Another important tool is use of social media effectively for differenet segments with different messages and creative work. Especially for Generations Y and Z, using the correct content with correct social media channel brings success for many brands. This can be used for healthy living purpose by policy makers, universities, schools and health professionals. Lastly, for emotional health many new approaches such as mindfulness are available. By using books, videos or going to trainings, people can learn to stay in "now" which reduces anxiety and negative feelings.

REFERENCES

Anderson, W. T., & Golden, L. (1984). Life-style and psychographics: A critical review and recommendation. *Advances in Consumer Research. Association for Consumer Research (U. S.), 11*, 405–411.

Ardell, D. B. (1979). The nature and implications of high level wellness, or why 'normal health' is a rather sorry state of existence. *Health Values, 3*(1), 17–24.

Ardell, D. B. (2002). What is wellness? *The Institute of Rehabilitation and Research.* Retrieved from http://www.ilru.org

Bozkurt, F. (2015). *Sağlıklı yaşam ve pazarlama.* İstanbul: Beta Yayınları.

Bozkurt, F., & Ergen, A. (2014). *Promoting healthy lifestyle for sustainable development. In Handbook of Research on Developing Sustainable Value in Economics, Finance, and Marketing*. Hershey, PA: IGI Global.

Chen, M. (2009). Attitude toward organic foods among taiwanese as related to health consciousness, environmental attitudes, and the mediating effects of a healthy lifestyle. *British Food Journal, 111*(2), 165–178. doi:10.1108/00070700910931986

Cohen, M. (2010). Wellness and the thermodynamics of a healthy lifestyle. *Asia-Pacific Journal of Health, Sport and Physical Education, 1*(2), 5–12. doi:10.1080/18377122.2010.9730326

Corbin, C. B., & Pangrazi, R. P. (2001). Towards a uniform definition of wellness: A commentary. *President's Council on Physical Fitness and Sports Research Digest, 3*(15), 1–8.

Corbin, C. B., Welk, G. J., Corbin, W. R., & Welk, K. A. (2008). *Concepts of physical fitness: active lifestyles for wellness.* Boston: McGraw Hill.

Diener, E. D., Emmons, R. A., Larsen, R. J., & Griffin, S. (1985). The satisfaction with life scale. *Journal of Personality Assessment*, *49*(1), 71–75. doi:10.120715327752jpa4901_13 PMID:16367493

Eikemo, T. E., Bambra, C., Huijts, T., & Fitzgerald, R. (2016). The First Pan-European Sociological Health Inequalities Survey of the General Population: The European Social Survey Rotating Module on the Social Determinants of Health. *European Sociological Review*, *33*(1), 137–153. Retrieved from https://watermark.silverchair.com/jcw019.pdf

Frijns, M. (2010). *Determinants of life satisfaction: a cross-regional comparison* (Unpublished final thesis). Maastricht University, School of Business and Economics, Master of Science in International Business Concentration.

Gil, J. M., Gracia, A., & Sanchez, M. (2000). Market segmentation and willingness to pay for organic products in Spain. *The International Food and Agribusiness Management Review*, *3*(2), 207–226. doi:10.1016/S1096-7508(01)00040-4

Institute of Medicine (US) Committee on Health and Behavior, Research, Practice, and Policy. (2001). *Health and Behavior: The Interplay of Biological, Behavioral, and Societal Influences*. Washington, DC: National Academies Press. Retrieved from https://www.ncbi.nlm.nih.gov/books/NBK43743/doi:10.17226/9838

Kickbusch, I. (2012). 21st century determinants of health and wellbeing: A new challenge for health promotion. *Global Health Promotion*, *19*(3), 5–7. doi:10.1177/1757975912454783 PMID:24802779

Korkut-Owen, F., & Demirbaş Çelik, N. (2018). Lifelong healthy lifestyle and wellness. *Psikiyatride Güncel Yaklasimlar*, *10*(4), 440–453.

Korkut-Owen & Owen, D.W. (2012). İyilik hali yıldızı modeli, uygulanması ve değerlendirilmesi. *Uluslararası Avrasya Sosyal Bilimler Dergisi*, *3*(9), 24–33.

Küçükemiroğlu, O. (1997). Market segmentation by using consumer lifestyle dimensions and ethnocentrism: An empirical study. *European Journal of Marketing*, *33*(5/6), 470–487. doi:10.1108/03090569910262053

Miller, G. D., & Foster, L. T. (2010). *Critical synthesis of wellness literature*. University of Victoria. Retrieved from http://www.geog.uvic.ca/wellness

Myers, J. E., Sweeney, T. J., & Witmer, J. M. (2000). The wheel of wellness counseling for wellness: A holistic model for treatment planning. *Journal of Counseling and Development*, *78*(3), 251–266. doi:10.1002/j.1556-6676.2000.tb01906.x

Naz, S. (2015). Relationship of life satisfaction and job satisfaction among pakistani army soldiers. *Journal of Business Research-Turk*, *7*(1), 7–25. doi:10.20491/isader.2015115749

Palmore, E., & Luikart, C. (1972). Health and social factors related to life satisfaction. *Journal of Health and Social Behavior*, *13*(1), 68–80. doi:10.2307/2136974 PMID:5025756

Pavot, W., & Diener, E. (1993). Review of satisfaction with life scale. *Psychological Assessment*, *5*(2), 164–172. doi:10.1037/1040-3590.5.2.164

Pirinççi, E., Rahman, S., Durmus, A. B., & Erdem, R. (2008). Factors affecting health-promoting behaviours in academic staff. *Public Health*, *122*(11), 1261–1263. doi:10.1016/j.puhe.2008.04.006 PMID:18849056

Reeves, M. J., & Rafferty, A. P. (2005). Healthy lifestyle characteristics among adults in the united states, 2000. *Archives of Internal Medicine*, *165*(8), 854. doi:10.1001/archinte.165.8.854 PMID:15851634

Seven Dimensions of Wellness. (n.d.). Retrieved from https://wellness.ucr.edu/seven_dimensions.html

Shin, D. C., & Johnson, D. M. (1978). Avowed happiness as an overall assessment of the quality of life. *Social Indicators Research*, *5*(1-4), 475–492. doi:10.1007/BF00352944

Strine, T. W., Chapman, D. P., Balluz, L. S., Moriarty, D. G., & Mokdad, A. H. (2008). The associations between life satisfaction and health related quality of life, chronic illness, and health behaviors among U.S. community-dwelling adults. *Journal of Community Health*, *33*(1), 40–50. doi:10.100710900-007-9066-4 PMID:18080207

Tambağ, H., & Öz, F. (2013). Evaluation of the psychoeducation given to the elderly at nursing homes for a healthy lifestyle and developing life satisfaction. *Community Mental Health Journal*, *49*(6), 742–747. doi:10.100710597-013-9602-x PMID:23400690

The Dahlgren-Whitehead Rainbow. (n.d.). Retrieved from http://www.esrc.ac.uk/about-us/50-years-of-esrc/50-achievements/the-dahlgren-whitehead-rainbow

Walker, S., Noble, K., Sechrist, R., & Pender, N. J. (1987). The Health-Promoting Lifestyle Profile: Development and Psychometric Characteristics. *Nursing Research*, *36*(2), 76–81. doi:10.1097/00006199-198703000-00002 PMID:3644262

Westgate, C. E. (1996). Spiritual wellness and depression. *Journal of Counseling and Development*, *75*(1), 26–35. doi:10.1002/j.1556-6676.1996.tb02311.x

Wiley, J. A., & Camacho, T. C. (1980). Lifestyle and future health: Evidence from the alameda county study. *Preventive Medicine*, *9*(1), 1–21. doi:10.1016/0091-7435(80)90056-0 PMID:7360725

World Health Organization. (n.d.). *Definition of Health*. Retrieved from http://www.who.int

Yasobant, S. (2016). Physical health promotion through modern technologies: challenges to concerns. In Handbook of Research on Advancing Health Education through Technology. Medical Information Science.

Yusuf, S., Hawken, S., Ounpuu, S., Dans, T., Avezum, A., Lanas, F., ... Lisheng, L. (2004). Effect of potentially modifiable risk factors associated with myocardial infarction in 52 countries (The INTERHEART study): Case-control study. *Lancet*, *364*(9438), 937–952. doi:10.1016/S0140-6736(04)17018-9 PMID:15364185

KEY TERMS AND DEFINITIONS

Emotional Health: Being free from emotional/mental illnesses such as clinical depression.

Emotional Well-Being: A person's ability to cope with daily circumstances and to deal with personal feelings in a positive, optimistic, and constructive manner.

Healthy Lifestyle: Way of life enhanced with activities, interests, and opinions that will help the individual reach optimal health.

Intellectual Health: Being free from illnesses that invade the brain and other systems that allow learning.

Intellectual Well-Being: A person's ability to learn and to use information to enhance the quality of daily living and optimal functioning.

Life Satisfaction: A judgmental process in which individuals assess the quality of their lives on the basis of their own unique set of criteria.

Physical Health: Being free from illnesses that affect the physiological systems of the body, such as the heart and the nervous system.

Physical Well-Being: A person's ability to function effectively in meeting the demands of the day's work and to use free time effectively.

Social Health: Being free from illnesses or conditions that severely limit functioning in society, including antisocial pathologies.

Social Well-Being: A person's ability to interact with others successfully and to establish meaningful relationships that enhance the quality of life for all people involved in the interaction (including self).

Spiritual Health and Spiritual Well-Being: The integration of one's spirituality with the other dimensions of life, thus maximizing the potential for growth and self-actualization.

Chapter 12
The Social Mandate to Deal With Mental Health:
A Comparison Between Interventions in a Mental Health Center, a School, and a Psychoanalytic Office

Alberta Mazzola
Independent Researcher, Italy

ABSTRACT

The chapter aims to explore the construct of mental health in a psychoanalytic perspective with a psychosocial approach. In particular, the chapter studies mental health by analysing traces to detect social mandate characterizing different mental health agencies. The highlighted hypothesis could be interpreted as that social mandate is a clue of local cultures about mental health, which determine fantasies about mental health issues, grounding on symbolizations shared by professionals, users, and community. The chapter introduces three clinical experiences of interventions, carried out in different contexts: a public mental health service, a public middle school, a psychoanalytic private office. All the presented experiences concern mental health field, even though they are characterized by different features in terms of subjects, methods, professionals, users, and organizations involved. The chapter explores those differences in order to focus on transversal issues.

DOI: 10.4018/978-1-7998-1185-5.ch012

INTRODUCTION

The wide concept of Mental Health could be considered deeply related to the concept of Well-being, which is even more wider than the first one. For instance, Merriam-Webster dictionary (n.d.) indicates Well-being as *the state of being happy, healthy, or prosperous* and the Cambridge dictionary's definition is (n.d.): *the state of feeling healthy and happy.* All the previous definitions about Well-being include the concept of Health. But what is Health, and in particular, what is Mental Health? Not a question with a simple or unambiguous answer. This chapter aims to focus on the concept of Mental Health, to explore it by studying different points of view about this topic.

It will be proposed, in particular, to consider Mental Health as a complex topic, historically and locally characterized, a culturally determined object. Getting to the heart of the epistemological matter, this chapter is not going to study Mental Health as a natural object, but as a cultural one. It is not going to take Mental Health as an object passible of being measured with examinations that could be replicated in any time and space, regardless the analyser's involvement. Whereas the chapter is going to explore the concept of Mental Health as a cultural construction, based on symbolizations which are shared in a particular social context, historically and territorially determined, which means characterized by local cultures. In this epistemological perspective, the analyser's point of view it's not something irrelevant or something which should be controlled to clean examination field. Contrariwise researcher's evolvement could be considered as a clue. For instance researcher's fantasies and feelings could be treated as a trace to explore issues' symbolizations in shared local cultures.

In this chapter's perspective, Mental Health is founded on local culture. Namely local cultures found different symbolization about Mental Health in Rome, in Tonga, or in Bangkok.

The author lives and works in Italy, in Rome, she is a Clinical Psychologist and Psychoanalyst, specialist in Psychological Intervention for the Person, Organizations and Communities, with professional experiences in different contexts and organizations dealing with Mental Health.

According with the previously introduced epistemological framework, the initial question can be rearranged as: how could the concept of mental Health be defined?

On 30 March 2018, on its official website, World Health Organization (WHO) describes Mental Health as:

Mental health is an integral and essential component of health. The WHO constitution states: Health is a state of complete physical, mental and social well-being and not merely the absence of disease or infirmity". An important implication of this definition is that mental health is more than just the absence of mental disorders or disabilities. Mental health is a state of well-being in which an individual realizes his or her own abilities, can cope with the normal stresses of life, can work productively and is able to make a contribution to his or her community (World Health Organization, 2018).

WHO's definition of Mental Health implies multiple elements which compose a complex concept:

- Mental Health does not coincide with the *absence of mental illness* but it's something more (and it's not exactly defined);
- Mental Health concerns the individual (*realizing his or her own abilities*) and the relations with his/her coexistence contests (*to make a contribution to his or her community*).

WHO identifies a multifactorial concept, composed by individual and relational factors. In accordance with that, this chapter will provide a Psychosocial perspective.

Both in Literature and in internet it is possible to find several interesting works about interventions based on a psychosocial approach. Those psychosocial interventions combine a psychological perspective, mainly concerning an individual target, and social perspective, generally aiming to determine actions on a community level. Whereas, the theoretical and methodological perspective here provided it's something different from that. We assume a Psychosocial perspective not only for interventions but also for analysing phenomena. We aim to explore phenomena concerning the relation between the individual and the social context.

In this perspective, Mental Health is not considered as an individual feature, as an object existing in nature but as a social construction, based on symbolizations that are shared in a particular cultural context. Common symbolizations ground people's fantasies and actions in those contexts they share. Let's think, for instance, to Mental Health agencies' users and professionals, they share symbolizations about what Mental Health agencies are and what they do.

This chapter aims to analyse the concept of Mental Health by studying the social mandate charactering agencies supposed to deal with it.

In particular, this chapter intends to contribute to the debate on Mental Health, focusing on a question: how is Mental Health perceived by professionals working in different agencies with the mission of deal with it and by their users? The highlighted hypothesis is that users' demand could be considered as a trace of socially shared symbolizations about Mental Health, on which fantasies about agencies' and professionals' utility and social mandate are built on.

The chapter will introduce three experiences of psychological intervention within different organizational contexts in Rome. The first one is a psychoanalytic work with a young woman who turns to the professional because of her anxiety problems.

The second experience refers to a psychosocial project pursuing school inclusion, carried out by a non-profit organization, with middle school classrooms, through walks to explore street art in surrounding urban suburbs. The last one is a psychotherapeutic work with a woman, demanded by a psychiatrist to test her supposed dissociative disorders.

What do these interventions have in common? Experiences so different from each other by subject, method, professionals, users and organizations involved, can all fall into the category of interventions to support Mental Health. The chapter aims to explore those differences in order to identify transversal issues. The highlighted hypothesis is that what seems to characterize Mental Health is precisely the complexity of concept itself that includes a heterogeneity of professional practices and social meanings. This could sound obvious but it is not if you consider diffused cultural trends in sciences, which are globally widespread, such as Evidence-based medicine. Evidence-based medicine refers to an epistemological approach which treats phenomena as objectivable, looking for invariants, supposed to be always valid regardless geographical or historical conditions, namely regardless of local cultures (Bower & Gilbody, 2005).

Evidence-based approach is pervasive in Mental Health field too, determining professional practices grounded on a medicalization process of psychic and relational phenomena, looking for individual invariants. Often, this perspective lead to identify Mental Health with the absence of diagnosis of mental disorders.

Whereas in this chapter's perspective, Mental Health could not be detected by identifying solely individuals as unit of analysis. Contrariwise it is crucial to re-inscribe individuals into relational dynamics and social coexistence system they belong to. In accordance with this unit of analysis's definition, we need to settle specific methodologies that allow to study relationships between individuals and changing social contexts of coexistence.

Hence, this chapter intends to explore heterogeneity by referring to different cultures evoking professional practices and shared meanings in Mental Health field.

It seems necessary to focus cultural premises concerning Mental Health professional practices as a clue to detect how local cultures ground specific object of intervention. Therefore the chapter intends to focus on users' and professionals' interpretations about Mental Health and about social mandate to deal with it. These interpretations can be considered as a trace of shared symbolizations which determine common representations of agencies' function, influencing users' demands and provided services.

Furthermore, the chapter intends to analyse social mandate turned to Italian Mental Health agencies by studying institutional documents and also by providing an historical perspective on Italian Mental Health system's development.

BACKGROUND: A LEAD THROUGH COMPLEXITY

This paragraph aims to presents theoretical categories useful to analyse Mental Health construct, as a lead through complexity.

Throughout the chapter, the analysis will proceed basing on an Evidential Paradigm (Ginzburg, 1986). When we refer to the concept of "paradigm", we are implying a connection with an overall conceptual construction (Kuhn, 1970), determining a particular epistemology, grounding a specific research tradition.

We refer to qualitative research perspective, aiming to detect social, individual and situational phenomena by analysing details, inconspicuous aspects, small clues, revealing something bigger and submerged (Demetrio, 1992). Qualitative research's aim is idiographic, focusing on the particular, pursuing to deepen knowledge about the specific case study, instead of looking for general laws (Coggi & Ricchiardi, 2005). The goal is not to reach an "absolute truth", but to get closer to a deeper understanding of investigated phenomena (Caronia, 1997), by studying clues and detecting traces.

In a methodological perspective, we could assert that this chapter practices inductive investigation procedures, namely knowledge originates from the observation of specific collected data. This way to proceed is highlighted in *Myths, emblems and clues* (1986), where Carlo Ginzburg analyses three examples to study their conjectural methods: Giovanni Morelli, an Italian art critic; Sigmund Freud, father of psychoanalysis; Conan Doyle's fictional character, Sherlock Holmes. All the three cases proceed by detecting infinitesimal traces, which lead to the comprehension of a deeper and otherwise unattainable reality. Pictorial marks (for Morelli), clues (for Sherlock Holmes) or symptoms (for Freud) are treated as traces revealing wider phenomena.

Furthermore, the chapter is based on psychoanalytic approach, psychosocially oriented. In accordance with this theoretical framework, the chapter aims to explore Mental Health not through an individualistic perspective but through a relational point of view.

As we previously said, the chapter proposes to consider Mental Health as a complex topic, historically and locally characterized. Mental Health is treated as a culturally issue, not as an object existing in nature by itself. We are not going to take Mental Health as an object passible of being measured with examinations replicable in any time and space, regardless the analyser involvement. Whereas we are going to analyse the concept of Mental Health as a cultural construction, based on symbolizations which are shared in specific social contexts, determined by history and territory, which means determined by local cultures.

Furthermore the chapter proposes to consider Mental Health issues, not as a characteristic of the individual but as the precipitate of collusive systems' failure. Individuals could take decision to react to pain related to collusive systems' failure, turning a demand to agencies symbolized as competent with specific issues.

The concept of collusive systems' failures refers to social systems of coexistence grounding on collusive assets, which fail. This perspective is based on the Theory of Collusion, a psychological psychoanalytic oriented model about emotional dynamic determining social relationships, conceived by Renzo Carli and Rosa Maria Paniccia (2003). In accordance with this model, social construction of reality begins by setting emotional meaning to different aspects of social experience, creating emotional symbolizations shared with people who participate to the same context. Colluding, from the Latin "cum-ludere", properly refers to this process of shared emotional symbolization (Carli & Paniccia, 2003).

In accordance with a psychoanalytic perspective, it's possible to assert that we proceed by constructing events through emotional symbolization of specific aspects of reality. In other words, we can identify reality through emotions concerning our way to symbolize reality's aspects. Furthermore this way to emotionally symbolize events is related to specific local cultures we participate to. Hence we should not presume events evoke emotions, whereas we assert emotions found events' construction. Otherwise, if this highlighted hypothesis is wrong, we wouldn't detect the complex common sense construction, that we could define as a collusive process, functioning in prescribing and protecting emotional system shared in a specific social context.

Individuals could experience a discrepancy between subjective feelings and common sense prescribed emotions. Such kind of experience could entail complex emotional reactions, often felt as painful, and could imply feelings like guilt, shame, social isolation or adaptation inadequacy.

Furthermore, reconsidering Mental Health within this perspective, it is possible to reinterpret individual's requests for psychological support and psychological distress as the precipitate of collusive systems' failure, which concerns the individual experience of a discrepancy between subjective emotions founding reality and common sense prescribed feelings. In accordance with this perspective, collusive process indeed work to socially share emotions grounding experienced events (Carli & Paniccia, 2012).

Hence we could reckon how can psychoanalytic psychotherapy specifically contribute to the debate on Mental Health? A psychoanalytic psychosocially oriented approach could provide criteria to clinically analyse contexts where Mental Health interventions are set, by detecting their peculiar local cultures grounding on collusive systems. In particular, we refer to interventions based on the Analysis of Demand model, whose objective and method concern the development of competence to detect emotions experienced in relations, using them as a trace, as a resource to explore problems encountered within those relations founding on specific collusive systems (Carli & Paniccia, 2003).

Moreover, we propose to focus how the individual, with his subjective decision, defines his state or experience as normal or pathological. Indeed Mental Health professional intervenes only if individual subjectivity comes to the decision to consult him. Therefore medical diagnosis is secondary to a sort of important subjective diagnosis acted by an individual who decides to define himself as diseased (Canguilhem, 1998). Absence of absence of pain is transformed in presence of illness, which could be object of diagnostic procedures. This symbolic process deeply marks the relationship between citizens and Mental Health system. Indeed this symbolic process founds on local culture based on a collusive system which requires an act of "proclaiming himself" as diseased, as a reaction to pain. Through this symbolic and emotional process the individual become "a user". Indeed becoming a user is requirement to establish a relation with Mental Health system. In a collusive dynamic, individual and coexistence context, share symbolic dimension setting the relationship with Mental Health agencies.

Coexistence context's social mandate entail mental diseased person identification, as an individual who because of his "different" behaviour contributes to the failure of conformist social systems.

Social mandate requires diversity isolation and institutionalization, to protect collusive system holding social relations founded on common sense emotions.

Social system protect common sense establishment, by requiring that "non-compliant" individuals are assigned to specialized professional organizations. As far as possible, Mental Health agencies are required to seek the *restitutio ad integrum* of those deviating from common sense people (Carli, Paniccia, Caputo, Dolcetti, Finore, & Giovagnoli, 2016). Individual affected by *mental disorders*, as defined as a result of a diagnostic process, they are not "aware" of emotions violating common sense. Otherwise if this awareness is active, then we are faced with "common emotional disorders", therefore with a request for *psychological distress*. In Mental Health assistance system, this difference grounds a distinction between psychiatric and psychological intervention (Carli & Paniccia, 2012).

Finally, we want to highlight possible developments regarding Mental Health system: agencies required with the social mandate of take care of Mental Health, could focus problems in social coexistence, besides diseases by working on demand, local cultures and coexistence issues. Analysing users' demand means dealing with recurrent critical social events and problems, some of which are indications of social emerging emergencies (Vari, 2014).

THREE EXPERIENCES OF INTERVENTION IN THREE DIFFERENT AGENCY DEALING WITH MENTAL HEALTH

This paragraph introduces three clinical experiences in Mental Health field, aiming to explore differences in order to identify transversal issues. In particular, the analysis focus on social mandate which characterize different agencies dealing with Mental Health. Indeed the analysis will consider institutional documents and users' demand, as traces to explore local culture about Mental Health and about organizations dealing with it.

The clinical experiences we are going to present, are carried out by the author, with the role of psychologist, in collaboration with different teams. All the interventions we are going to introduce take place in Rome in 2017-18. They are set in different context: a public Mental Health Service, a psychoanalytic private office, a non-profit organization actualizing a project with a public middle school in the territory of a roman suburb. The data we are going to present are collected by analysing literature and reported clinical experiences, in accordance with a psychoanalytic approach, psychosocially oriented, based on the Analysis of Demand model (Carli & Paniccia, 2003).

A Psychosocial Perspective On A Public Mental Health Service Intervention

To present first intervention, which takes place in a public Mental Health Center, it is necessary to introduce Italian public Mental Health services' current organization, besides providing an historical perspective of its development.

Mental Health Center (for brevity, we will call it CSM, using the Italian acronym) is the organism that on behalf of the Department of Mental Health (for brevity, we will call it DSM) and the Local Institution for Healthcare, up to the Ministry of Healthcare, has the mandate to accept and to filter citizens' requests. The purpose of CSM is to *promote and protect health, both on an individual and a collective level*, for resident population and people standing in its own territory, to allow the best quality of life as possible, by providing services for *prevention, therapy, rehabilitation* (Ministero della Salute, 2006). On its official website, Local Institution for Healthcare defines Mental Health as a fundamental area of intervention, aiming to combine actions addressed to *support social inclusion* and actions addressed to *take care of psychic distress, psychiatric disorders and disabilities* (ASL Roma1, n.d.).

In the previous lines, it's possible to spot traces (in italics) of Local Institution for Healthcare's purposes. In particular:

- promote and protect Health, both on an individual and a collective level;

- support social inclusion;
- take care of psychic distress, psychiatric disorders and disabilities.

These definitions show differences about the object of intervention: “individual and collective Health” should not be considered the same concept of “psychiatric disorder”, they are different constructs. The concept of “psychiatric disorders” evokes a purely *individual* issue, whereas the concept of “individual and collective Health” refers to a social dimension, evoking *relations* and *coexistence contests.*

“Psychiatric disorders” and “individual and collective Health” could be considered as traces of different shared symbolizations about Mental Health Services’ scope.

Organization determines specific goals, which could be considered as traces of organizational social mandate, since social mandate founds on symbolizations about organization’s function shared by professionals, users and community it lies in.

Specific symbolizations about organization’s social mandate and purposes lead to determine specific goals and to define specific strategies and devices to reach those goals, according with the organization’s scopes.

Different symbolizations lead differences in term of paradigms, methodologies and tools for interventions. In a wider perspective, they lead differences in term of representations about professionals’ work and relationship with organizations’ users (Mazzola, 2018).

It is possible to highlight once again how the notion of Mental Health is wide, complex and composite. It includes several and different constructs, coexisting in a heterogeneous category. In depth, mental disorder and individual or social distress represent two of the objects included in Mental Health category, despite the differences characterizing them.

Mental disorders evoke an individual perspective, with a focus on a person’s idiosyncratic patterns and traits. Psychiatry provides theories and tools appropriated to deal with this topic.

On the other hand, the construct of individual and social distress evokes a relational perspective, with a focus on local context of coexistence. Psychology and Psychoanalytic Psychotherapy provide dedicated methodologies to deal with this issue.

What does this difference could be considered as a trace of? To inquire this question we propose to analyse agencies assigned to deal with Mental Health in an historical perspective, from asylum’s existence to actual Mental Health services assets’ development.

In Italy in 1978, Law No. 180 is approved, promoting a complete reform of psychiatric assistance, determining the progressive replacement of psychiatric asylum with a radically new model of territorial Mental Health service system.

Law's approval takes place under the pressure of deinstitutionalization movements diffused in Trieste and in other areas of Italy. At the time of the promulgation of the law, turnover of patients is minimal.

Law No. 180 aims to promote a cultural change, by asserting that even in psychiatric field Mental Health system must found its bases on person's rights to healthcare, contrariwise the assessment of social dangerousness. In accordance with Law's issued values' asset, treatments turn to a voluntary basis. Law No. 180 establishes that no one can be hospitalized in psychiatric hospitals. Despite, in case of hospitalization needed, since Psychiatric asylum are removed, the Psychiatric Diagnosis and Treatment Services of general hospitals carry out clinical treatments.

A law, which dates back to 1904, previously ruled mental Health system in Italy, focusing on a specific social need, which is "protect society from mental disorders".

Process of hospitalizations started after a psychiatric certification and a commissioner's order to alienate civil rights to diagnosed person. Mental Health care was administered by local districts, each of them refers to their own asylum. Law No. 180 starts a process leading to asylums removal, on a national scale. By the end of the '90s, with all asylums' closure, new Mental Health services are introduced, with the aim to ensure mentally diseased people shall conduct their lives in an inclusive social context.

After Law 180's approval, it begins a long lasting process of wide Mental Health system's reorganization, involving administrative and institutional levels. New provisions are introduces on a national and regional basis, new regulatory frameworks are established to progressively determine Mental Health Departments' responsibilities, provided services, settled goals and procedures, involved professionals, determined targets and intervention standards.

In March 1999, Italian Ministry of Health announces the successful final closure of all public asylums. This event could be considered as the ending stage of a poignant cycle, more than two decades lasting. Italian Mental Health system reform represents a long and complex course, with a high historical and symbolical impact on Italian society on different levels, since it evokes heated debates among professionals, family members, administrators, politicians, involving Italian public opinion in a broad sense.

In 1981, Local Departments of Mental Health are established, as institutes entitled to rule territorial district on a technical, administrative and managerial level, programming and providing services, projects and activities.

Residential and housing groups are enhanced to provide accommodation addressed not only to previously hospitalized users but also to new users, never hospitalized before, turning Mental Health services because of precarious living conditions or involved in family conflicts. Mental Health agencies' aim includes rehabilitation, training and socialization, actualized through recreational and leisure activities such as expressive workshops, literacy courses and schooling.

In the mid of the '80s the number of cooperatives involved in Mental Health work placement grow and their range of competences and activities is gradually extended. In the following years, cooperatives increasingly focus on interventions aiming to promote empowerment for people with handicaps and disabilities or affected by addiction problems or social marginalization. Cooperatives work develop in a social entrepreneurship perspective. Cooperatives' social purposes meet Mental Health Departments' ones. Thus in the '90s Departments run a significant work to support Mental Health services' users to fully exercise their citizenship rights, namely as workers. Mental Health Departments and cooperatives' scope connection leads to enlarge cooperatives' business, providing new services and activities addressed to Mental Health services' users. Cooperatives' offer extends to rehabilitation and empowerment programs, with different specific focuses, such as accommodation, work, education and training, social inclusion, network building, self-help groups.

In 1975-1976 the first CSM was established with the purpose of supporting previously hospitalized patients and dealing with new users' crisis. CSMs run as day centers and work to reduce hospitalized patients' number and to shorten hospitalization's duration. It is interesting to highlight that CSMs are introduced before the national reform (Law 180), when asylums are still working. Hence for a while two different organizational and cultural assistance models operate at the same time (IDeaSS Italy, n.d.).

Law No. 180 is considered a worldwide example as a symbol of culture revolution in its field, since it radically changes Mental Health care and assistance methods. It is indicated as the first law in the world which bans asylums, representing a symbolic victory for people who worked for it, determining a huge cultural heritage, entailing nowadays living trains.

In accordance with Carli and Paniccia's work, we propose a psychosocial interpretation of Italian Mental Health system development.

In the '60s, '70s and in the beginning of the '80s italian asylum system collapses. At the same time, an emerging culture spreads. Growing values of equality and minorities protection condemn every act of diversities institutionalizing or marginalization. Meanwhile in that historical period Psychiatry attempts to actualize Mental disorder affected people's reintegration to social and familiar context. A new category it is introduced: "the psychiatric operator", which transversally includes psychiatrists, psychologists, nurses and all mental health professional workers, all together involved in pursuing users' social reintegration. Hence analysing Mental Health services development it is possible to remark that ideological base grounds social reintegration process, determined as attempted outcome. Social reintegration process was based on values rather than dedicated methodologies and differentiated contributions of various professional perspectives, entailing the lack of formalized techniques grounded on specific theories. Hence ideological tension replaces professional technicality.

In the mid of the '80s until the end of the '90s, social reintegration is at first juxtaposed and then replaced by psychotherapies, addressed to new users (as common emotional disorders affected users) and, when it is possible, addressed to traditional psychiatric users. Psychotherapy shows an increasingly clear and specific attempt to take care of mental disorders defined by using DSM psychiatric nosography categories. A pervasive return of technicality occurs, concerning not psychiatric movement but Psychotherapy. Both in Mental Health agencies and in professionals' orientation we see behavioural techniques gradually prevailing over psychoanalytic and systemic approach. Contrariwise the highlighted hypothesis is that a complex phenomenon, as social reintegration is, could not be chased by applying techniques pursuing interventions addressed to specific and limited objects, such as behaviours. Indeed psychoanalytic perspective with a psychosocial approach proposes categories to reinterpret social reintegration phenomenon as a psychosocial intervention within users' relation with coexistence context, where problems defined as mental distress emerge (Carli & Paniccia, 2011).

Furthermore this chapter aims to study Mental Health in a relational and psychosocial perspective grounded on psychoanalytic models, by focusing the area of Mental Health agencies. As we said, the highlighted hypothesis is that users' requests could be considered as traces of social mandate founded on symbolizations shared in local cultures. According with this focus we could inquire: what kind of requests users turn to Mental Health agencies?

Let's introduce a case study, set in a public Mental Health service: a CSM sited in Rome.

A woman turns to CSM because she got episodes of amnesia and disorientation. She asks for neurological examination, to check for the presence of dementia. A CSM psychiatrist visits her and, after excluding dementia, demands her for a psychological visit to verify the presence of dissociation disorder. When the CSM psychologist meets her for the first time and asks about her request, the woman starts crying and telling about her sentiments of anxiety and sadness. The psychologist, who is the author of this chapter, treats the woman's request with the Analysis of Demand approach. The woman reports problems within relations with her coexistence contests. Throughout a psychotherapeutic work, it was possible to reinterpret woman's demand. In this case, the woman emotionally denied her desire in relations, in which she acted with a sacrificial approach. At one point her relational pattern seems not to work anymore for her and she feels disoriented, both in a figurative way (emotionally) and in a proper one (with episodes of amnesia). She feels powerless facing problems with her family and at work and she feels assailed by sentiments of anxiety and sadness. The woman's demand to take care of her relations in crisis is turned to a CSM through a request to check a medical problem (amnesia). We could say the woman *medicalize* her issue, since she transform an emotionally complex relational problem in a request treatable through a medical approach.

Analysing CSM users' requests, it's possible to highlight recurring events like the clinical situation just introduced: in several other encountered cases, CSM receives demands to deal with relational problems, through requests of checking medicalized symptoms.

Not only the woman treats her issue as a symptom, but also CSM psychiatrist does (checking for dementia), properly according with his area of competence and in accordance with the determined goal of dealing with Mental Health, interpreted as mental disorders.

CSM users and professionals seem to share fantasies about CSM as an agency dealing with medical problems. Regarding medical problems, we intend to refer to individual related issues, which are liable of diagnosis and treatments, better if it's a pharmacological one not concerning emotional users' and professionals' subjectivity involvement.

It's worth to report a difference among *individual* and *subjective* level.

Merriam-Webster (n.d.) defines individual as "being an individual or existing as an indivisible whole", where individual is defined as *a particular being or thing as distinguished from a class, species, or collection: such as a single human being as contrasted with a social group or institution.* Instead *subjective* is defined as *relating to the essential being of that which has substance, qualities, attributes, or relations; characteristic of or belonging to reality as perceived rather than as independent of mind.*

It's possible to underline differences among two different constructs: on the one hand, individual as a whole, isolated from a species; on the other hand subjective with relations and perceptions, we could say with emotionally involvement.

According with the highlighted hypothesis about professionals' and users' symbolizations as a trace of social mandate, we could identify CSM as Mental Health agency dealing with individual problems treatable by medicalized approach, in accordance with the purpose of taking care of mental disorders. Whereas, CSM also got the scope of dealing with individual and social distress, which evokes social mandate to deal with users' request as result of relationships and coexisting contexts in crisis, with a focus on users' emotional distress about it.

Furthermore we could say that person who choose to turn Mental Health agency a request for psychological distress is the one who decide to take charge of a problem shared by coexisting system participants (Carli, 2015). As we previously said, we propose to define Mental Health issues not as a characteristic of individual but as precipitate of collusive systems' failure. Individuals could take decision to react to pain concerning coexistence collusive systems' failure, turning a demand to agencies symbolized as competent with specific issues.

We outline a possible development of CSM social function: it could be useful to work on a cross analysis about individual requests reported in a determined territory, to provide a social interpretation about local emerging issues, in order to plan interventions not only for individual treatment but for collective prevention too.

A PSYCHOSOCIAL PERSPECTIVE ON A PSYCHOANALYTIC PRIVATE OFFICE INTERVENTION

Moving to another context, what kind of requests are turned to a psychoanalytic psychotherapist working in a private office?

Let's introduce a case study, set in a psychoanalytic psychotherapeutic private office, located in Rome.

A woman turns psychotherapist because of her feelings of anxiety. She says she is worried about her academic career, since she is afraid not to take last university exams. Throughout a psychotherapeutic work based on Analysis of Demand approach, it is possible to re-interpret the client's demand, who presents issues with her familiar and university contexts. She wondered about her life according with what she expected others would consider the right way for her, but at one point this strategy doesn't work anymore, since she feels a growing anxiety approaching her graduation. She is afraid for her future and feels paralyzed by the idea of taking a choice, facing her resources and her limits to identify desires and chase them.

As for CSM, analysing psychotherapeutic private office clients' demand, it is possible to trace recurring events. Psychoanalytic private office clients' demands often concern emotions perceived as wrong, unacceptable or problematic. These requests found on symbolizations of emotions as something dangerous and to be treated in private, in a confidential and discreet treatment context. Comparing with CSM users' demands, the psychotherapeutic requests are not symbolized as grave because medicalized symptoms, but because idiosyncratic.

In a different way comparing with CSM, the request are often at individual level, too. While, as we said, in CSM the unit of analysis is individual with his own medicalized symptoms, in psychotherapeutic private office social context seems to disappear and everything is an intimate place where to bring personal sentiments. Furthermore emotions could be disconnected by relational context which they are related to. Hence psychotherapeutic private office could be symbolized as a place out of time and space, as a metaphor for inner space, where to fix problems with personal feelings and emotions. These symbolizations could be shared in collusion by professionals and clients, evoking for both of them different related fantasies, such as some of the more widespread: fantasies about a place where to face limitless client's inner world ruled by frightening feelings; fantasies about professional's emotional neutrality (all the field is dedicated to customer's inner word); fantasies about not reportable or analysable professional's procedures because of an emotional nature of the work (perceived in opposition to a rational way to proceed); and so on. Moreover, we may consider psychotherapeutic literature, where there are many contents analysing psychotherapeutic setting of interventions, on the contrary it's hard to find professional contributes on social impact. The topic doesn't seem to provoke a particularly heated debate within the scientific community, if compared to other themes, such as the psychoanalytic setting and its variations. The unit of analysis is one again focused inside the office, detached by the context it lies in.

Document analysis provides other traces about psychotherapeutic private office's social mandate. Searching for Italian laws ruling psychotherapeutic private office's activity, it's possible to discover there are not many documents but the Article No. 41 of the Constitution of the Italian Republic:

Private economic enterprise shall be free. It may not be carried out against the common good or in such a manner that could damage safety, liberty and human dignity. The law shall provide for appropriate programmes and controls so that public and private-sector economic activity may be oriented and co-ordinated for social purposes (Senato della Repubblica, 1948).

Therefore, psychotherapeutic private office, as private economic enterprise, should be *oriented for social purposes* and *shall provide for appropriate programmes and controls.*

What kind of programmes and controls are determined for psychotherapeutic private office's activity?

It is possible to refer to the Art. No. 2229 of the Italian Civil Code (1942) declaring that intellectual professions' exercise requires registration in dedicated registers or lists. Verification of registration requirements, list maintenance and disciplinary power over register's members are delegated to professional associations, under State supervision.

Hence the Constitution of the Italian Republic determines psychotherapeutic private office's activity must aim at social purposes and its activity must be ruled and controlled, switching level, by professional's behaviour.

Also on a legal level, norms concerning contexts (office and its social purposes) are juxtaposed with individual (professional and his behaviour).

Furthermore according with the highlighted hypothesis about professionals' and clients' symbolizations of Mental Health agencies as a trace of social mandate, we could identify psychotherapeutic private office as an agency deputed to deal with individual issues, too. Psychoanalytic psychotherapeutic office is symbolized as an intimate place taking cover from the social context. A place where to fix troubles with personal feeling and emotions, symbolized as idiosyncratic and problematic for the person who turns the request. We suppose psychotherapeutic private office professionals' social mandate is properly to deal with private individual issues.

Whereas, focusing on a psychosocial perspective, it's possible to propose an implied psychotherapeutic private office's social function in developing clients' relationships in coexisting context by working with the person who turns a psychotherapeutic request.

A PSYCHOSOCIAL PERSPECTIVE ON A NON-PROFIT ORGANIZATION INTERVENTION AT SCHOOL

Introducing the third case study, we propose a shift in terms of intervention's target, moving from individual to context. If in the previous two clinical situations, psychological interventions were carried out after an individual's request, in this case a clinical intervention is developed as psychosocial project addressed to a roman public middle school and its classrooms.

Regional district administration wanted to finance projects facing schools' dropout problems.

A non-profit organization composed of psychologists proposes a project whose aim is to develop relation between school and the area in which it is located. The project is based on a reinterpretation of dropout phenomenon, as a student's reaction to sentiments of isolation and uselessness felt within the relation with school coexistence context. The assumption is: if at school it's possible to get interesting activity, you want to get there. The project aim to work with school, at school and in school time, to explore students' interests related to a common object: territory, which school and students' family share. The territory we are talking about is a roman suburb, where most of the students live and where school is sited.

This intervention was carried by a team composed by the author and three colleagues, all of them psychologists. Every professional works with one classroom composed by 15-25 students aged 10-12. On a first stage, the project aims to explore students' interests and connections between interests and territory. Later, all the classrooms work to create a thematic map, linking emotional relevant places with point of interest to discover, planning territory exploratory walks that every classroom takes on its own. In the end, all the groups together plans a final event where the 4 classrooms meets and share their works. Teachers and families are invited to come to the final event to share their thoughts and stories about territory. As we said, every classroom choose a theme to elaborate. The chosen topic are: street art, history, trade and craft, classroom's story, in the surrounding suburb. Indeed the project's main aim is not to work on themes, but to intervene on students' relationship with classmates and the wider coexistence context at school, throughout working on themes.

The project's purpose is to develop relation between school and territory in order to develop the relation between students and school coexistence context, to contrast sentiments of isolation and uselessness, founding dropout phenomenon.

Hence it's possible to underline that this intervention lies in Mental Health field, by a reinterpretation of the construct. Indeed this project proposes a reinterpretation of Mental Health as an issue concerning coexistence system, rather than only related to problematic individuals. Dropout phenomenon is not solely a matter of students, it is actually a matter of sentiments connected to relations in coexistence contests, invoking schools, families and actors sharing a specific territory.

Dropout phenomenon is treated as a trace of risk of social isolation, which requires prevention interventions, according with WHO's definition of Mental Health, previously showed in this chapter: *Mental health is a state of well-being in which an individual realizes his or her own abilities, can cope with the normal stresses of life, can work productively and is able to make a contribution to his or her community* (World Health Organization, 2018).

Within this intervention, psychologists assume a psychosocial perspective to propose a reinterpretation of Mental Health interventions as prevention of social isolations.

CONCLUSION

Throughout this chapter, we explored the construct of Mental Health in a psychoanalytic and psychological perspective with a psychosocial approach. In particular, the chapter analyses the construct of Mental Health by studying different organizations aiming to deal with it. The chapter introduces three clinical experiences of Mental Health interventions, actualized in different contexts. It's highlighted how the three proposed experiences represent different ways to regard to Mental Health, showing different users' and professionals' interpretations, defining different kind of interventions. Throughout the chapter we look for traces to detect social mandate characterizing different Mental Health agencies. The highlighted hypothesis is that social mandate is a trace of local culture about Mental Health, which defines fantasies about Mental Health issues, founding on symbolizations shared by professionals, users and community.

The chapter intended to explore differences between Mental Health agencies and their local cultures in order to identify transversal issues. The highlighted hypothesis is that what seems to characterize Mental Health is precisely the complexity of the concept itself which includes a heterogeneity of professional practices and social meaning.

After all, we could say Mental Health is actually a social mandate to intervene. With the purpose of planning interventions aimed to take care of Mental Health, it is important to focus on social mandate, which is locally, historically and culturally connoted.

The first clinical experience introduces CSM local culture, whose social mandate identify a Mental Health agency dealing with individual problems treatable with a medicalized approach, according with the scope of taking care of mental disorders. Whereas CSM purpose of taking care of individual and social distress evokes social mandate to deal with users' request as a result of relationships and coexisting contexts in crisis, with a focus on users' emotional distress about it.

The second clinical experience is set in a psychoanalytic psychotherapeutic private office. It emerges symbolizations about a decontextualized context. In psychotherapeutic office's local culture, the social context seems to disappear and everything is an intimate place where to bring personal feelings detached by the relational context which they are connected to. Thus the office can be defined as a private economic initiative which, according to the Italian Constitution, must be addressed for social purposes. Social function of a psychoanalytic office may seem given for granted but it is not. We suppose psychotherapeutic private office professionals' social mandate is to take care of problems with personal feelings and emotions.

Comparing psychoanalytic psychotherapeutic private office and CSM, it's possible to remark that the requests are often at an individual level in both cases. While, as we said, in CSM the unit of analysis is individual with his own medicalized symptoms, in psychotherapeutic private office the focus is individual with his own idiosyncrasy.

In first and second case, we see interventions addressed to individuals, even though the unit of analysis is the relation between individual and social context. The third case introduces a new difference: the intervention is address on a social level. It's a psychosocial intervention carried out by a non-profit association and addressed to 4 classrooms in a public middle school. The project aims to develop relation between students and school coexistence contexts, to contrast sentiments of isolation and uselessness, founding dropout phenomenon. The association, composed by psychologist, work on the social mandate providing a new interpretation of it: facing dropout, means facing social isolation, as a preventive Mental Health intervention.

In conclusion, all the introduces experiences are based in Mental Health field although they show differences in terms of professionals and teams, targets, goals, tools and context of intervention. However it's possible to underline a transversal dimension: local cultures defines social mandates which determine users' requests and professional's goals of interventions.

Through the analysis of different Mental Health organizations' social mandate, it seems possible to draw a broad and heterogeneous scenario, including the diagnosis for individual to development of knowledge on problems of coexistence systems in crisis.

We could conclude highlighting that what seem to characterize crosswise Mental Health field is the amount of demands dealing with grave sentiments determining intervention's request addressed in first person or for another person.

Indeed Mental Health could be considered as a complex issue concerning local cultures which means concerning coexistence and social level although it relapses on an individual level. We remark that it is important for professionals and agencies dealing with Mental Health to analyse social mandate and users' requests, in order not to settle automatic procedures but to plan organizational developments oriented to social impact.

REFERENCES

ASL Roma1. (n.d.). *Dipartimento di Salute Mentale* [Mental Health Department]. Retrieved May 14, 2019, from https://www.aslroma1.it/azienda-dipartimentieri/dipartimento-di-salute-mentale

Bower, P., & Gilbody, S. (2005). Stepped care in psychological therapies: Access, effectiveness and efficiency. *The British Journal of Psychiatry*, *186*(1), 11–17. doi:10.1192/bjp.186.1.11 PMID:15630118

Canguilhem, G. (1998). Il normale e il patologico [The Normal and the Pathological] (M. Porro, Trans.). Torino: Einaudi. (Original work published 1966)

Carli, R., & Paniccia, R. M. (2003). Analisi della domanda. Teoria e tecnica dell'intervento in psicologia clinica [Analysis of Demand. Theory and technique of intervention in clinical psychology]. Bologna: Il Mulino.

Carli, R., & Paniccia, R. M. (2011). La cultura dei servizi di salute mentale in Italia. Dai malati psichiatrici alla nuova utenza: l'evoluzione della domanda di aiuto e delle dinamiche di rapporto [The culture of Mental Health Services in Italy. From psychiatric patients to new users: The evolution of the aid demand and the dynamics of the relationship]. Milano: FrancoAngeli.

Carli, R., & Paniccia, R. M. (2012). Malattia mentale e senso comune [Mental illness and common sense]. *Rivista di Psicologia Clinica, 2*, 201 - 206. Retrieved from http://www.rivistadipsicologiaclinica.it

Carli, R., Paniccia, R. M., Caputo, A., Dolcetti, F., Finore, E., & Giovagnoli, F. (2016). La relazione che organizza il contesto sanitario: Domanda dell'utenza e risposta dei servizi sanitari, nel territorio e nell'ospedale [The relationship which organizes the healthcare context: Users' demand and response of healthcare services, in the territory and the hospital]. *Rivista di Psicologia Clinica, 1*, 7–44. doi:10.14645/RPC.2016.1.608

Caronia, L. (1997). Costruire la conoscenza [Building knowledge]. Firenze: La Nuova Italia.

Coggi, C., & Ricchiardi, P. (2005). Progettare la ricerca empirica in educazione [Planning empirical research in education]. Roma: Carocci Editore.

Demetrio, D. (1992). Micropedagogia. La ricerca qualitativa in educazione [Micropedagogy. Qualitative research in education]. Firenze: La Nuova Italia.

Ginzburg, C. (1986). Miti, emblemi e spie [Myths, emblems and clues]. Torino: Einaudi.

IDeaSS Italy. (n.d.). *From the asylum to territorial services for mental health.* Retrieved May 14, 2019, from http://www.triestesalutementale.it/english/doc/BrochureTriesteENG.pdf

Individual. (n.d.). In *Merriam-Webster's dictionary.* Retrieved from https://www.merriam-webster.com/dictionary/individual

Italian Civil Code. (1942). Retrieved May 14, 2019, from https://www.brocardi.it/codice-civile/libro-quinto/titolo-iii/capo-ii/art2229.html

Kuhn, T. S. (1970). Logic of Discovery or Psychology of Research? In I. Lakatos & A. Musgrave (Eds.), *Criticism and the Growth of Knowledge* (pp. 1–22). Cambridge, UK: Cambridge University Press. doi:10.1017/CBO9781139171434.003

Mazzola, A. (2018). Psicoterapia nei contesti: Quale rapporto tra il mandato dei servizi di salute mentale e le domande ad essi rivolte? Resoconto di un intervento in un CSM [Psychotherapy in contexts: What relationship between MentalHealth Services and their users' demands? Report of a clinical intervention in a MentalHealth Center]. *Rivista di Psicologia Clinica, 1*, 66–84. doi:10.14645/RPC.2018.1.716

Ministero della Salute. (2006). *I servizi di salute mentale* [Mental Health services]. Retrieved May 14, 2019, from http://www.salute.gov.it/portale/temi/p2_6.jsp?id=168&area=salute%20mentale&menu=rete

Senato della Repubblica. (1948). *La Costituzione della Repubblica Italiana* [The Constitution of the Italian Republic]. Retrieved May 14, 2019, from http://www.senato.it/application/xmanager/projects/leg18/file/repository/relazioni/libreria/novita/XVII/COST_INGLESE.pdf

Subjective. (n.d.). In *Merriam-Webster's dictionary*. Retrieved from https://www.merriam-webster.com/dictionary/subjective

Vari, R. (2014). Centro di Salute Mentale: La relazione 'individuo/ambiente di convivenza/Servizio' nell'intervento clinico per le malattie mentali [Mental Health Center. The relationship 'individual/ social coexistence milieu/Service' in the clinical intervention for mental illness]. *Rivista di psicologia clinica, 1,* 154-185. Retrieved from http://www.rivistadipsicologiaclinica.it

Well-being. (n.d.). In *Cambridge dictionary*. Retrieved from https://dictionary.cambridge.org/dictionary/english/well-being

Well-being. (n.d.). In *Merriam-Webster's dictionary*. Retrieved from https://www.merriam-webster.com/dictionary/well-being

World Health Organization. (2018). *Mental health: strengthening our response.* Retrieved May 14, 2019, from https://www.who.int/news-room/fact-sheets/detail/mental-health-strengthening-our-response

Chapter 13
Personal and Professional Well-Being Among Early Childhood Teachers:
Are They Related?

Sanja Tatalović Vorkapić
https://orcid.org/0000-0002-9170-8455
Faculty of Teacher Education, University of Rijeka, Croatia

Renata Čepić
Faculty of Teacher Education, University of Rijeka, Croatia

ABSTRACT

Early childhood teachers' work satisfaction is an essential prerequisite for their work attainments and quality work outcomes. At the same time, besides their professional well-being, their personal well-being is of utmost importance, which raises the question about the nature of their relatedness. Therefore, this study was aimed to explore the personal and professional well-being among Croatian early childhood teachers. A total of 179 early childhood teachers from the Kindergarten "Rijeka" have participated in this research. Results showed that early education teachers were moderately satisfied with their work. Similarly, results about their personal well-being demonstrated moderate to high levels of optimism, positive emotions, flow, and life satisfaction. Correlation analyses revealed significant positive relationship between high levels of all personal well-being dimensions and high level of work satisfaction. Additionally, it was determined that older and highly experienced early childhood teachers are significantly less satisfied with work and less optimistic.

DOI: 10.4018/978-1-7998-1185-5.ch013

INTRODUCTION

Focusing on the well-being of all participants within the complete educational system is not only a necessity but also the main aim of educational curriculums all over the world. Croatian national curriculum of an early and preschool care and education (2014) emphasized that the well-being of children of an early and preschool age is the main purpose for the educational work in kindergartens. Analyzing the significant determinates of children's well-being, it was determined that the well-being of their teachers showed to be the most significant one, which is clearly emphasized in the statement of McCallum and Price (2010): *"Well teachers, well students"*. The preservation of the teachers' well-being is crucial when trying to achieve a high quality of the educational process. Therefore, early childhood teachers' work satisfaction is an essential prerequisite to their work attainments and quality work outcomes. At the same time, besides their professional well-being, their personal well-being is of utmost importance, which raises the question about the nature of their relatedness, since total well-being of teachers is a multidimensional concept (McCallum, Price, Graham & Morrison, 2017). One of the well-known definition of the educator's well-being is that well-being is *"the positive emotional state resulting from the harmony between all the environmental factors on the one hand and the personal needs and expectations of the educators on the other"* (Aelterman, Engels, Van Petegem & Verhaeghe, 2007).

Therefore, this study aimed to explore the personal and professional well-being among Croatian early childhood teachers. Personal well-being in this study presents the set of several significant positive characteristics of early childhood educators. So, personal well-being is operationalized and defined by an early childhood teachers' optimism, positive emotions, flow and life satisfaction. On the other side, their professional well-being is measured by their work satisfaction. Since, there is a lack of similar researches in our country, especially in the field of an early and preschool care and education, it is very contributing to run this study in Croatia. Acquired data should result in practical implications for educator's work improvement from the aspect of positive psychology at the workplace. Therefore, this study points out the importance of research in the field of an early and pre-school education and contributes to improving the educators' profession. Expanding the scientific knowledge to early education teachers about their professional and personal well-being, and exploring and taking into account the empirical evidence as the basis for quality work, work achievements and quality of work outcomes in the field of an early and pre-school education could be improved.

BACKGROUND

The satisfaction of the employees' work in a specific working organization is a prerequisite for work attainment and the quality of work outcomes. Having an educators' profession in mind, their satisfaction is a prerequisite not only for the quality of work outcome, but the effects that they have on an optimal psychical development of children within the frame of implicit pedagogy. With that, the satisfaction of an educator becomes more significant. The teacher is the result of his/her "cumulative autobiography" – he/she acts on the basis of his/her constructs, beliefs, understanding of human beings, learning, professional growth, and development (Čepić & Kalin, 2017). This is why it is very important to analyze the beliefs of an educator and understand how educators professionally progress and which requirements contribute to that growth/progress, and encourage it. Observing practice, or observing educators in an educational work environment where they are surrounded by children, parents, professional associates, outside factors and many different unusual situations, a question arises, how much does his/her satisfaction affect his/her behavior and satisfaction in a working organization, and how much does it affect his/her life satisfaction in general. It is important how much the educator radiates positive thoughts, positive behavior, attitude and activity on a child, the parents and everyone they meet and are in contact with. In a large part, all stated above contributes to the quality in an educational practice. Some studies imply that adults are like a mirror to the children, an example that unknowingly affects their findings, behavior and actions (Tatalović Vorkapić, 2012, 2015, 2017). Sometimes they are not even aware of this. While talking to the parents, they often listen to their stories of how their child mimics his educator or another adult he/she is in contact with. Often times they witness a game in which little girls imitate behaviors, use a familiar word they heard before. Sometimes by acting a certain way towards the children, they can, unknowingly, positively or negatively influence the mood of those children. That is why it is of utmost importance that an educator is positive, optimistic, satisfactory with his/her life, and the workplace. The relation of life satisfactory and working organization through an educator's implicit pedagogy affects his/her educational work and satisfaction. Considering the aim of this research and the focused variables, contemporary theoretical and empirical cognition will be shown on the following: positive thoughts, or optimism, positive emotions, flow, life satisfaction and work satisfaction within a good work organization.

Optimism and Early Childhood Educators

By the end of the seventies, researches have shown that the way we think is mostly positive, rather than negative or realistic, which was named as the Pollyanna principle

(Martlin & Stang, 1978). Today it is known that three types of positive thinking exist – self-efficacy, hope and optimism. Optimism is a general expectation that more good things than bad will happen to us in life. Optimists never give up on their goals despite the obstacles that may get in their way (Rijavec, Miljković & Brdar, 2008). They are persistent, tenacious and believe in a positive outcome when found in adverse life situations. Optimists expect, and wish for good and positive things to happen, and explain the cause of negative events as something temporary – something that will pass. Unlike them, pessimists are always negative when thinking about the outcome of an event. Optimists are often persistent in achieving their goal, seldom give up, are tenacious and consistent. They are more successful than the pessimists are. They achieve success in education, at the workplace and in sports. They never waste time or motivation. Research have shown that optimists endure a lesser amount of stress and its intensity, as opposed to pessimists (Carver & Scheier, 1999; Chang & Sanna, 2003; Brdar & Bakarčić, 2006).

The way people see and perceive a cause for a certain event in life, Seligman (1998) named as *explanatory style*. He does not consider optimism as a personality trait, but a style of explaining the cause of certain events. An optimistic person finds the cause of negative events in external factors as something current. A pessimist views a situation as something permanent, internal and long term. Some researchers link the consequences of an optimistic explanatory style with success in college, work productivity (Schulman, 1995), success in sports (Rettew & Reivich, 1995) as well as rarely getting sick and greater belief in the possibility of stopping potential health problems (Peterson & De Avila, 1995). Contrary to this, the consequences of pessimistic explanatory style are linked with symptoms of depression (Robins & Hayes, 1995).

Dispositional optimism is genetically conditioned, (Plomin et al., 1992) and is influenced by childhood experiences as well. Those experiences are linked to trust and a safe attachment (Carver & Scheier, 1999). With the development of explanatory style, a genetic role exists, the one of the parents. With their behavior, they influence to a great extent the development of the explanatory style in children. An optimistic parent explains negative events in a way in which the child will not have a feeling of guilt, but rather in a way, which will make the child, feel good. The contrary is with the parents of pessimistic explanatory style. They interpret negative and bad situations to their child in a pessimistic way. They explain mistakes made by their children as their laziness and *"incompetence"* (Seligman et al., 1995).

Optimism can be taught in other ways besides from the parents in early childhood. A big influence on the child comes from the early childhood educator. Due to their parents' work, children spend a large part of the day in establishments for early upbringing and education of the child. The educator is the person who, through strategy of planning and leading the educational process, transfers their values, attitudes and ways of thinking to the children and presents the child's behavioral model. That is why it is of utmost importance of educators' behavior towards children, and the way he/she transfers positive emotions as well as the negative ones.

When children, within a family or an educational establishment, constantly meet with positive examples, the chances of adopting optimism and hope from their parents' who use other upbringing styles increases (Raboteg-Šarić, Merkaš & Majić, 2011). A longitudinal research conducted in Finland, with the aim of exploring the influence of the temperaments and upbringing attitudes of mothers on the developments of dispositional optimism during 21 years have demonstrated that unfriendly educational attitudes of mothers predict pessimism (Heinonen et al., 2005). Optimism is positively correlated with a series of other indicators of psychosocial well-being. These are life satisfaction and self-esteem, while it is negatively correlated with depression, anxiety and the extent of experience of stress (Ciarrochi et al., 2007; Scheier et al., 2001; Snyder, Rand & Signom, 2005; Mijočević & Rijavec, 2006).

Positive Emotions and Life Satisfaction Among Early Childhood Educators

Barbara Fredrickson (1998, 2001), with the basis of the Broaden-and-Build theory of positive emotion, highlights that the role of positive emotions exist and is connected to the capability of people to broaden their momentary thought-action repertoires and build their enduring personal resources. Contemporary psychological studies showed that positive emotions improve cognitive activity (Buckley & Saarni, 2009). In one of the studies (Isen, 2002), it was demonstrated that the children who were in a happy mood succeeded in solving the tasks much better than the children who were not induced in such a mood. This and similar studies showed that positive emotions act successfully on solving different problems because they activate thought processes of higher order, as well as creativity. What is known about a good mood is that we remember things connected to it longer than the things we learned under the influence of negative emotions (Miljković & Rijavec, 2009). Emotions are integral part of the educational process (Prosen, Smrtnik Vitulić & Poljšak Škraban, 2011), and they could significantly affect the climate in the educational group or classroom, as well as the children's learning outcomes (Hosotani & Imai-Matsumura, 2011).

Life satisfaction relates to a global evaluation of one's personal life. It makes the cognitive component of subjective well-being (Penezić, 2006). All good and bad aspects of life, including physical hedonism, are included in subjective well-being. *"Life satisfaction is a measure of the subjective well-being of an individual. It can be measured with the help of four components that determine it. These include general satisfaction, satisfaction of certain areas, and the components of positive and negative affective states."* (Rijavec, Miljković & Brdar, 2008:49). Within their work, it is very important for an educator to be satisfied because that is what makes the results of the work much better. Conducted researches speak to that as well. Life satisfaction of early childhood educators (N=295) was explored by Tatalović Vorkapić & Lončarić (2013). The authors of this research pointed out to a great importance and influence of life satisfaction of an educator to the quality of their work and function in a preschool establishment, what was confirmed in further studies (Tatalović Vorkapić & Čepić & Šekulja, 2016; Tatalović Vorkapić & Peloza, 2017). The authors also highlighted the importance of satisfaction, which directly influences on the quality of the learning process and teaching children, because a satisfied educator with high levels of all personality traits except neuroticism contributes a great deal to the high level of subjective well-being. It was established that openness and conscientiousness only have indirect positive effects on life satisfaction, reducing the sense that it diminishes achievements of everyone personally. Koller-Trbović and associates (1996) explored how satisfied are the educators with their personal lives in different life situations, caused by the war, as well as the time after the war in Croatia. They highlight the importance of the research in order to advance the profession, their work and life conditions, and health preservation. Škrinjar emphasizes (1994) the need to attach importance and care for the employees who have the responsible and important job of working with children who are having difficulties in development and can therefore wear the person down. With this research the assumption was that the educator's satisfaction of personal and professional life is a big aspect in the functioning of the professional work. Researchers have assumed that the person who is satisfied with his/her personal life in all areas, healthy and happy, but responsible, competent and capable as well, contributes to a large degree to a good work environment with children and co-workers at the workplace. The aim of the research was to question how the educator functions, and what are his/her needs at the workplace in order to strengthen the profession. The results of the research show that the dissatisfaction of the educator in his/her private life is significantly correlated with the satisfaction at work. Satisfaction of the educator is connected with the working effect. The dissatisfaction of the educator is also correlated with the assessment of previously negative happenings not having strengthen the educators to react better in future situations. The researchers highlight that the educators and their dissatisfaction put themselves into a relation with a passive outlook towards the problems, which cause them: dissatisfaction, rage, anger and the inability to adjust. All stated has a bad and negative impact on the children they are working with and care about. The conclusion of the authors was that it is very important to invest in educators so their work with children with special needs may improve as well. In the Croatian research by Brkić & Rijavec (2011) the aim was to establish whether differences exist in the sources of stress, coping strategies and the life satisfaction between the teachers of children from 1st to 4th grade (N=84) and the teachers of children from

5th to 8th grade (N=96). It was determined that there was no significant difference in the sources of stress, coping strategies or in life satisfaction. The results of the multiple regression analysis have shown that coping with the problem and coping with the emotions are important predictors of life satisfaction. The teachers who deal with the stress by choosing to deal with the problem (problem-oriented strategy) with a positive attitude have better life satisfaction, while the ones who deal with stress by choosing to deal with emotions (emotions-oriented strategy) have lesser life satisfaction. From all stated above, it can be concluded that optimism in people significantly affects their life satisfaction.

Flow And Early Childhood Educators

Csikszentmihalyi (1978, 1988, 1997, 2006) run studies with people who worked on something that gives them pleasure, but are not rewarded for it. Not materialistically, with money, nor with praise. All respondents engaged in different activities. For example, mountaineering, chess, painting etc. He found out that all of them have the same positive pleasant experience, called the flow. One of its characteristics refers to incorporating the activity and the consciousness within the individual. A person engaging in an activity that presents challenge to that individual causes the inclusion of all the skills and capabilities that that individual possesses. Also, the individual is preoccupied with the activity he/she is engaging at that moment. It can be concluded that the activity appeared spontaneously, and automatically the individual has a feeling of satisfaction, preoccupation with this activity. The other characteristic of flow includes a clear goal and feedback to the individual as proof that he/she is completely preoccupied with the activity. The clearer the goal the individual strives for, the faster he/she will get to the feedback and the flow will be stronger. The individuals who experience flow do not have the sense of time or, in other words, in those moments of flow they lose track of time. The state of comfort gives the individual a sense of satisfaction which can be named as the third characteristic of flow. Therefore, flow is characterized by: the merging of the activity and the consciousness, clear goals and feedback, complete focus on the activity, the feeling of control over the situation, loss of self-awareness, and the change in the perception of time, enjoying the activity by itself (Nakamura & Csikszentmihalyi, 2002). In addition, a state of flow ensues when a big, above-average interest, skill and abilities exist (Delle Fave & Massimini, 2004). Activities cause flow. For some it is a routine activity, while for others that same activity is a challenge. Over thirty years of research have shown that there is a relation between flow and positive experiences and well-being (Nakamura & Csikszentmihalyi, 2002). The longer the state of flow exists during a day, the better the quality of their experience – creativity and more positive emotions. For many years researches have proven the existence of a relation between flow and positive experiences as well as well-being. In everyday life, the more we experience the state of flow, the better our quality of experience, the better our creativity and positive emotions we will have. The assumption about the educators experiencing a greater level of flow than some other professions, is a prerequisite of high, both professional and personal, well-being of the educator, which is established in the Croatian research as well (Tatalović Vorkapić & Gović, 2016).

Good Working Organization – Positive Psychology At Work

The working organization has the feature of a complex system whose various parts are connected and functionally harmonized in a way in which they create a steady structure and act as a whole. The organization has certain features, which are: a harmonized effort of members in accomplishing common goals; division of labor; differentiation of parts, hierarchy of position. Many researchers think that today we are dealing with great changes in the structure of the working organization. Thus Toffler (according to Baloch & Kareem, 2007), a famous futurologist, optimistically sees a new employee as: independent, flexible, educated and skilled. The challenges met by every working organization, and the employee him/herself are: the diversity of work force (age, gender, race); globalization; the life/family conflict – work that relates to harmonizing a career and a family; decrease of work force; lifelong learning; the advancement of technology. A considerable amount of every day is being spent in the workplace. It is of utmost importance for the employees' to feel good, and are satisfied and happy. Studies show that experiencing positive emotions considerably affects the work satisfaction (Warr, 1999). While satisfied, the employees are better at solving tasks, making decisions, have a developed creativity, are good towards others, more positive, ready to help, have better understanding for others, are more sympathetic and tolerant (Isen, 2002). Satisfaction of life is in a direct relation with mental health and life satisfaction (Turner & Burling, 2002). Therefore, it is important to know how to increase satisfaction. Positive psychology suggests a solution, or gives its contribution to it. The approach to work is very important and should be based on strengthening human strengths, positive psychological capital and positive leadership.

The claim of Gallup's researchers Buckingham & Coffman (1999) which they reached after including 80 000 managers from more than 400 companies worldwide is based on the ideas that everyone has his/her specific talents, traits and virtues. It is surely important to recognize and use one's talent and traits in his/her work. The best managers are aware of this and are led by it in the workplace, which helps them achieve impressive results. Their guiding light is to assert and derive strong traits with people, as well as develop and strengthen their potentials, while ignoring the weak and bad points of every individual.

At the same time, it has been studied, which factors mostly contribute to satisfaction at work. So, five factors have been determined (Buckingham & Coffman, 1999):

1) *work conditions* (safety at the workplace, salary, policy of the enterprise) – it can be concluded that when the mentioned work conditions are met, the employee feels good at his workplace, works better and more efficient;
2) *the behavior of the immediate manager* (respecting the employees, trust, understanding and development) – it can be concluded that when it comes to positive interpersonal relations, the employee feels appreciated by the management which greatly contributes to increasing working effect;
3) *team/colleges* (the possibility of cooperation, common goals, trust) – teamwork and collegiality contribute to better work through the satisfaction of all employees;
4) *management* (trust in the enterprise's mission and the competence of management) – it is important for improvement and further guidelines of the working organization;
5) *personal commitment to the enterprise* (pride of belonging, intention to stay the lifetime) – in the end it presents a sort of a peak of satisfaction from the employee to the working organization.

The studies show that when it comes to working organizations, which dedicate the importance of developing talents, a positive influence on life satisfaction and behavior in a working organization that is positive is made (Cameron et al., 2003). Many experts believe that the questions of organizational learning are of great importance for the development of quality in educational establishments (Čepić & Krstović, 2011; Čepić, Tatalović Vorkapić & Ružić, 2016). Organizational learning as a complex and unstructured form of learning implies dealing with the professional development of individual as well as organizational goals in an integrated way in order to respond to the challenges of organizational learning. The increase of quality of upbringing and education depends on the professional development of the educator. Professional growth does not occur in vacuum and it is important that it includes other elements in a broader context (such as professional identity, environmental impacts, social circumstances of development and motives for participating in professional development), which can also have an impact on the institutional practice (Čepić & Kalin, 2017).

Therefore, in educational situations, the importance of articulating and verifying educator's values, beliefs, and attitudes is of utmost importance, as they contribute to a better understanding and development of their professionalism and professional identity, as well as to ensuring children's well-being (Čepić & Kalin, 2017). Thoughts and assumption is that if we are satisfied and fulfilled at work, we will be satisfied after the work as well. Also, if we are satisfied at work, the work effect will be better and more productive. This is included in researches that have been conducted. Jeleč Kaker (2009) has conducted a research of the levels of satisfaction of work and the level of burnout in the workplace of social workers (N=57) employed in the Slovenian healthcare. The results have shown dissatisfaction with salary, working conditions, benefits, advancement and rewarding. Social workers are satisfied with communication skills, superiors, colleges and characteristics of work. The participants show a middle level of exhaustion and cynicism and a high level of professional effectiveness. Statistically, the most prominent relation, negative at that, was between cynicism and characteristics of work, exhaustion and working conditions, while there was no significant relation found between professional effectiveness and satisfaction of the workplace. The presence of a high level of correlation between cynicism, exhaustion and work characteristics and working conditions suggests the need for a quality and continuation in tracking of the problem of burnout and (un)happiness of work among the social workers in the healthcare. Therefore, it is completely understandable that many working organizations highlight the work satisfaction as a very important factor. Ilona Boniwell (2008) states ways to increase work satisfaction and encourage positive processes, which are based on the principles of positive psychology. They are: *"Bringing diversity into work, encouraging intrinsic motivation, encouraging creativity, strength-based approach, team development, meta perspective, flow and employee participation, open atmosphere, strengthening and self-organization."* (according to Rijavec & Miljković, 2009:14).

MAIN FOCUS OF THE CHAPTER

Issues, Controversies, Problems

Having in mind the importance of positive psychology in educational work of educators in kindergartens, it is very important to examine their work satisfaction. Thus, the aim of this research is to examine the relation between work satisfaction and certain variables of well-being among educators of preschool children, such as their flow, positive emotions, optimism and life satisfaction. Therefore, the issues of this research are to examine:

1) the work satisfaction of early childhood educators in kindergarten.
2) the well-being of early childhood educators operationalized based on their flow, positive emotions, life satisfaction and optimism.

3) the relation between work satisfaction and all the variables of well-being of early childhood educators (flow, positive emotions, life satisfaction and optimism) and socio-demographic variables (age, work experience).

Based on the theory and former cognition of positive psychology at the workplace and through literature the following hypothesis are set:

1) Considering the lack of former researches, a moderate level of work satisfaction of early childhood educators is expected.
2) Considering the former studies have shown higher levels of all variables of well-being early childhood educators, higher level of the same variables is expected in this research.
3) A significant positive relation between the work satisfaction and all variables of well-being of early childhood educators is expected.

Research Methodology

Participants

The research was conducted on a sample of N=179 early childhood educators from the Kindergarten "Rijeka" in the city of Rijeka, Croatia, exactly from four different centers for preschool education. All the participants were female, with the average age of M=43.40 years (SD=10.91) in the range of 25 to 64 years (from the total of N=197 participants, this question was answered by N=152), with the average work experience of M=20.30 (SD=12.12) in the range of 1 to 46 years (from the total of N=197 participants, this question was answered by N=172). In the complete sample, N=171 (95%) of the participants is employed, of which N=41 (41%) in nursery groups, while N=116 (69.5%) of the participants are in mixed kindergarten groups. As for the distribution of age and work experience, the results of Kolmogorov-Smirnov's test for age (K-Sz= =0.123; $p<0.05$) and work experience (K-Sz=0.007; $p<0.05$) have shown that they significantly differ from the normal distribution. Following these findings, no preconditions for applying parametric statistics have been achieved.

Measures

In this research, a set of standardized questionnaires were applied, which measured the following variables: satisfaction of working organization, flow, positive emotions, optimism and life satisfaction.

Employee perceptions of quality of management practices measured by the *13 Core items Inventory* (Buckingham & Coffman, 1999; Harter & Creglow, 1999) adapted by Rijavec, Miljković and Brdar (2008) was used. Determined Cronbach alpha in this research is at the satisfactory level α=0.843. The questionnaire consisted of 12 items. Example of item: *"I know what's expected of me at work."*

The Flow Questionnaire for measuring early childhood educators' flow has been applied (Csikszentmihalyi, 1975; Csikszentmihalyi & Csikszentmihalyi, 1988) adapted by Rijavec, Miljković and Brdar (2008). With The Flow Questionnaire, the Cronbach alpha coefficient was set at α=0.768. The questionnaire was consisted of 12 items. Example of item: *"I was completely absorbed in the work."* The questionnaire examined the level of flow of the participants-educators at work.

*The Positive and Negative Affective Schedule (*Watson, Clark & Tellegen, 1988), adapted by Rijavec, Miljković & Brdar (2008) was applied for measuring emotions among early childhood educators. It consists of 20 items. The participants evaluate to what extent they are described by various words describing positive and negative affective states. The evaluations could be requested for passed days, present moments or in general. The participants evaluate on the scale of 1-5. (*1= not at all or very little; 2= slightly; 3= moderately; 4= quite; and 5= very*). Example of item: *"Please mark the following adjectives with how you GENERALY feel*: for example *"Excited"*. The results of the study by measuring different emotional states, positive and negative are as follows: for the set of positive emotion items equals α = 0.867, and for the set of negative emotional items equals α = 0.896.

The Satisfaction with Life Scale (SWLS; Diener et al., 1985), adapted by Rijavec, Miljković & Brdar (2008) was used for measuring life satisfaction among early childhood educators. It consists of 5 items, 4 of which are affirmative and one negating, but in compliment to the meaning of the scale. An example of item from the questionnaire is: *"I am satisfied with my life."* In the research conducted by Rijavec, Miljković & Brdar (2008) on the students of the faculties in Rijeka and Zagreb, Cronbach alpha coefficient of life satisfaction of the educators equaled α=0.72 while in this research, with the educators from the Kindergarten "Rijeka", it equaled α=0.843 which shows a satisfactory level of reliability.

The Life Orientation Test Revised (LOT-R, Scheier et al., 1994) adapted by Rijavec, Miljković & Brdar (2008) was applied for measuring early childhood educators' optimism. This questionnaire was consisted of 6 items which characterize clarity and simplicity. After recording the claims, the estimates are added up. One item example is: *"In uncertain times, I usually expect the best."* In this research, which referred to the optimism of an educator of preschool children, it was established that the Cronbach alpha coefficient equaled α=0.710, what is satisfactory.

Likert's scale of 5 degrees by registering the appropriate numeric value depending on how much they agree or disagree with a statement (*1 = totally disagree; 2 = partially disagree; 3 = maybe, I agree and disagree; 4 = partially agree; 5 = completely agree*) has been used for subjects' evaluations on all questionnaires except PANAS.

Procedure

After an official appeal to the Kindergarten "Rijeka" with the request to conduct a research by the Faculty of Teacher Education in Rijeka the approval of the principal of the kindergarten was obtained. A part of this research was conducted within the frame of a graduate thesis by Jasna Crnčić under the title: *"Positive psychology at work – How do the educators perceive their satisfaction of work in kindergartens?"*. The memo contained the purpose, the aim of the research as well as the contact information of the researchers along with a short description of the research. The same memo contained the proposed possibility of reporting the results of the research in a verbal or written form, if the institution desired it.

The gathering of data was conducted via the survey of an adequate sample in the Kindergarten "Rijeka". Filling out the questionnaire was conducted individually during the educators' brakes with a written explanation of the aim and the purpose of the research. Filling out the questionnaire was anonymous, voluntarily and confidential. The written instructions were as follows: *"Taking part is anonymous and voluntarily. Please answer the question genuinely. The filling of the questionnaire takes about 10 minutes. Who does not want to participate in filling in the questionnaires, please return the blank poll. Thank you for your understanding and cooperation."* It is emphasized that the ones who really want to, because of the importance of a correct i.e. honest answer in order for the data to be credible fill the questionnaires.. For the purposes of the research, no personal information of the educators were used, and the results were analyzed at a CPO level. The filling of the questionnaires took about ten minutes. A total of 245 questionnaires were distributed. In the processing of results, a computer program SPSS.20 was used. In the statistical data processing, a descriptive and correlation statistical analyses were conducted.

SOLUTIONS AND RECOMMENDATIONS

Early Childhood Educators' Satisfaction With Work – Professional Well-Being

The first research problem referred to the examination of satisfaction with work of the educators in kindergarten. The arithmetic mean of the satisfaction was determined of M=3.62 (SD=0.68), in the range of 1.69 to 4.92. Regarding the professional well-being, results showed that early education teachers were moderately satisfied with their work. Very few studies have been made about the satisfaction with work of educators. Kim & Loadman (1994) state the results of the meta analysis which showed that only 2% of research about satisfaction of the educators' work is conducted on the scale of special education or kindergarten.

The research run by Šimić-Šašić, Karin & Lapić (2011), in which participated 92 educators from the Croatian kindergartens, demonstrated that educators were moderately satisfied with their work (M=3.70), (SD=0.65). Moreover, 50% of the educators are *satisfied*, 11.96% are *totally satisfied*, and 38.04% are *somewhat satisfied* with their work. Similar results with the gained values were established in this research which confirms the moderate level of satisfaction of work as an educator. Recently, authors state that the interventions directed towards strengthening the commitment to work are more efficient than the interventions directed towards relieving stress and preventing burnout at the workplace (Maslach, 2003), so this has to be taken into account while planning future activities directed towards the quality of our educational system, so that the capable teachers/educators would retain in it.

For example, the authors Čepić & Pliško-Seferagić (2016) conducted a research on the sample of 178 educators from 9 kindergartens in the Istrian County with the goal of examining the quality of the teaching process in kindergartens from the perspective of the educators. Results have shown that in further actions directed towards the development of the "inside quality" in kindergartens need more attention especially toward improving of communication within the establishments, strengthening the cooperation between the educators and decreasing the bureaucracy. Results of correlation analysis showed that the higher number of employed workers in a kindergarten, years of working experience and a higher number of children in a group generates less satisfaction of educators in the working environment, while a more proactive style of leadership from the principal leads to a greater satisfaction. It has been shown that institutional measurements of stimulating positively correlate with financial results and results of learning.

A research conducted by Peko and colleagues (2009) was dealing with the examination of how primary school teachers (N=180) and pedagogues (N=85) view the quality of school management, and analyzed the relation between variables: management, school environment, organizational efficiency and work satisfaction. Based on the correlated analysis, a statistically significant and positive correlation of all examined variables was established. Therefore, a high and significant correlation of value between perception of organizational efficiency and the school environment was established, which confirms the data from other researches about the connection of those variables (Domović, 2003). This means that it is of great importance that the educational employees of all profiles are satisfied of the working organization because they work with more quality and stimulus, have better environment and mood. It can be concluded that there is a correlation between the attitude of a worker and working effectiveness, which is confirmed by the Peko & associates' research (2009), as well as this one.

Early Childhood Educators' Personal Well-Being

The second problem of the research refers to the examination of well-being of educators via their life satisfaction, optimism, flow, positive emotions and negative emotions. In Picture 1 we can see the established average values of stated variables which are the basis of an educators' personal well-being. Results have shown that the level of life satisfaction M=3.89 (SD=0.75) in the range of 1.40 to 5.00; level of optimism M=4.02 (SD=0.66) in the range of 1.83 to 5.00; and the level of flow M=4.06 (SD=0.52) in the range of 2.25 to 5.00. As for the emotions which are most experienced by the educators in the workplace, total levels of positive emotions M=37.72 (SD=5.81) in the range of 16-50 were established, as well as the total levels of negative emotions M=15.07 (SD=5.64) in the range of 10-36. The established results point to a moderate level of personal well-being of the educators, with a significantly larger presence of positive emotions as opposed to negative emotions. Therefore, the results about their personal well-being demonstrated moderate to high levels of optimism, positive emotions, flow and life satisfaction. Furthermore, when comparing the received results of this research with the results of similar research conducted by Tatalović Vorkapić & Jelić Puhalo (2016), this research shows a higher level of life satisfaction with the educators from Kindergarten "Rijeka", which points out to the importance of the place of work variable. Also, in the same research (Tatalović Vorkapić & Jelić Puhalo, 2016) a lower level of optimism has been established as opposed to this research, which brings into light the type of sample of educators participating in the research, since these participants were from war-stricken counties of Croatia.

Finally, comparing the established results referring to the flow of the educators, with the research from Tatalović Vorkapić & Gović (2016) a similarity in the gained findings is visible. It can be assumed that a higher level of flow within the workplace of the educators due to creativity, the possibility of activity choice, affection towards the work, sensibility towards the children and a free choice of work they do and enjoying the work that gives them the possibility of freedom and innovativeness. Namely, the author Csikszentmihalyi, in his book "*Flow*" (2006) notes that work can be a pleasure, even the most pleasurable part of life.

The Relationship Between Professional And Personal Well-Being Among Early Childhood Educators In Croatia

The third problem of the research refers to the examination of the relation of work satisfaction with all variables of well-being with educators (flow, positive emotions, life satisfaction and optimism) and with socio-demographic variables (age and work experience). Considering the fact that no prerequisites of appliance of parametric

Table 1. Correlation matrix between work satisfaction, flow, positive emotions, life satisfaction, optimism, age and work experience

	Flow	Positive emotions	Life satsfaction	Optimism	Age	Work experience
Work satisfaction	**0.413****	**0.384****	**0.387****	**0.350****	**-0.205***	**-0.215****
Age	0.127	-0.105	-0.084	**-0.227****	1.000	**0.938****
Work experience	0.120	-0.080	-0.125	**-0.234****	**0.938****	1.000

*p=0.05; ** p=0.01

statistic have been made, a nonparametric statistic has been made my calculating the Spearman's coefficient of correlation, and coefficients and statistical significance were established, as shown in Table 1. Correlation analyses revealed significant positive relationship between high levels of all personal well-being dimensions and high level of work satisfaction. In other words, the more the educators are satisfied with their work, the more flow they have, the more they experience positive emotions at work, the better their life satisfaction is, and have significantly higher optimism.

Additionally, it was determined that older and highly experienced early childhood teachers are significantly less satisfied with work and less optimistic. It is assumed that his is due to exhaustion, losing interest for work or disinterest because of worse materialistic conditions or even saturation. A satisfied educator is more positive, cheerful, ready to cooperate, communicative, aspire to change, learning, changing ones' own practice, and all of that is positively held on the educational practice. An educator who loves the work, is preoccupied with progress and ambition, certainly has his/her goals he/she wants to achieve and work for. Of course, for all of this, he/she has a way, a strategy and a plan. As for the desire of achieving the goal, problems and unforeseen situations are necessary. Precisely in the work of upbringing and educating there is a series of changeability and unpredictability. In order to overcome and get rid of the negativity, it is very important that the educator has a positive attitude, way of thinking and acting. Also to have hope and optimism which will help cope with stressful and unpredictable situations, and at the same time alleviate the way to the planned and imagined goal. An educator who has a cheerful spirit, acknowledges a good relationship, is of a positive attitude greatly influences the development of positive attitude, hope and positive way of thinking. All of the above is the best and most appropriate way of developing optimism within the children of preschool years. Therefore, it is assumed that the educators with positive thoughts and an optimistic outlook and the feeling of satisfaction with their life influence all of that to others around them. Contrary to this, negative emotions and attitudes act in a depressing and disincentive ways, stop and prevent the realizing of the intended goal, which decreases the chances that a person will be satisfied with his/her life (Halama, 2010).

Research have shown that the people who are satisfied with their lives have better marriages, accomplish better social relationships, are more resistant to stress, are more effective in the workplace, are healthier and emotionally more stable (Diener et al., 2002; Hills & Argyle 2001; Lyubomirsky 2001; Brajša- Žganec & Kaliterna Lipovčan, 2006). Since personal and professional well-being of early childhood teachers is generally at moderate level in this study, lifelong learning programs should be aimed at the content that enhances their overall well-being.

FUTURE RESEARCH DIRECTIONS WITH CONCLUSIONS

The research aim was to question the satisfaction of educators in a working organization in which they work, as well as to analyze the relation between their professional well-being and variables of personal well-being (life satisfaction, optimism, flow and positive emotions) and socio-demographic variables (age and length of service).

Summed up, it was established that the employers are moderately satisfied with their work, and they show a heighten level of well-being in relation to all individual variables. Considering the correlation analysis, it was established that their professional and personal well-being are considerably positively related, and that their satisfaction at work and optimism are considerably higher with younger educators and ones with shorter length of service.

When interpreting the received data it needs to be taken into account that the results might be different if the sample of examinee's was from other parts of Republic of Croatia, and not only from the city of Rijeka, specifically from the city's kindergartens. Namely, the specificity of some kindergartens, in this case it were the kindergartens under the local city administration, probably had an influence on the received results when talking about life satisfaction of the educator. If the private kindergartens in the city of Rijeka were included, it is assumed that different results would be given. There is an assumption that in other cities in the Republic of Croatia there is also a difference in the satisfaction of educators working in kindergartens. This means that the next research should be conducted on a much larger, random and therefore a representative sample, which would allow the generalization of the results of the research.

The results which established the relation between age and life satisfaction might be different than the existing ones if some other variables were included, such as: marriage status, physical health, number of friends, self-respect and appreciation which, by the theoretical frames of Rijavec, Miljković & Brdar (2008) considerably influence the level of life satisfaction. Also, it would be desirable for the future researches to add length of work experience along with different age groups (probationer, educators from 10 to 30 years of work experience and educators over 30 years of work experience – the ones nearing retirement) include the students from the Early and preschool education and include the variable of the reason of choosing that study. That would possibly give more precise results on their level of optimism and life satisfaction.

No matter the stated disadvantages of this study, this paper shows the importance of research in the preschool upbringing and education area. It is a good "way", a direction for improvement, development of the educators and their profession. The future of educational work, improvement of quality and its development in a professional sense, depends primarily on the engagement of the educator and the expert teams of preschool establishments. The educator him/herself is the carrier of change and progress. It is up to him/her how much he/she will be appreciated, accepted and respected. That is why we hope this study will be encouragement to educators to continue experimenting, learning by doing, exploring their own practice and attain a lifelong education so they would gain the necessary competences. Educators should take part in planning and making decisions more often, and take bigger responsibility for their own professional development and learning. If we aim towards the question of *How do we professionally develop?*, most of the experts will agree that we learn above all from practice, reflections of practice and in practice. Analyzing early childhood educators' practice and the results of practice in relation to set assumptions and solving problems through reflection educators develop knowledge which is a result of action and their professional competence. Although there is no miracle recipe, we must highlight that the professional growth of an educator cannot be ignored and underestimated as well as being based on simplified, rationalist or bureaucratic models which negate the complex character of organization and practice and a part of the educators autonomy. Only by everyday exploration of the practice, connection among the kindergartens, and sharing experience can we improve the existing state and quality of the profession of the educational system. All of this combined will contribute to raising the social reputation and quality of work of an educator as well as securing optimal working conditions.

We hope that this paper will contribute to further researches in the area of preschool education and broadening new cognitions of the area. The research can help professional associates with coming up with educational workshops, reflections and supervisions which can contribute to profession strengthening of an educator. Among the key factors in the development of successful educational establishments are surely the improved autonomy and strengthening of the educators. Establishing such a climate and culture in which the professional development of an educator would take place via the mutual cooperation, conversation, search for constructive solutions collectively and mutual learning. Ideas and information should arise from the ones with something to contribute, no matter their position within the organization. Educational establishments should create management structures which enable the inclusion and decision making of the educator, because the educators are the ones affecting the change in their establishments. A great importance in all this lies in the principle whose role is to actively cooperate in the assessment of the current state of affairs, and contribute to the planning of the future and directing changes and innovations in kindergartens to the satisfaction of the works of all its employees.

ACKNOWLEDGMENT

We would like to thank all early childhood educators and parents who agreed to participate in this study and Jasna Crnčić for her support in research. Also, we would like to thank Lovro Lisjak on his professional support in translating the chapter. This work has been supported in part by the Faculty of Teacher Education and in part by University of Rijeka under the project „*Children's well-being in transition periods: the empirical validation of ecological-dynamic model*", no. uniri-drustv-18-11.

REFERENCES

Aelterman, A., Engels, N., Van Petegem, K., & Verhaeghe, J. P. (2007). The well-being of teachers in Flanders: The importance of a supportive school culture. *Educational Studies*, *33*(3), 285–297. doi:10.1080/03055690701423085

Argyris, C., & Schön, D. A. (1978). *Organizational Learning: A Theory of Action Perspective*. San Francisco, CA: Josse.y-Bass.

Baloch, Q. B., & Kareem, N. (2007). Book Review: *The third wave. Journal of Managerial Sciences*, *1*(2), 115–143.

Boniwell, I. (2008). *Positive psychology in a nutshell* (2nd ed.). London: PWBC.

Brajša-Žganec, A., & Kaliterna Lipovčan, Lj. (2006). Kvaliteta življenja, životno zadovoljstvo i sreća osoba koje profesionalno pomažu drugima. *Društvena istraživanja*, *4-5*(84-85), 713-728. Retrieved from http://hrcak.srce.hr/10874

Brdar, I., & Bakarčić, S. (2006). Suočavanje s neuspjehom u školi: Koliko su važni emocionalna kompetentnost, osobine ličnosti i ciljna orijentacija u učenju? *Psihologijske Teme*, *15*(1), 129–150.

Brkić, I., & Rijavec, M. (2011). Izvori stresa, suočavanje sa stresom i životno zadovoljstvo učitelja razredne i predmetne nastave. *Napredak, 152*(2), 211– 225. Retrieved from http://hrcak.srce.hr/file/123100

Buckingham, M., & Coffman, C. (1999). *First, Break all the Rules: What the world's greatest managers do differently*. New York: Simon & Schuster.

Buckley, M., & Saarni, C. (2009). Emotion regulation: Implications for positive youth development. In R. Gilman, E. S. Huebner, & M. J. Furlong (Eds.), *Handbook of positive psychology in schools* (pp. 107–118). New York, NY: Routledge.

Cameron, K. S., Dutton, J. E., & Quinn, R. E. (2003). *Positive Organizational Scholarship*. San Francisco: Berrett-Koehler.

Carver, C. S., & Scheier, M. F. (1999). Stress, coping, and self-regulatory processes. In L. A. Pervin & O. P. John (Eds.), *Handbook of personality: Theory and research* (pp. 553–575). New York, NY: Guilford Press.

Čepić, R., & Kalin, J. (2017). *Profesionalni razvoj učitelja: status, ličnost i transverzalne kompetencije*. Rijeka: Učiteljski fakultet Sveučilišta u Rijeci.

Čepić, R., & Krstović, J. (2011). Through lifelong learning and learning organisations towards sustainable future. *International Journal of Innovation and Learning, 10*(2), 195–213. doi:10.1504/IJIL.2011.041797

Čepić, R., & Pliško-Seferagić, L. (2016). Poticanje razvoja infrastrukture kontinuiranog učenja: izazov za odgajatelje. In N. Tatković, M. Radetić-Paić, & I. Blažević (Eds.), Kompetencijski pristup kvaliteti ranog i predškolskog odgoja i obrazovanja (pp. 281-294). Medulin: Dječji vrtić Medulin i Fakultet za odgojne i obrazovne znanosti Sveučilišta Jurja Dobrile u Puli.

Čepić, R., Tatalović Vorkapić, S., & Ružić, S. (2016). Samovrednovanje kvalitete procesa učenja na individualnoj, timskoj i organizacijskoj razini iz perspektive učitelja. *Školski vjesnik, 65*, 11-21.

Chang, E. C., Sanna, L. J., & Yang, K.-M. (2003). Optimism, pessimism, affectivity, and psychological adjustment in US and Korea: A test of a mediation model. *Personality and Individual Differences, 34*(7), 1195–1208. doi:10.1016/S0191-8869(02)00109-5

Ciarrochi, J., Heaven, P. C. L., & Davies, F. (2007). The impact of hope, self-esteem, and attributional style on adolescents' school grades and emotional well-being: A longitudinal study. *Journal of Research in Personality, 41*(6), 1161–1178. doi:10.1016/j.jrp.2007.02.001

Csikszentmihalyi, M. (1975). *Beyond boredom and anxiety*. San Francisco: Jossey Bass. Row.

Csikszentmihalyi, M. (1978). Attention and the holistic aproach to behavior. In K. S. Pope & J. L. Singer (Eds.), *The stream of consciousness* (pp. 335–358). New York: Plenum. doi:10.1007/978-1-4684-2466-9_13

Csikszentmihalyi, M. (1997). *Finding Flow*. New York: Basic Books.

Csikszentmihalyi, M. (2000). *Beyond boredom and anxiety. Experiencing flow in work and play*. San Francisco: Jossey-Bass. (Original work published 1975)

Csikszentmihalyi, M. (2006). *Zanesenost [Flow]*. Zagreb: Naklada Slap. (in Croatian)

Csikszentmihalyi, M., & Csikszentmihalyi, I. S. (1988). *Optimal Experience: Psychological studies of flow in consciousness*. Cambridge, UK: Cambridge University Press. doi:10.1017/CBO9780511621956

Delle Fave, A., & Massimini, F. (2004). Bringing subjectivity into focus: optimal experiances, life themes and person-centred rehabilitation. In P. A. Linley & S. Joseph (Eds.), *Positive Psyhology in Practice* (pp. 581–597). London: Wiley & Sons.

Diener, E., Emmons, R. A., Larsen, R. J., & Griffin, S. (1985). The Satisfaction with Life Scale. *Journal of Personality Assessment*, *49*(1), 71–75. doi:10.120715327752jpa4901_13 PMID:16367493

Diener, E., Lukas, R.E. & Oishi, S. (2002). Subjective Well-Being. The Science of Happiness and the Satisfaction. Part III. *Emotional-Focused Approaches*, 63-73.

Domović, V. (2003). *Školsko ozračje i učinkovitost škole*. Jastrebarsko: Naklada Slap.

Fredrickson, B. L. (1998). What good are positive emotions? *Review of General Psychology*, *2*(3), 300–319. doi:10.1037/1089-2680.2.3.300 PMID:21850154

Fredrickson, B. L. (2001). The role of positive emotions in positive psychology: The broaden-and-build theory of positive emotions. *The American Psychologist*, *56*(3), 218–226. doi:10.1037/0003-066X.56.3.218 PMID:11315248

Halama, P. (2010). Hope as a mediator between personality traits and life satisfaction. *Studia Psychologica*, *52*(4), 309–314.

Harter, J. K., & Creglow, A. (1999). A meta-analysis and utility analysis of the relationship between core employee opinions and business outcomes. In M. Buckingham & C. Coffman (Eds.), First, break all the rules (pp. 255-267). New York: Simon & Schuster.

Heinonen, K., Räikkönen, K., & Keltikangas-Järvinen, L. (2005). Dispositional optimism: Development over 21 years from the perspectives of perceived temperament and mothering. *Personality and Individual Differences*, *38*(2), 425–435. doi:10.1016/j.paid.2004.04.020

Hills, P., & Argyle, M. (2001). Happiness, introversion-extraversion and happy introverts. *Personality and Individual Differences*, *30*(4), 595–608. doi:10.1016/S0191-8869(00)00058-1

Hosotani, R., & Imai-Matsumura, K. (2011). Emotional experience, expression, and regulation of high-quality Japanese elementary school teachers. *Teaching and Teacher Education*, *27*(6), 1039–1048. doi:10.1016/j.tate.2011.03.010

Isen, A. M. (2002). A role of neuropsychology in understanding the facilitating influence of positive affect on social behavior and cognitive process. In C. R. Snyder & S. J. Lopez (Eds.), *Handbook of positive psychology* (pp. 528–540). New York: Oxford University Press.

Jeleč Kaker, D. (2009). Zadovoljstvo poslom i sagorijevanje na poslu socijalnih radnika u zdravstvu u Republici Sloveniji. *Ljetopis Socijalnog Rada*, *16*(3), 537–549. http://hrcak.srce.hr/47814

Kim, I. & Loadman, W. E. (1994). *Predicting teacher job satisfaction.* ERIC Document Reproduction Service No. ED 383707.

Koller-Trbović, N., Žižak, A., & Tasić, D. (1996). Zadovoljstvo odgajatelja osobnim životom u promijenjenim okolnostima. *Kriminologija & Socijalna Integracija*, *4*(2), 120–126.

Lyubomirsky, S. (2001). Why are some people happier than others? The role of cognitive and motivational processes in well-being. *The American Psychologist*, *56*(3), 239–249. doi:10.1037/0003-066X.56.3.239 PMID:11315250

Maslach, C. (2003). Job burnout: New directions in research and intervention. *Current Directions in Psychological Science*, *12*(5), 189–192. doi:10.1111/1467-8721.01258

Matlin, M. W., & Stang, D. J. (1978). *The Pollyanna principle. Selectivity in language, memory, and thought*. Cambridge, MA: Schenkman.

McCallum, F., & Price, D. (2010). Well teachers, well students. *Journal of Student Wellbeing*, *4*(1), 19–34. doi:10.21913/JSW.v4i1.599

McCallum, F., Price, D., Graham, A., & Morrison, A. (2017). *Teacher wellbeing: A review of the literature.* The University of Adelaide.

Mijočević, I., & Rijavec, M. (2006). Optimistični i pesimistični eksplanatorni stil i školski uspjeh u višim razredima osnovne škole [Optimistic and pessimistic explanatory styles and school performance in the higher forms of elementary school]. *Odgojne Znanosti*, *8*(2), 347–360.

Miljković, D., & Rijavec, M. (2009). Važnost pozitivnih emocija u odgoju i obrazovanju [The Significance of Positive Emotions in Education]. Napredak, 150(3-4), 488-506.

Myers, D. G., & Diener, E. (1995). Who is happy? *Psychological Science*, *6*(1), 10–19. doi:10.1111/j.1467-9280.1995.tb00298.x

Nacionalni kurikulum za rani i predškolski odgoj i obrazovanje. (2014). *Ministarstvo znanosti, obrazovanja i sporta* [The National Framework Curriculum of the Pre-school Education. Ministry for science, education and sport: Republic of Croatia]. Retrieved from http://www.azoo.hr/images/strucni2015/Nacionalni-kurikulum-za-rani-i-predskolski-odgoj-i-obrazovanje.pdf

Nakamura, J., & Csikszentmihalyi, M. (2002). The concept of flow. In C. R. Snyder & S. J. Lopez (Eds.), *Handbook of positive psychology* (pp. 89–105). New York: Oxford University Press.

Peko, A., Mlinarević, V., & Gajger, V. (2009). Učinkovitost vođenja u osnovnim školama. *Odgojne Znanosti*, *11*(2), 67–84.

Penezić, Z. (2006). Zadovoljstvo životom u adolescentnoj i odrasloj dobi. *Društvena istraživanja, 15*(4-5), 643-669. Retrieved from hrcak.srce.hr/10864

Peterson, C., & de Avila, M. E. (1995). Optimistic explanatory style and the perception of health problems. *Journal of Clinical Psychology*, *51*(1), 128–132. doi:10.1002/1097-4679(199501)51:1<128::AID-JCLP2270510120>3.0.CO;2-1 PMID:7782467

Plomin, R., Scheier, M. F., Bergeman, C. S., Pedersen, N. L., Nesselroade, J. R., & McClearn, G. E. (1992). Optimism, pessimism and mental health: A twin/adoption analysis. *Personality and Individual Differences*, *13*(8), 921–930. doi:10.1016/0191-8869(92)90009-E

Prosen, S., Smrtnik Vitulić, H., & Poljšak Škraban, O. (2011). Teachers' Emotional Expression in Interaction with Students of Different Ages. *Center for Educational Policy Studies Journal*, *1*(3), 141–157.

Raboteg-Šarić, Z., Merkaš, M., & Majić, M. (2011). Nada *i* optimizam adolescenata u odnosu na roditeljski odgojni stil. *Napredak, 152*(3 - 4), 373 – 388. Retrieved from hrcak.srce.hr/file/123149

Rettew, D., & Reivich, K. (1995). Sports and explanatory style. In G. M. Buchanan & M. E. P. Seligman (Eds.), *Explanatory style* (pp. 173–185). Hillsdale, NJ: Lawrence Erlbaum Associates, Inc.

Rijavec, M., & Miljković, D. (2008). Pozitivna psihologija na poslu [Positive psychology at work]. Zagreb: IEP – D2.

Rijavec, M., Miljković, D., & Brdar, I. (2008). Pozitivna psihologija [Positive psychology]. Zagreb: IEP-D2.

Robins, C. J., & Hayes, A. M. (1995). An appraisal of cognitive therapy. In M. J. Mahoney (Ed.), *Cognitive and constructive psychotherapies* (pp. 41–65). New York: Springer.

Scheier, M. F., Carver, C. S., & Bridges, M. W. (1994). Distinguishing optimism from neuroticism (and trait anxiety, self-mastery, and self-esteem): A re-evaluation of the Life Orientation Test. *Journal of Personality and Social Psychology*, *67*(6), 1063–1078. doi:10.1037/0022-3514.67.6.1063 PMID:7815302

Scheier, M. F., Carver, C. S., & Bridges, M. W. (2001). Optimism, pessimism, and psychological well-being. In E. C. Chang (Ed.), *Optimism and Pessimism: Implications for theory, research, and practice* (pp. 189–216). Washington, DC: American Psychological Association. doi:10.1037/10385-009

Schulman, P. (1995). Explanatory style and achievement in school and work. In G. McC. Buchanan & M. E. P. Seligman (Eds.), *Explanatory style* (pp. 159–171). Hillsdale, NJ: Lawrence Erlbaum Associates.

Seligman, M. E. P. (1998). *Learned optimism*. New York: Pocket Books.

Seligman, M. E. P., Reivich, K., Jaycox, L., & Gillham, J. (1995). *The Optimistic Child*. Boston, MA: Houghton Mifflin.

Šimić Šašić, S., Klarin, M., & Lapić, L. (2011). Percepcija odgovornosti, društvenog statusa i zadovoljstvo poslom kod odgojiteljica. *Magistra Iadertina, 6,* 17-32. Retrieved from http://hrcak.srce.hr/87329

Škrinjar, J. (1994). *Profesionalna opterećenost i sindrom burnout djelatnika u ustanovama za rehabilitaciju osoba s težom mentalnom retardacijom* (Disertation). Zagreb: Fakultet za defektologiju, Sveučilište u Zagrebu.

Snyder, C. R., Rand, K. L., & Sigmon, D. R. (2005). Hope Theory: A Member of the Positive Psychology Family. In Handbook of Positive Psychology. Oxford University Press.

Tatalović Vorkapić, S. (2012). The significance of preschool teacher's personality in early childhood education: Analysis of Eysenck's and Big Five Dimensions of personality. *International Journal of Psychology and Behavioral Sciences*, *2*(2), 28–37. doi:10.5923/j.ijpbs.20120202.05

Tatalović Vorkapić, S. (2015). How much personality is important in educational context? In *International Conference EDUvision 2015: "Modern Approaches to Teaching Coming Generation"* (pp. 75-83). EDUvision, Stanislav Jurjevčič. Retrieved from http://eduvision.si/Content/Docs/Zbornik%20prispevkov%20EDUvision%20 2015.pdf

Tatalović Vorkapić, S. (2017). Personality and Education: Contemporary issues in Psychological science about Personality in Teacher Education. In C. Martin & D. Polly (Eds.), *Handbook of Research on Teacher Education and Professional Development Professional Development* (pp. 163–186). IGI Global.

Tatalović Vorkapić, S., Čepić, R., & Šekulja, I. (2016). Are there any differences in personality traits and life satisfaction between preschool and primary school teachers? *Journal of Research in Childhood Education*, *30*(3), 361–373. doi:10.1080/02568543.2016.1179236

Tatalović Vorkapić, S., & Gović, A. (2016). Relationship between flow and personality traits among preschool teachers. *Metodički obzori, 11*(1), 24-40. Retrieved from https://hrcak.srce.hr/168804

Tatalović Vorkapić, S., & Jelić Puhalo, J. (2016). Povezanost osobina ličnosti, nade, optimizma i zadovoljstva životom odgojitelja predškolske djece [The connection of personality traits of pre-school teachers with their hopes, optimism and life satisfaction]. Napredak, 157(1-2), 205-220.

Tatalović Vorkapić, S., & Lončarić, D. (2013). Posreduje li profesionalno sagorijevanje učinke osobina ličnosti na zadovoljstvo životom odgajatelja predškolske djece? [Does Professional Burnout Mediate the Effects of Personality Traits on Life Satisfaction among Preschool Teachers?]. *Psihologijske Teme*, *22*(3), 431–455.

Tatalović Vorkapić, S., & Peloza, I. (2017). Exploring the personality traits and well-being among pre-school and primary school teachers in Croatia. *Current Issues in Personality Psychology*, *5*(1), 21–31. doi:10.5114/cipp.2017.65830

Turner, N., Barling, J., Epitropaki, O., Butcher, V., & Milner, C. (2002). Transformational Leadership and Moral Reasoning. *The Journal of Applied Psychology*, *87*(2), 304–311. doi:10.1037/0021-9010.87.2.304 PMID:12002958

Warr, P. (1999). Well-being and the workplace. In D. Kahneman, E. Diener, & N. Schwarz (Eds.), *Well-being: The foundations of hedonic psychology* (pp. 392–412). New York, NY: Russell Sage Foundation.

Watson, D., Clark, L. A., & Tellegen, A. (1988). Development and validation of brief measures of positive and negative affect: The PANAS Scales. *Journal of Personality and Social Psychology*, *47*(6), 1063–1070. doi:10.1037/0022-3514.54.6.1063 PMID:3397865

Chapter 14
The Role of AYUSH in Mental Well-Being

Ranjit Kumar Dehury
https://orcid.org/0000-0002-3926-9459
University of Hyderabad, India

Rajeev Kumar
Indian Institute of Technology, Kharagpur, India

ABSTRACT

Mental wellbeing was the centerpiece of the Indian system of medicine. Many healthcare issues are resolved by the peace of mind and brain stimulating processes. Of late, Government of India adopted many systems of medicines that are complementary to the modern allopathic medicines and named it AYUSH system of medicine. In this Ayurveda, Yoga, Homoeopathy, Siddha, Unani, Swa-rigppa, and additional healing systems are represented. There is also a great need for psychological wellbeing due to the rapid increase in stressful life situations. The current modern medical care is not adequate to provide mental health services in the society. At the same time, many indigenous and AYUSH system have come into action and solve the problem the best way it possible. The chapter focuses on the role of AYUSH system in catering to mental wellbeing in India. The policies of the government of India are to promote mental health and wellbeing in society. The specialties of various systems of medicine in curing the mental health conditions have been elaborated.

DOI: 10.4018/978-1-7998-1185-5.ch014

BACKGROUND

The AYUSH services are used by Indian population very widely over a period of time. The Care and cure is assured in many aspects of healthy life in the population which otherwise deprived from the modern biomedical system of medicine. The modern biomedical system of care is very costly and difficulty to reach by masses in India. The faith of people is always with the AYUSH system of medicine due to its services in millennia of Indian culture and society. The AYUSH services are always targeted in a holistic manner and there is less barriers to access by the people for the services. The Indian system of medicine look at various mental health ailments with harmony in the system which causes less side effects and cure for many diseases. The body and mind are taken as a whole while prescribing medicines in most of the cases. So, there would be cure at mental level.

The World Health Organization defined traditional medicine as the combination of the knowledge, skills, and practices based particularly on the theories, beliefs, and experiences which are indigenous to different cultures irrespective of explicable or not, and helping in management of health, prevention, diagnosis, improvement or treatment of both physical and mental illness (World Health Organization, 2000). The use of traditional medicine in various mental ailments is widely practiced in the world for the benefit of the patients. In India different system of traditional medicines were in use since ancient times with proven results for cure and prevention of mental health ailments. The traditional medicine services were usually accessible to the members of the society widely across time. So, these are the first line of treatment for the community even in unorganized community for mental health services. Moreover, the social and cultural cohesion among members of the society help in dealing with many issues of mental health in the community itself instead of modern day hospital facility which help in recovery of many mental health conditions.

The therapeutic cure of each system of medicine is also well documented by the practitioners of the respective particular system. Many of the practitioners receive training in informal way without going to formal training in the designated institutes in ancient time. The knowledge also transmitted from one generation to other very first in the informal way of training and capacity building by proper handholding. Many of the knowledge are tacit in nature and can be learn by close observation and treatment by the healers. Latter on with the help of codified ancient knowledge many things transmitted easily through generations. These treatment procedures are also many a time evidence based and the method to capture evidence is quite different from the modern laid down guidelines.

Latter on with the trust of the people and requirement of alternative system or complementary system governments start adopting these methods in the system of common public services. It has been found that there is also need of curative system for all mental health ailments. Whereas, the modern system has limited medication for limited mental health ailments. Which necessitates the requirement of alternative system of medicines to provide full coverage for wide rang mental health conditions. At this juncture, the alternative systems comes into picture with their age old curative actions which thy otherwise practiced in the process of cure along with winning the trust of the community.

A large number of people take alternative medicines exclusively or along with the modern biomedicine for many acceptable reasons like faith and cultural acceptability, low cost, and firm belief on the systems of medicine. Moreover, India have starkly very low number of specialists available in the field of psychiatric which provide systematic modern biomedicines for cure of mental health cases (Thirthalli, J., Zhou, L., Kumar, K., Gao, J., Vaid, H., Liu, H., ... & Nichter, M. (2016).

Methodology

This study reviewed various types of reports like existing policies of AYUSH, various guidelines of AYUSH services implementation, and reports of AYUSH systems of medicine in different states and central government. The literature reviewed policy and programme documents, and un-published grey literatures in the form of notes and reports at relevant sections. This is a secondary analysis to elaborate the existing policies and implementation of AYUSH services, and its' loopholes in implementation in mental health services. The opinion and experience of AYUSH care providers are also taken into consideration while treating mental health cases in the respective places. This article describes the existing policies and procedures of mental health services in hospital and community by providing AYUSH medicines in mental health. The details of efficacy of each system of medicine is explained in various sections based on evidences found in literatures directly and indirectly relating to their system. The scientific studies were taken from indexed databases like PubMed, Scopus, and Web of Sciences. The evidences were found out for various mental health ailments and explained the situation and readiness to incorporate those in the mental health programs. The philosophy of each alterative system of medicine is discusses based on the context of mental health services. Ethical approval was not required as all data are used from secondary sources. However, the opinions and arguments of implementing staffs have been gathered without harm to them.

FINDINGS

Mental Health policy in India

Mental Health policy 2014 in India has a vision for improvement of mental health conditions. The policy primarily focus on promotion of mental health care, prevent mental health illness, accelerate recovery of mental illness, and de-stigmatization of mental health conditions. Additionally, it focus on the inclusion of various socio-economic groups for the treatment of mental health. Steps are also taken for increase in accessibility and affordability of quality mental health services throughout the life of a person in the community. The important goals are reduction of distress and disability among mental health patients. The reduction of premature mortality caused by mental health need to be addressed according to the policy. A country wide campaign can be initiated for better understanding of the mental health conditions which would allow creation of awareness in the nation. The creation of stewardship and leadership are desparately needed at various level of governance like national, state, and district levels (Ministry of Health and Family Welfare, Government of India (2014).

There are various acts in India from time to time enacted for the creation of good health in the community. Among them acts and regulations like Mental Health Act-1987, National Mental Health Programme-1982, District Mental Healthcare Mode, District Mental Health Programme-1995, Persons with Disabilities Act-1995, Right to Persons with Disabilities Bill-2002, Mental Healthcare Bill-2013, National Mental Health Policy- 2014, and The Rights of Persons with Disabilities Act- 2016 played crucial roles and responsibility (Kaur, R., & Pathak, R. K. (2017).. All these acts and regulations have their own advantage and weakness in the implementation process. However, still optimal mental health services are not achieved in the community due to poor implementation and lack of adequate resources at various levels.

The policies usually consists of a set of values well organized, having principles and objectives for the improvement of improving health along with reduction of disease. (Whiteford HA, Degenhardt L, Rehm J, Baxter AJ, Ferrari AJ, Erskine HE. Charlson FJ, Norman RE, Flaxman AD, Johns N, Burstein R, Murray CJ. Vos T (2013). Whereas, a specific program is all about setting interventions with specific objective to promote the health along with prevention, treatment and rehabilitation. The program also well monitored and evaluated for further improvement and funding purpose (6. Mental health policy, plans and programmes—updated version 2 (2005) [6]. All these transformative aspects in mental health program implementation played a role for transforming the society in achieving desired targets. The vision by the policy would lead to take strong steps in building capability of mental health through various programs in the community. Over a period of time stewardship is supposed to be there for creation of health care facilities in grass roots level.

Mental health issues including suicide considered to be serious problem globally. As usual India is the largest country for adolescent population which group need more attention for mental health. Evidences found that there preventive care can be provided by peers to the population of mental health adolescents (Roy, K., Shinde, S., Sarkar, B. K., Malik, K., Parikh, R., & Patel, V. (2019). Among the age group of 10-23 years almost 22.9% people live with years lived with disability (YLD). The problems have significant effect on the individual, their family and society at large.

Historical Development of AYUSH System in India

Ancient india have its own system of medicine deeply entrenched in the sciences of Vedas where atharva veda deals with Ayurveda and healing art for the mankind. In British India though there was many people depend on the Indian system of medicine still then very less patronage was there from the British India government. Only princely states provide some shorts of patronage that to trusted few on the provision of medical care relating to indigenous systems. However, people use indigenous medicines at their own trust and resources including mental health. The Government of India through high level committees like Bhore (1946), Mudaliar (1961), and Srivastava Committee (1975) try to reform the health care system in which additional effort were also exerted for improvement of Traditional Complementary and Alternative Medicine for the care of common people in an institutionalized manner [1-3]. Whereas, the National Health Policy (1983) envisaged a phased integration of indigenous medicine with modern medicine for both preventive and cure of various diseases at grass roots level which also include healthy living [4]. With the aim to improve the alternative systems of medicine government create a separate wing known as Department of Indian System of Medicine and Homeopathy (ISM&H) in 1995. The department latter on renamed as AYUSH for stronger emphasis in the year 2005 with more focus to cater many people in the community. In the year 2005, the National Rural Health Mission (NRHM) tried to mainstream AYUSH in many parts of the country in which a lot of AYUSH health centers were opened for the wide spread services of the population with the help of doctors, medicines, and procedures of the respective AYUSH system of medicine [5-7]. The NRHM focuses more on many non-communicable diseases to be cured at AYUSH centers in the county which also focus on mental health. Mental Health conditions are a serious concern at the grass roots level where availability of psychiatrist is highly constrained. However, in 2014 the real change happen when Ministry of AYUSH was established to independently take decisions without much consultation with the ministry of Health and Family Welfare for the propagation of alternate medical systems. The ministry have additional work of stressing on medical education, quality control, drug standardization, and research and development for the wider dissemination of services [8].

Further, the National Health Policy 2017 (NHP-2017) focused more on independent functioning of AYUSH centers in the county for wide rang e of services along with challenging disease conditions which are otherwise difficult to cure in the current biomedical systems. The NHP-2017 make targets for achieving good health including mental and spiritual health among the population within a time fram. It also make provision of funds for functioning of various programs in india with a defined target and time line.

Role of AYUSH System in Mental Health in India

AYUSH system played an important role in serving mental health cases at various level. This is palpable from the trust of the community and evidences gathered by various scientists and clinicians or healers. There is also an ongoing process of evolution of the treatment procedures in alternative system of medicines along with proved and established processes. All the evidences are documented in ancient scripture, and ethnographic evidences in the community. Though clinical trial and many other systemic issues are still exists in gathering evidences, still many aspects in bits and pieces are already proved in the system. AYUSH system is recognized by World Health Organization for cure of many diseases. Indian government also recognize the AYUSH system as a proper interventions for various health conditions including mental health specialization. Various research wings of AYUSH ministry like Central Council for Research in Homoeopaty (CCRH), and Central Council for Indian Medicine (CCIM) invest in conducting research in mental health to address the steepening issues in mental health in India. Further, a lot of investment happen in provision of manpower, medicines and hard infrastructure in provision of mental health services to patients in public health services.

Ayurveda

Ayurveda has its origin in Vedas more than 5000 years ago dealing with art of healing. It classify Tridosha (ie, three bioforces, vata, pitta, and kapha) which is embedded in the theory of humor in the body for maintenance of healthy life. Medications usually involves natural substances, special diets regimen, purification rituals, and some surgical procedures for cure. Mental health uses many of these procedures for prevention and cure in the society by adopting various prosedures (Thirthalli, J., Zhou, L., Kumar, K., Gao, J., Vaid, H., Liu, H., ... & Nichter, M. (2016).

Mental illness and mental health found in Indian texts like the Atharva Veda and other Vedic texts along with traditional system of medicines of Siddha, Unani, and Ayurveda where the detailed explanation is found on mental health and disorders. Latter on the mental hospital found 'chemical revolution' in psychiatric management which is a measure departure from the existing treatment of mental conditions especially in early part of nineteenth century (Sundaram, S.K., Kumar, S. (2018). Ayurveda stil played a big role in management of mental health in India by catering to masses despite the presence of modern-day psychiatric in different hospitals.

Studies shows that there is link of gastrointestinal system and mental health in Ayurveda which is also linked with depression. These age old findings also corroborate with the modern biomedical concept of health. Major Depressive Disorder (MDD) is associated with gut dys-regulation which ultimately linked with mental health (Steer, E. (2019). So, when treatment of mental conditions are taken into condition the entire gastrointestinal system is given importance in addition to preventive care.

The control of various dermatological diseases according to ancient medicine systems (e.g. Ayurveda, Yoga, and Unani) are practice of meditation, exercises, and related practices. The branch of psychodermatology takes care of many dermatological problems by keeping the mind healthy. The integrated approach to skin disease involves taking care of mind, skin and psychological stress (Shenoi, S. D., & Prabhu, S. S. (2018). Thias care and cure is very evidenced from the scientific data and have good impact on the health care system.

Ayurvedic psychiatry help a lot in treatment of many diseases relating to psycho-social concern. It also supplement allopathic and vernacular concerns it high degree of pragmatism (Lang, C. (2018). So, mental health concerns are addressed in the course of time in various branches of traditional medicines to get cure. The specialized branches of Ayurveda have fair dealings with the emerging concerns.

An six day intensive program having holistic instruction and experience in the sphere of mind-body practices usually develop to a remarkable and sustained shift in the overall perception of self-awareness which is part of favorable well-being (Mills, P. J., Peterson, C. T., Pung, M. A., Patel, S., Weiss, L., Wilson, K. L., ... & Chopra, D. (2018). All these proven evidences shows that the Ayurveda have propor regimen for the treatment of the diseases of mental health origin. The systems also help in achieving many aspects of the diseases as an early response.

Neuropsychiatric and neurodegenerative disorders like Alzheimer's disease, Parkinson's disease, schizophrenia, epilepsy, depression and anxiety are posing serious concerns in the society. Whereas, Ayurveda is having solution for treatment along with various nootropic herbs having multiple bioactivities in different disorders. Scattered information is available pertaining to traditional Ayurvedic remedial options for various mental disorders (Sharma, R., Kabra, A., Rao, M. M., & Prajapati, P. K. (2018). Ayurvada helps in cure of many diseases of old age and related to mental health with sharp menthod of treatment in the system. There is also holistic approach for care and cure which is evident from the system of medicine.

Siddha

The Siddha system is contemporary of Ayurveda and mostly flourished in south India. Many of the procedures relating to practice of medicine is similar to the ancient Ayurveda and mostly found in Tamil literature. So, the diagnostic and treatment follows concepts of mind for cure. Siddha help in care and cure of largely south Indian people with the treatments mostly aligned with herbal systems of medicine. The Indian systems of medicine mostly take care of many aspects of care among the mental health patients which is evident from the studies. There are established methods for cure of mental health diseases and certified by the concerned board for the cure of patients. The contribution of Siddha as a system of medicine towards the care and cure of mental health cases is immense. People of certain region also impose faith on the methods of cure without having any detrimental effects.

Yoga

Yoga embodies the unification of a person's consciousness with universal consciousness for achievement of goal of life with a healthy living. There is absolutely no intervention of pharmaceutical regimen for the health of a person. Rather various postures (Asanas), breathing control mechanisms (Pranayama), and Meditation procedures (Dhyana) are adopted as practices to get cure or maintenance of health (Thirthalli, J., Zhou, L., Kumar, K., Gao, J., Vaid, H., Liu, H., ... & Nichter, M. (2016). There are many findings confirm the cure or relative wellbeing of patients by practice of Yoga in different cases and particularly mental health cases.

A therapeutic review of Neti kriya confirm that many disease conditions relating body and mind were cured and especially help in many disease of respiratory tract. Jala neti (Nasal water irrigation) help in enhancing presence of mind, intelligence and improve vision (Meera, S., Rani, M. V., Sreedhar, C., & Robin, D. T. (2019). All these aspects help in mental wellbeing of a person in different situations. Energy is gatyered by practicing Yoga which is very useful in maintenance of health for long period of time in the case of human being. Yoga is not just practices in India but also spread in the entire globe for the benefit of the people in various countries. The mental health remain good among the Yoga practicing people.

In United States of America practice of Yoga practices with special focus on mindfulness helps in safe and effective intervention for paediatric groups. Evidence also found that yoga can control mental health issues among the adolescent populations

(Stephens, I. (2019). All these achievements of yogic practice help in solving many issues of Adolescent groups.

Laughter Yoga (LY) is found to be useful for cure of symptoms of depression within short term period. The LY also help in reduction of residual mood, anxiety and stress symptoms among adults. The LY can be used as a method to reduce depression and improve quality of life (Bressington, D., Mui, J., Yu, C., Leung, S. F., Cheung, K., Wu, C. S. T., ... & Chien, W. T. (2019). The form of Yoga may differ but the effects are always found to be positive if practiced in life for improvement of mental health.

The Mind-body exercises in the form of Yoga offer good cure for the rheumatoid arthritis (RA) patients which leads to improvement of both physical and mental health. In adult worker participating in Yoga have better physical function and mental health can be created by the practice (Greysen, H. M., Hong, O. S., & Katz, P. (2019).

The Yoga is becoming a popular approach for the improvement of the quality of life (QoL) among women with breast cancer as a supplementary care practice in addition to the modern medicine. A meta-analysis was done to assess yoga-specific effects relative to other physical exercise intervention (eg, aerobics) with breast cancer. The study found that yoga is effective as other exercise interventions in improving the QoL of women (El-Hashimi, D., & Gorey, K. M. (2019). The quality of life can be improved even among the patients with critical conditions by practice of Yoga. These thighs are now ad days very popular in different hospitals as additional methods of care due to efficacy.

A study has been conducted among the patients with chronic hemodialysis those suffer from an increased cardiovascular disease, deconditioning, fatigue, sleep disturbances, anxiety and depression, and decreased health related quality of life. Here Yoga is reported to have positive effects over distress and functional performance among the chronic diseases. Interestingly Yoga help in improvement in quality of life, reducing pain, reducing fatigue, solving sleep disturbance, and improving physical functions (Kauric-Klein, Z. (2018). Overall yoga found to be a complementary methods of treatment for the people having many diseases. Mental health and Yoga help in improvement of the system to a great extent.

Naturopathy

The very science of naturopathy advocates for effective use of five fundamental materials like earth, water, fire, air, and ether (space). There is strong advocate of use of these concepts both internally and externally and requirement of changing lifestyle and diet for cure. Pharmacological medications are not advocated for use and practice of spirituality is highly encouraged. Naturopathy provide a scope for going natural. Our system always finds a natural concept to remain healthy both physically and mentally. There are trainers suggests how to go natural way of life. For cure of many ailments. The nature provides many methods without biomedicine for care and cure in the society. The natural processes are always helping in many aspects of human being for the care and cure.

Homoeopathy

Homoeopahy as a system put primacy on mental symptoms for cure and care. Many diseases show mental symptom due to various reasons and can be cured by interventions of medications having cure for mental diseases. The mental symptoms guide a lot to achieve cure in different form in homoepathy. The usual mental conditions like hallucination, depression, illusion, outburst, excessive happiness or sorrow, craving for something, headstrong etc. are some of the important conditions for interventions by homoeopatic drugs.

Contrary to the biomedical model of health homoeopathy considers entire body in a holistic manner and provide services in a broader view with much responsibility. Homoeopathy takes care of the physical, mental and emotional aspects of people for cure. Whereas, other alternative practices like yoga, hypnotherapy and meditation put primacy on 'functional' spiritual practices in which the responsibility in fixed on the person for individual care (Bell, F. (2000).

Evidences found that homoeopatic drugs improve 'sensation of well-being', and support the working of ultra-high dilution effects which otherwise cannot be proved by the existing laboratory methods (Kuzeff, R. M. (1998).

A study found that the sleep disorders among alcoholic is reduced by taking homoeopathic medicines. The homoeopathy treatment can be used to help clients in breaking the cycle of alcohol dependence (Rogers, J. (1997). There are many more diseases can be cured by the method of homoeopathy especially of mental diseases for complete cure. This is trusted methods of treatment in hundreds of countries for the treatment of several diseases. Today the diseases have different concerns for cure and homoeopathy help in many of cases.

Unani

Unani methods way back to the practice of medicines and teaching of Hippocrates and Galen in medicine which is also known as Greco-Arabic (Unan means Greece) medicine.

Though it is established in the Middle Age with the patronage of Arabian and Persian kingdoms and their doctor, but latter on Mughals make it their court medical system with sufficient patronage. So, it become a part of Indian medicine and people adopt it with enormous faith. Unani system of medicine based on the idea of various humours like blood components, phlegm, and both yellow and black bile. It usually adopt similar process like regimental therapeutic procedures, special diets regimen, medicines from available herbs and surgery (Thirthalli, J., Zhou, L., Kumar, K., Gao, J., Vaid, H., Liu, H., ... & Nichter, M. (2016).

The Unani medicine is very ancient and tested by Greek civilization almost 2500 years ago. The Unani medicine aims for near no disease condition in leading a healthy life. The Unani medicine advocate clean and fresh water, clean air and consumption of fresh food for maintenance of disease free life. There is also requirement of maintenance of balance on body and mind for metabolic activity to maintain the evacuation of wastes. The system of medicine largely advocate for promoting health, preventing disease and achieving cure through various regiments and diet therapies (Lone, A. H., Ahmad, T., Anwar, M., Sofi, G., Imam, H., & Habib, S. (2012).

In medicine systems like Ayurveda, Unani, or Chinese traditional medicine the imbalance of different 'elements' and factors for disease are important. Rectification of those imbalances pave the way to cure (Bhuiyan, P., Khatun, Z., Jahan, S., Morshed, T., Rahman, S., Afsana, N. A., ... & Rahmatullah, M. (2013).

There is lack of treatment of patients due to various causes in psychotherapy. Whereas, almost four-fifth of population of India in one way or other depend on Ayurvedic and Unani systems of medicine along with religious treatments consisting of prayers, fasting and various witchcraft and magical rituals (Bagadia, V.N., Shah, L.P., Pradhan, P.V., Gada, M.T. (1979). The faith of Indian people is obvious for the systems of medicines. The cure and care is beyond doubt for mental health conditions.

Malankholia (Melancholia) a condition having mental health concerns like constant grief, fear and dubious aggression is cured by Unani medicines and regimen. This has been well explained in ancient book of "Kitab Al-Havi." The detailed management of diagnosis and treatment of melancholia has been described in the Unani system of medicine by this the suffering of humanity can be mitigated to a great extent (Ahmed, N. Z., Alam, A., Khalid, M., Sheeraz, M., & Qamri, M. A. (2015). Many mental health conditions are well explained in the treaties for cur eof mental health conditions.

Sowa-Rigpa

Sowa-Rigpa is a method of cure well known as the science of healing and otherwise called Amchi medicine. It's also well known as Tibetan medicine which is recognized by government of India for its efficacious cure and provision of services to a section of Indian society. The system of medicine is practiced mostly in Himalayan region by both Tibetan and Indian people especially by tribal and Bhot people. This system adopts many nuances of Ayurveda by adopting predominantly the pharmacological (herbal) interventions (Thirthalli, J., Zhou, L., Kumar, K., Gao, J., Vaid, H., Liu,

H., ... & Nichter, M. (2016). There are many codified method of cure for mental health conditions.

The policies of the government of India are to promote mental health and wellbeing in society is discussed thoroughly.

The specialties of various systems of medicine in curing the mental health conditions have been elaborated.

REFERENCES

Ahmed, N. Z., Alam, A., Khalid, M., Sheeraz, M., & Qamri, M. A. (2015). An Insight on Malankholia (Melancholia): Unani Perspective. *Medical Journal of Islamic World Academy of Sciences, 109*(2459), 1–7.

Bagadia, V. N., Shah, L. P., Pradhan, P. V., & Gada, M. T. (1979). Treatment of mental disorders in India. *Progress in Neuro-Psychopharmacology, 3*(1-3), 109–118. doi:10.1016/0364-7722(79)90075-4 PMID:401334

Bell, F. (2000). The complex'whole': Exploring homoeopathic and spiritual considerations. *The Australian Journal of Holistic Nursing, 7*(1), 31. PMID:11898219

Bhore Committee Report Government of India. (1946). *Report of the Health Survey and Development Committee* (vol. 2). Delhi: Manager of Publications.

Bhuiyan, P., Khatun, Z., Jahan, S., Morshed, T., Rahman, S., Afsana, N. A., & Rahmatullah, M. (2013). *Use of Quranic verses, amulets, numerology, and medicinal plants for treatment of diseases: a case study of a healer in Narsinghdi district.* Bangladesh: American-Eurasian Journal of Sustainable Agriculture.

Bressington, D., Mui, J., Yu, C., Leung, S. F., Cheung, K., Wu, C. S. T., ... Chien, W. T. (2019). Feasibility of a group-based Laughter Yoga intervention as an adjunctive treatment for residual symptoms of depression, anxiety and stress in people with depression. *Journal of Affective Disorders, 248*, 42–51. doi:10.1016/j.jad.2019.01.030 PMID:30711868

El-Hashimi, D., & Gorey, K. M. (2019). Yoga-Specific Enhancement of Quality of Life Among Women With Breast Cancer: Systematic Review and Exploratory Meta-Analysis of Randomized Controlled Trials. *Journal of Evidence-Based Integrative Medicine, 24*.

Government of India. (n.d.). *National Rural Health Mission e meeting people's health needs in rural areas: framework for implementation. 2005-2012.* Ministry of Health and Family Welfare. Available from: http://www.nrhm.gov.in/images/pdf/about-nrhm/nrhm-framework-implementation/nrhmframework-latest.pdf

Greysen, H. M., Hong, O. S., & Katz, P. (2019). The Association Between Yoga Use, Physical Function, and Employment in Adults With Rheumatoid Arthritis. *Holistic Nursing Practice, 33*(2), 71–79. doi:10.1097/HNP.0000000000000296 PMID:30747775

Kaur, R., & Pathak, R. K. (2017). Treatment Gap in Mental Healthcare Reflections from Policy and Research. *Economic and Political Weekly, 52*(31).

Kauric-Klein, Z. (2018). Effect of yoga on physical and psychological outcomes in patients on chronic hemodialysis. *Complementary Therapies in Clinical Practice.* PMID:30712744

Kuzeff, R. M. (1998). Homeopathy, sensation of well-being and CD4 levels: A placebo-controlled, randomized trial. *Complementary Therapies in Medicine, 6*(1), 4–9. doi:10.1016/S0965-2299(98)80050-2

Lang, C. (2018). Translation and purification: Ayurvedic psychiatry, allopathic psychiatry, spirits and occult violence in Kerala, South India. *Anthropology & Medicine, 25*(2), 141–161. doi:10.1080/13648470.2017.1285001 PMID:28480739

Lone, A. H., Ahmad, T., Anwar, M., Sofi, G., Imam, H., & Habib, S. (2012). Perception of health promotion in Unani herbal medicine. *Journal of Herbal Medicine, 2*(1), 1–5. doi:10.1016/j.hermed.2012.02.003

Meera, S., Rani, M. V., Sreedhar, C., & Robin, D. T. (2019). A review on the therapeutic effects of NetiKriya with special reference to JalaNeti. *Journal of Ayurveda and Integrative Medicine.*

Mental health policy, plans and programmes—updated version 2. (2005). *Mental health policy and service guidance package.* World Health Organization.

Mills, P. J., Peterson, C. T., Pung, M. A., Patel, S., Weiss, L., Wilson, K. L., ... Chopra, D. (2018). Change in sense of nondual awareness and spiritual awakening in response to a multidimensional well-being program. *Journal of Alternative and Complementary Medicine (New York, N.Y.), 24*(4), 343–351. doi:10.1089/acm.2017.0160 PMID:29216441

Ministry of AYUSH, Government of India. (2015). Available from: http://www.indianmedicine.nic.in/

Ministry of Health and Family Welfare Government of India. (2011). Available from: http://www.mohfw.nic.in/

Ministry of Health and Family Welfare, Government of India. (2014). *New Pathways New Hope*. National Mental Health Policy of India. Retrieved from https://mohfw.gov.in/sites/default/files/34711242651412939786%20%281%29.pdf

Ministry of Health and Family Welfare, Government of India. (1983). *National Health Policy 1983*. New Delhi: MoHFW. Available from: http://www. communityhealth.in/~commun26/wiki/images/6/64/Nhp_1983.pdf

Ministry of Health and family Welfare, Government of India. (2002). *National Health Policy 2002*. New Delhi: MoHFW. Available from: http://mohfw.nic.in/WriteReadData/l892s/18048892912105179110National%20Health%20policy2002.pdf

Mudaliar Committee Report Government of India. (1961). Report of the Health Survey and Planning Committee. New Delhi: Ministry of Health.

Rogers, J. (1997). Homoeopathy and the treatment of alcohol-related problems. *Complementary Therapies in Nursing & Midwifery*, *3*(1), 21–28. doi:10.1016/S1353-6117(97)80030-3 PMID:9432423

Roy, K., Shinde, S., Sarkar, B. K., Malik, K., Parikh, R., & Patel, V. (2019). India's response to adolescent mental health: A policy review and stakeholder analysis. *Social Psychiatry and Psychiatric Epidemiology*, 1–10. PMID:30607452

Sharma, R., Kabra, A., Rao, M. M., & Prajapati, P. K. (2018). Herbal and holistic solutions for neurodegenerative and depressive disorders: Leads from Ayurveda. *Current Pharmaceutical Design*, *24*(22), 2597–2608. doi:10.2174/1381612824666180821165741 PMID:30147009

Shenoi, S. D., & Prabhu, S. S. (2018). Psychodermatology: An Indian perspective. *Clinics in Dermatology*, *36*(6), 737–742. doi:10.1016/j.clindermatol.2018.08.013 PMID:30446197

Srivastava Committee Report Government of India. (1975). Health series and medical education: a programme for immediate action: a report of the group on medical education and support manpower. New Delhi: Ministry of Health and Family Planning.

Steer, E. (2019). A cross comparison between Ayurvedic etiology of Major Depressive Disorder and bidirectional effect of gut dysregulation. *Journal of Ayurveda and Integrative Medicine*, *10*(1), 59–66. doi:10.1016/j.jaim.2017.08.002 PMID:30655102

Stephens, I. (2019). Case report: The use of medical yoga for adolescent mental health. *Complementary Therapies in Medicine*, *43*, 60–65. doi:10.1016/j.ctim.2019.01.006 PMID:30935556

Sundaram, S. K., & Kumar, S. (2018). Tracing the development of psychosocial rehabilitation from its origin to the current with emphasis on the Indian context. *Indian Journal of Psychiatry*, *60*(6), S253–S256. PMID:29527057

Thirthalli, J., Zhou, L., Kumar, K., Gao, J., Vaid, H., Liu, H., ... Nichter, M. (2016). Traditional, complementary, and alternative medicine approaches to mental health care and psychological wellbeing in India and China. *The Lancet. Psychiatry*, *3*(7), 660–672. doi:10.1016/S2215-0366(16)30025-6 PMID:27209157

Whiteford, H. A., Degenhardt, L., Rehm, J., Baxter, A. J., Ferrari, A. J., Erskine, H. E., ... Vos, T. (2013). Global burden of disease attributable to mental and substance use disorders: Findings from the Global Burden of Disease Study 2010. *Lancet*, *382*(9904), 1575–1586. doi:10.1016/S0140-6736(13)61611-6 PMID:23993280

World Health Organization. (2000). *General Guidelines for Methodologies on Research and Evaluation of Traditional Medicine*. Geneva: World Health Organization.

Chapter 15
Spirituality and Well-Being in a Successful Life

Bhanu Prasad Behera
National Institute of Science and Technology, India

ABSTRACT

Life on earth is about evolving spiritually. Spirituality is not only about meditation and prayer. Life itself is a property of the spirit. Life is about growth, experience, and learning. There are several dimensions that help us to perform our spiritual practices to become internally free and stable. Spiritual wellbeing is a highly personal and universal experience. Spiritual wellbeing is an integral part of emotional, physical, and mental health. Spirituality has positive effects on our lives. It gives peace, freedom, and happiness; helps in treating stress, depression, anorexia; etc. Spiritual wellbeing helps in making relationships better, enhancing personal value, maintaining better work-life balance, understanding the personal value, time to spend alone, finding inner peace, finding job satisfaction, maintaining active lifestyle, balancing and controlling life, better health and longer life, a strong spiritual community, and better connection between people.

INTRODUCTION

Spiritual wellbeing helps in making relationship better, enhance personal value, maintain better work-life balance, understand the personal value, time to spend alone, finding inner peace, finding job satisfaction, maintaining an active lifestyle, balancing and controlling life, better health and longer life, a strong spiritual community and better connection between people.

DOI: 10.4018/978-1-7998-1185-5.ch015

BACKGROUND

Spiritual knowledge enables a person to have a clear vision, make quick and accurate judgements and feel relaxed, and all these saves his time and energy so that he can now spend some time usefully with his family and friends. Spirituality gives a deep religious experience in the sense that it enables the Soul to be linked with the Supreme Soul (Raj-Yoga meditation, n.d). But the method is scientific and is based on rational understanding. People irrespective of their religion, may benefit from this treasure of wisdom, using their own language and terminology as people generally do in science and as also they do something in religions when they use different names, such as Parmatma, Allah or Jesus etc. Spiritual wellbeing also enables a person to stabilize in the real nature of the self and thereby, to experience deep peace.

MAIN FOCUS OF THE CHAPTER

Sujoy (2018), Life on earth is about evolving spiritually. Spirituality is not only about meditation and prayer. Life itself is a property of the spirit. Life is about growth, experience and learning. There are several dimensions which help us to perform our spiritual practices to become internally free and stable. Spiritual wellbeing is a highly personal and universal experience. Nowadays humanity is searching for peace, love, unity, understanding etc in spite of material prosperity, scientific and technological advancement – spirituality is the missing dimension of life. Spiritual wellbeing is an integral part of emotional, physical and mental health. Spirituality has positive effects on our lives. It gives peace, freedom and happiness, helps in treating stress, depression, anorexia etc. Spiritual wellbeing helps in making relationship better, enhance personal value, maintain better work-life balance, understand the personal value, time to spend alone, finding inner peace, finding job satisfaction, maintaining an active lifestyle, balancing and controlling life, better health and longer life, a strong spiritual community and better connection between people.

Ravi Shankar (2008); Development of and tackle with people in the society, the first thing you use is Sama. "Sama means in a peaceful and understanding way". When that does not work out then you go to the second method as the rescue. The Second method is Dana, Dana means forgiving, creating a space. When people don't recognize your generosity in allowing them space, then the third principle comes into picture i.e. Bheda. Bheda means to create discrimination, make a difference, and intentionally create a gap. If someone is at loggerheads with you, first discuss with him. All the problems arise due to lack of communication. If you communicate properly, talk to him with love, evenness starts. When that does not work out, then with the same love you just ignore him.

If someone makes a slip-up, then ignore their mistake. Don't take notice. Allow them to realize for themselves. Your generosity, your letting go should make people realize their mistake. If they do not notice even then, then you start using difference, Bheda. Bheda creates differences. It two persons are there, and then you be partial to one person because by doing that the other person will realize the mistake he has done. Now even if he doesn't come to the way then use the fourth method-Danda, take a stick and make them realize (Danda) The same four methods also apply to our inner life as well. However, in inner life it's not one after the other. Sama is the equanimity in the mind inside. But observing equanimity becomes difficult for many people.

Dana suggests discarding something, that disturbs you, that which cannot put you in equanimity. What is it that disturbs you? A guilt feeling of doing one thing wrong or an egoistic feeling of getting done one thing nice. Both these feelings, this whole mind, with all its merit and demerits give it away, surrender, Dana. Dana, that is surrender. Surrender is the most misunderstood word in the world today. Surrender is not slavery. Surrender is something which you cannot force upon someone. Surrender happens out of love, gratitude and trust. When there is fear drop the fear. The dropping of the fear happens with the trust, and that is surrender. If doubt still remains, do nothing and just watch, breathe, meditate. That will clear your doubts. There is no other way to come out of your doubt. Dana (giving), the second aspects of inner growth, is very important. Giving includes forgiving also. Without surrender and without love, your meditation will be dry. Although you can learn various techniques for meditation but Bheda, separate the imperishable from the perishable. The human body is so hollow and so empty. We never realized before that inside our body there is so much emptiness. The whole body can be place into a little envelope. When one is watching the body, pleasant sensation arises; unpleasant sensation arises, as you watch they all disappear. The third thing that one can do is differentiate between the permanent and the impermanent. One must disassociate himself from the sensation. Bheda means seeing the permanence and the impermanence. This very body is impermanent and, with every attention to it. One becomes a glow of consciousness. It is not the body, it is the glow, it is the consciousness. It is the Chetan, Chitta that is coming out of every pore of the body.

Then comes Danda, means support. Determination and commitment are Danda. Your spiritual discipline is Danda. The mind is like a vine (creeper), it needs support. Listening to spiritual discourses, satsangs, practices in Guru's presence are all the support, the Danda. Spirituality liberates us from all the negative and irrational attitudes and asks us to give up defeatist mentality, to build up our confidence, to be in high spirits and to march forward. It makes us aware that our society has given us a lot and that we owe some responsibility towards society and without discharging it, we can never even be liberated.

Spiritual knowledge enables a person to have a clear vision, make quick and accurate judgements and feel relaxed, and all these saves his time and energy so that he can now spend some time usefully with his family and friends. Spiritual gives a deep religious experience in the sense that it enables the Soul to be linked with the Supreme Soul. But the method is scientific and is based on rational understanding. People irrespective of their religion, may benefit from this treasure of wisdom, using their own language and terminology as people generally do in science and as also they do something in religions when they use different names, such as Parmatma, Allah or Jesus etc. Spiritual wellbeing also enables a person to stabilize in the real nature of the self and thereby, to experience deep peace.

Thus it gives mental relaxation and releases a person from stress and tensions. This experience of peace opens new avenues of happiness, strengthens one's conscience and inwardly guides a person to change his behavior and to become a better person. The practice of this positive thinking and the taste of peace and bliss save a person from wastage of time and energy on negative thoughts. This makes him more efficient. Spirituality also enhances one's concentration, detachment, imagination, self-control, etc, for in this practice, one detaches the mind from one's sense organs and withdraws it from one's gross and physical environment and focuses it on the self and God, and one voluntarily controls his thoughts.

The Spiritual Insights

Insight is the spiritual wisdom which is the missing dimension in our present life. It helps us to understand one's innate self. So that he identifies his inner powers and capabilities which are at his disposal to determine the implications of the changes that are happening around us. There are two aspects of us: the innate self and the acquired self. The innate self is otherwise known as soul, atma, spirit, which is the essence and storehouse of all values. It performs all the mental activities through three main faculties- the mind, the intellect and the sub-consciousness. The acquired self is whatever we have acquired after coming to this world: the ego, beliefs, body, relationships, position, wealth, skills, possessions, achievements etc. We are so conscious of the acquired self that all our actions and resources are concentrated around physical development. Hence, developing the real human resource is neglected, due to lack of awareness of our innate potential.

In order to develop the innate resources, we have to understand the inner mechanism of the three faculties which perform all the mental activities- the mind, the intellect and the sub-consciousness or sanskaras or the personal management information system. If we know how to manage ourselves on the basis of the information or the wisdom then our life will be better organized. Applying the insights means to understand how the mind works and how to change our mindset, understanding our thinking mechanisms and our decision making processes.

One should aim to be peaceful the whole day. Being peaceful not only makes us feel very comfortable but also helps to create a peaceful environment around benefiting all, improve our concentration resulting in improved work efficiency, enhance creativity and job satisfaction, provide greater space to understand, accept and accommodate others, thereby improving relationship, inspire others to work in a peaceful way, thereby creating a wave of transformation, radiate good vibrations to the body, keeping it healthier. Peace makes the body organs work more efficiently and helps to improve sleep.

Life is about growth, experience and learning, but sometimes we don't understand life-the things that happen to us or in some cases, that doesn't happen to us. But the essence is to evolve spiritually. Often we don't understand why bad things happen to us. Whether this refers to relationship problems or breakups, finances, career, health issues, addictions, depressions etc. We have to understand that bad thing happen to us only as lessons that we have to learn and experience, to grow and evolve spiritually. There are several attitudes which help us to sustain our spiritual practices, cultivate and maintain our values.

We are inspired by spirituality and purity of purpose when we maintain an attitude of detachment regarding the rewards of our good actions. This attitude also serves to immunize us from criticism and attempts to make us doubt ourselves and our abilities. Thus the influence of external pressure no longer distort our judgment about what is right. We develop our ability to take responsibility and discharge our duties wisely.

All kinds of values – universal or temporal including human, social, ethical, moral, spiritual, economic, etc are demonstrated by our actions (Karma). Values and spirituality are to be developed together because their relationship is inextricably interrelated and interdependent. So when spirituality is developed, values emerged and when values are developed, they increase spirituality.

Spirituality is about self- awareness. It means to have awareness of our own eternal spiritual identity and the kind of values we need to be living. It means to be clear about our inherent worth to be reflected in our daily life. The very purpose of spirituality is to make us more effective, by helping us to improve our thoughts, words and actions. Spirituality brings a sense of purpose for our living. Spirituality helps us to develop inner wellbeing and an understanding of two basic inner faculties the intellect and the mind. The intellect is our intelligence, our ability to focus and to see things clearly. The mind controls thoughts and emotions understanding how they operate helps us to start directing them. In the way, we also come to understand how we want them to perform. Thus change begins here, as we get to know ourselves at this level of our being, we will definitely experience inner positive change. These changes lead to personal growth. Spirituality helps us to manage the energy of thoughts in a constructive way and we start to see our problems in a different way. So spirituality takes us closer to our inner self, where we find a reservoir of qualities like peace, love, joy, beauty, knowledge etc to deal with the outside world. Spirituality does not refer to any particular religion nor does it refer to any religious rituals. It simply refers to one's rational belief in one's own identity as a metaphysical self which is basically different in nature from the body, including the brain, and from matter and all its forms. And since one's belief influences one's mindset, the term refers to one's outlook, attitudes, values, preferences, priorities, lifestyle, relationships, memory content and behavior, all based on the belief in the metaphysical self. The term 'Spirituality' refers also to a simple spiritual practice, such as meditation which is based on the aforesaid belief and which strengthens one's moral sense. Restores one's inner harmony, reforms and improves one's outlook and attitudes and also gives relaxing, uplifting, enriching and ecstatic super sensuous experiences.

SPIRITUAL WELLBEING BRINGS IMPROVEMENT IN THE BELOW ASPECTS OF A HUMAN PERSONALITY

Positive Attitude

Neuliep (1996) As per the traditional theory of management, Theory X; A normal human being intrinsically dislikes work and attempts to avoid it if he or she can do so. He also tries to avoid responsibility and has little ambition and needs security above all things and prefer to be directed and controlled by someone. Due to the dislike of work, workers should be subjected to control, direction, threat and punishment. But as per the neo-classical theory of management, the Theory Y; a normal human being does not dislike work because it may serve as a source of satisfaction to him.

Development of Self (n.d.); External control and threats are not always a necessary means for mobilizing human effort towards organizational goals. A normal human being tends to seek responsibility. Lack of ambition and avoidance of responsibility and importance of security are not man's intrinsic nature but these results from a negative experience and are acquired nature. The traits of imagination, creativity etc. are widely distributed in the population. But normally, one would feel happy if he can give expression to his creativity. Spirituality, on the other hand, gives a composite view of human nature. It says that in their pristine nature all the human soul is pure and has positive qualities but gradually their nature has become degenerated. It is a result of degeneration that they have acquired the negative traits of indolence, lack of sense of responsibility. It, therefore, tells us not to adopt a completely negative attitude towards human nature in general but to have a positive approach and to inspire workers to stabilize in their original nature through soul-consciousness. It emphasizes that a balance must be maintained between love and law and flexibility and firmness. We should consider the inherent dignity of every individual, and repose trust, for a soul as everyone is a child of God, the Divine. And yet, we should observe caution because everyone does not have the same degree of goodness since there has been degeneration in varying degrees. This view makes us more pragmatic and practical and also enables us to act with our belief in human dignity and to see the response to our belief and trust.

Healthy and Happy behavior

Viral (2019),If one treats others with hatred and with a bloated ego, hurting the self-respect and sensitivities of others, one cannot be a good human being or a good manager. One has, therefore, to have a positive view of human nature, the positive or negative beliefs determine our positive or negative attitudes and the positive attitudes, in turn, make our behavior healthy and happy. Further, since our positive beliefs and attitudes about human nature enable us to treat others as worthy human beings and to behave nicely with them, so we are able to use the full potential of the employees by giving them opportunities of participation and creativity in a self-controlled manner and with self- respect.

Change in Attitude Towards Wealth

Spiritual Wisdom tells us that, besides the gross wealth, there are other kinds of wealth, such as Spiritual Knowledge, virtue, blessings of others, earned through service and so on. These notions of wealth change our attitudes and outlook, resulting in a change in our behavior. One now considers one's thoughts, energy and time also as various kinds of money or precious treasures and tries to save these resources from unnecessary expenditure and from wastage. One tries not only to have a high quality of industrial products but also high quality of his conduct and actions.

Behavioral Change Due to the Spiritual Relationship

A person's behavior is always relation-oriented. the behavior of a mother towards her son, a husband towards his wife, a student towards a teacher and anyone towards another can be explained on the basis of the relationship as a major determinant. So, when a person is convinced that his basic relationship behind all other physical, or work relationship is that of 'Spiritual Brothers' because all are children of God, who is the Mother-Father of Mankind, then one's thought process changes. It brings a shift in the axis of behavior. It widens one's concern from his family towards society. One's love is no longer directed to a few but to all. This awakens in man the qualities of sympathy, service and fellow-feeling and puts his behavior on a new and a higher level.

Again, the Philosophy and Law of Karma and Re-incarnation give a person the essential awareness to avoid bad Karma and to be good in one's behavior, for, otherwise, one will have to suffer for one's bad behavior in this or the next life. Thus, Spiritual Knowledge guides a person not to increase a debt of negative Karma but to make efforts to get rid of the past karmic account.

Honesty, Integrity and Moral Values.

If a person does not have morality and principles, or high character and good conduct, he loses his image and can neither guide nor direct, nor even inspire others. So as a manager, a person is required not only to have certain managerial skills but he must be qualitatively also a good person in order to be a good manager. How can one expect control over others if one has no control over himself, i.e. his mind and his sense-organs? A good manager is one who is a man of good character so that people do not question his honesty, integrity and private or public life. Character is the strength of a person that enables him to stand and look into another person's eyes. It is this which establishes one's credibility among one's friends, relatives, neighbours, customers and employees. A man without character is cement without strength or a rusty piece of iron. How long can one run an industry if one cannot run one's life properly? Relying on a characterless person is like depending on a broken reed or trying to obtain juice from an already crushed sugarcane.

A characterless person is one who has deformed habits, is addicted to certain intoxicants, has a weakness towards certain person or objects, is a slave to certain sensual pleasures, has lack of control over himself and has no self-respect and also no regard for others. Such a person loses his energy, his will to stand difficulties, his efforts to maintain loyalties and individual dignity and he loses his wealth and vigor. Such a person ultimately becomes a liability for society. It is, therefore, rightly been said that if the character is lost, everything is lost.

Maintain Relations and Certain Balances

A good relationship works like a lubricant in the 'society' family' and 'workforce' whereas hostile relations work as dust, rust and friction and lead to break down of social dynamics. Thus it is the relationship which can make or mar the atmosphere at the workplace as also in the family and in the society as a whole. Some of the virtues that lead to building cordial and happy relationship are politeness, humility, appreciation, cooperation, talent, getting friendly etc. The reverse of these leads to estrangement, and enmity etc. At the workplace, the performance of employees is greatly influenced by their inter-personal relations at various levels. If there are no harmonious relations at the workplace, productivity suffers. Congenial social environment and interpersonal equations are utmost necessary for maintaining enthusiasm and devotion to work. Following some of the qualities that can maintain happy relations or can bring improvement in existing relations: Broadmindedness, Fellow-feeling, Sharing good things of life and not being selfish, avoiding too much of argumentation etc

Spirituality is based on the understanding that each and every one of us is an immortal soul and that the world is a global family. This awareness gives a new dimension and a better and stronger footing to our relationship. It adds a sense of permanence to our relationships and broadens our vision. It shatters the narrow outlook and we begin to focus on everyone as our own. Our bonds of love which, earlier, united us only with our physical relatives now expand and extend to all. This broader vision strikes at the roots of selfishness. The Spiritual wisdom lay great emphasis on friendliness (maîtri), forgiveness (kshma), Compassion(karuna), Cooperation (sahyoga), Contentment (santosh). Spirituality also gives its participants the habit of positive thinking and look upon the positive qualities of a person. It infuses in them the spirit to be so nice to everyone that they too feel inspired to become great. It brings about the reformation of character, revolution in one's outlook and bases relations on happy feelings.

Take Quick Decisions and Conflict Resolution

In planning, problem-solving, conflict - resolution, selection of proper persons for specific jobs and facing rapid changes that occur due to altered conditions, one needs to make a quick decision. In order to take a decision, a person generally needs to think of (a) the possible alternatives, (b). to think of the merits and demerits of each one of those alternatives, (c) to make a rational system- analysis, from the point of view of manpower and talents required, costs involved, quality etc (d).to calculate their compatibility, possibilities and advantages or disadvantages with reference to the present administrative, financial, technological and other kinds of setup (e).to consider what changes would any step require in approach, strategy,, tactics etc. and to consider such other factors. All these processes of consideration, comparison, calculation etc. have to be done quickly.

This presupposes a high degree of intuition, concentration and sophistication in one's thought –process and thought-content. Only a person with a high alert, active, imaginative, dynamic and innovative mind can have these. Moreover, Spirituality gives a person such a high degree of strength of will that one does not waver under different kinds of pressures and so he does not change judgments because of fears, favours or frigid and frivolous considerations. And despite this all, if in the result any such thing happens as is not encouraging, he does not lose the balance of his mind. Thus, in conclusion, one must have the following powers, qualities, state of mind and values in order to make quick and correct decisions. Spirituality improves the abilities like Intuition, Power to analyze, Mental composure and calmness, Freedom from prejudices, Power of perceiving and withstanding pressures and the ability to detach etc for self-actualization and self- stabilization.

Motivate and Inspire Others

Motivation is necessary to inspire willingness in workers for better performance so that they carry out efficiently and with enthusiasm, the activities allocated to them and also play an efficient part in administration.

Time Management

We have a limited time span of life and, therefore, if one wishes to achieve one's goals, one has to plan his efforts in such a way that time is not wasted. For making the best use of time and for managing it successfully, the following qualities or values are of immense help. Avoiding negative thinking, for it is wastage of time and energy, Doing things with great interest and not in a careless manner. Having full concentration, for it helps in achieving a maximum within minimum time, Proper coordination and communication, Proper distribution and allocation of work.

Maintain Discipline and Take Disciplinary Action

The organizations spend time, money and energy to achieve certain goals and organize personnel, materials and equipment for the purpose, cannot afford to overlook acts of gross indiscipline by employees. It cannot sit idle over reports of workers gossiping at the workplace during working hours, coming late, insulting colleagues, abusing seniors, damaging machines and equipment. One has to take disciplinary action against such persons. For this job following are some of the abilities, qualities needed.

Ascertaining the veracity of the report of acts of indiscipline, offering adequate opportunity to the accused to explain his conduct, Assessing the severity of the act of indiscipline, Observing impartiality, justice and proper procedure, Punishing the guilty where necessary with a touch of consideration and good wishes, using utmost restraint in remarks and actions. Spirituality gives a person the ability to be restrained. It provides a person with the ability to be free from prejudice and develops his ability to judge independently and to be kind and considerate and to make possible attempts to reform.

Levy (1996) Sigmund Freud makes a tripartite division of the self into Id, Ego and Superego. The 'id' is the primitive, undifferentiated basis of mental life. It is the fundamental, oldest and largest layer. It is the primary source of psychic energy. He says that Id is a chaos, a cauldron of seething excitement, Instincts fill it with energy. Its logic is that of emotion and not of reason. It knows no value, no morality. Id processes have no relation to the idea of time and are beyond any external influences. Due to this nature of Id, there is dormant unhappiness in our life. About Ego, Freud says that it grows out of Id. The processes of external stimuli or environment make it act as an executive of consciousness. Ego is only partly conscious. He calls the other part which is not conscious as pre-conscious, because though it is latent yet it can come to a conscious level. Because the state of consciousness is transitory in nature. An idea which is now at a conscious level may not be so a moment later, But it can come again to the conscious level due to certain stimuli. The Superego, in every individual, is a refined version of the Ego. It is watching, judging and punishing the individual. It persuades the impure to become pure and perfect. It also puts moral restrictions on the individual's desires and actions. The Libido is the unconscious dynamic urge. We always suspected that, behind the multitude of small, occasional instincts, there lies something much more serious and powerful. These instincts change their aim by displacement – by passing energy of one instinct to the other.

Freud concluded that there are two fundamental instincts 1. Eros or life instincts – whose basic aim is to preserve or to build up. 2. The other instinct is Thanatus or 'death instinct'. Which represents a tendency towards the dissolution of the living substances and its return to a state of inanimate matter. Libido is nothing but the total energy of Eros. Explaining further Freud says that Libido is the sexual energy but not in the literal sense nor has it to do with man's or woman's organs of reproduction. It is rather an affection in general. He considers Libido as the unifying source and Id is the greatest reservoir of Libido.

According to the Spiritual Perspective, 'Id' is the collection of a person's sanskaras that can be changed by realizing our real identity and practicing spirituality. In fact, the feeling of unhappiness and also the Narcissistic state etc are due to body consciousness and can be altered into happiness and spiritual love respectively by the practice of soul consciousness. The 'Id' or the reservoir of sanskaras was originally not anarchic or a cauldron of seething excitement but has become so due to a constant state of body consciousness over a long period of time. 'Ego' is a person's 'Conscious mind' and 'Superego' is his 'Conscience' or the moral voice of the original state of the self. Spiritual review of Childs Ego and Superego Freud says that 'Id' is that primal matrix from which the ego and Superego evolve by progressive differentiation. It primarily includes primary urges. So the kid is all

–'Id' however with the parental ego; the child's own ego bit by bit emerges. From the non secular perspective, it may well before mentioned that originally the kid encompasses a reservoir of its own sanskaras, however as he grows, comes into contact with others, observes, learns, adopts some ways that and rejects others and is influenced within the method, he builds his own ego and manifests it.

This type of learning, influencing and strengthening of his personal ego, exerts some hold over his Sanskaras (Id) conjointly and, curb the fantasies or remodeling the negative urges, he expresses himself the manner he has freshly learnt, accepted and adopted.

So, it cannot before mentioned that there was no ego within the child; the proper issue would be to mention that it began to surface bit by bit with value-added strength and new influences.

Organizations collapse once individuals don't seem to be ready to adopt new ways that and unable to alter from inside. As organizations are manufactured from individuals and once time demands a modification from them and that they don't seem to be willing to alter then survival becomes a haul. We have to be sensitive to the underlying feelings of the members of the team. It can't simply be assumed that everybody is sharing an equivalent level of commitment to alter. Normally, whenever time has demanded modification from individuals there are completely different classes of individuals with differing kinds of reactions towards modification. These are those who resist modification, Who attempt to bunk faraway from modification, Who tend to ignore modification, Who embrace modification and adapt it within the manner it comes. The ways that to alter may be distinguished into two parts: the exhausting manner and also the straightforward manner. The exhausting manner is wherever we have a tendency to force to alter. If we have a tendency to be slow to alter, world forces us to rethink and that we are forced into creating changes that don't seem to be continuously pleasant.

On the opposite hand, modification may be exhilarating once we take up the challenge of being pro-active and conceive to modification before time. The simplest time to alter is once we are growing, learning and at the height of our performance and also the level of satisfaction is high. People might resist modification because of the explanations that centre on the emotions of loss and grief that are fully fledged from the past changes- either there's the concern of the unknown and lack of understanding of the implications which are available in the long run or there's a scarcity of trust within the leaders who are asking them to alter and folks feel it's not a true syndrome. Some individuals assume that there's a threat to their values and that they might have to be compelled to compromise them. Some don't seem to be clear concerning |the method in order that they feel they'll be worse off with the modification process. Whereas some have terribly unpleasant past experience and are frightened of the modification method. The organization's direction is set on the idea of the facts obtained from the structure SWOT analysis therefore on get in the long run and reach out for those opportunities that are gap up. The insights facilitate to redefine the mission, vision statements and also the values become fuel to achieve out the vision.

However at an equivalent time the barriers cannot be unnoticed within the Key Result Areas and precautions have to be compelled to be taken to attain the vision. The methods adopted ought to be in alignment with the values to associate an implementation method that have to be compelled to be developed. It is necessary to own the correct mental position whereas coming up with for our future that is influencing us. The simplest mental position is that of a detached observer. Within the state of being a detached observer, we have a tendency to be ready to see ourselves and also the influences within our life.

The key to stability could be a balance. The method involves two major areas of balance: Foremost, the balance between the past and also the future and second the balance between exhausting thinking and soft thinking i.e., to be analytical, logical and rational however at an equivalent time be intuitive, inventive and affectional.

Step 1: SWOT

Emet (2017), SWOT analysis is an analytical tool ordinarily utilized in the strategic coming up with of a business. However it' s utilized in a distinct manner strategic coming up with the analysis of our personal strengths, weaknesses, opportunities and threats. Our personal strengths are those aspects of life that are dedicated and dealing well. Weaknesses are those aspects of life that don't seem to be therefore smart and are inflicting sorrow and discomfort to us. Threats are those things that have a tendency to be worrying concerning within the future, and opportunities are those changes which will be right there ahead. If solely we have a tendency to be ready to acknowledge them, so as to review ourselves, we've to adopt the mind-set of observation a very detached manner. It's necessary to be objective and unemotional through out the method. Applying the insights means to grasp how the mind works and the way to alter our mind-set, understanding our thinking mechanisms and our deciding processes. The mind could be a terribly powerful entity that imagines, thinks, feels forms ideas etc. each moment the mind creates thoughts: we are able to say that the mind is coming up with committee of the inner organization. The intellect is where the wisdom and willpower to take decisions are stored. This is the most crucial faculty which understands each and every thought and reasons and analyses, discriminates, evaluates, and then gives its decisions whether to carry out the practical actions or not.

All the actions get registered in the sub-consciousness or sanskaras as the records of the self in the form of experiences, tendencies, habits, traits, talents or memories and as a result, form our personality. Any record from the sub-consciousness can be traced within a fraction of a second and accordingly, the thought process starts. They are positive thoughts, necessary thoughts, negative thoughts and waste thoughts. Positive is value based thoughts which have no selfish intentions. The necessary thoughts are related to the day to day routine, work, profession, career, etc.; the negative thoughts are based on weaknesses, vices, evils, selfishness and complexities etc and the waste thoughts are mainly connected with the past happenings, events and upon which the mind keeps on worrying about the unknown.

The Power and Effect of Thoughts

As is the quality of our thoughts so are our feelings, attitudes, beliefs and behavior. The power and effect of our thoughts are such that we are responsible for our own thoughts, feelings and behavior. Thoughts have great power and we create our experiences by the thoughts we choose to think. Frequent repetition of the same type of thoughts creates our beliefs and attitudes. Positive thoughts generate energy and strength and negative thoughts rob us of the power and strength and make us feel tired and drained. Thoughts are like seeds that we plant in our mind and the more we hold on to a particular thought the more power we have to invest in it. what we believe comes true for us due to the thought power. It takes time to change and transform the old patterns of thinking. We have to have patience with our self.

The Intellect

Every thought the mind creates is sent to the intellect which will evaluate, judge, refine and make a decision upon if and when necessary. The intellect is gifted with the wisdom and will power which acts as a filter to take accurate decisions. So if we want to take the right decisions we need to have a good filter.

The problem is that there is some interference that is developed which alter the function and affect the will-power.

Step 2: Purpose

Life can be centered on work, money, power, family, society and there are many ways to make short term gains. By identifying our higher purpose and core values we can live from a principle centre that will lead us to long term effectiveness based on natural laws. The purpose of our life has to be understood from various perspectives. So that we are able to give meaning to our life and lead a meaningful life. For every successful and fulfilled human being, the shaping of a life worth living starts with identifying and then building on the purpose that each of us was born to fulfill. Our purpose affects the way we work, live, being in the world and the results we achieve. Purpose means to follow the intuition and do the things that really matter so that we use our resources and talents for the greater good and explore what is meaningful.

Step 3: Values

We must clarify the innate values and the acquired values which are most deeply connected to the purpose and how to use these values as the basis for choice, selection and decision making. Thus our value determines our worth. The value is true motivators and is important for achievements of the purposes in life. Each and every individual is blessed with a core value-system when he is born. But the values can either be chosen consciously from understanding or shaped unconsciously from conditioning. These include traditional influences of family, society, religion, education, media, sciences etc. by unconscious influences. Values are like moral compasses because they guide us in our actions on a day to day basis while being consistent with our purpose. Different types of values pulling in different directions lead to inner conflict and stress so we need to clearly define our priorities.

Step 4: Vision

The fifth step in this planning model is to have a clear vision. Vision means to develop a mental image of the purpose and values of what we are aiming for, in the form of a symbol for future success as a personal logo that will guide us for the future and remind us of what we are aiming to achieve. We create our own script by the quality of our vision.

Step 5: Barriers

The purpose of being aware of the barriers is that by comparing our vision with our present situation, we discover what is it that is going to come in my way. Before we embark on an adventure, it is important to anticipate what obstacles we will have to deal with on the way. The lulls are the times when we feel completely powerless, burnt out of energy, no motivation to move forward, and the undercurrents are the powerful streams of our own weaknesses driving us making us feel helpless. Hence we need to be realistic about the problems and limitations that exist in our lives in order to overcome them. We must not only be aware of the barriers presented by external circumstances or people, but we must also be aware of our own limitations. We have to be aware of our sanskaras and realize that we have to challenge assumptions about ourselves and the problems that exist in our life. Spiritual understanding helps us address these barriers and overcome them easily. In order to address these barriers, we have to change our attitude and perception towards it. Spirituality helps us to see these barriers as stepping stones to success. Instead of thinking about the problems, we start to think about the solutions. It enables us to expand our understanding that no situation lasts, forever. It is our own negative thinking that stretches the situation as far as we wish to. It is definite that we cannot change the adverse situation but we can definitely change our attitude towards it. Spirituality also gives a deep understanding about the eternal laws of nature, thus sometimes we have to leave it for time to heal and give full justice i.e. understanding the law of karma and developing the patience to wait and see.

Step 6: Key Result Areas

Key result area is something we refer to in a process of change in an organization. It is the areas which have been identified as key areas in which a change would lead to the effective overall change in the organization. When we can use this term in self-management, it refers to those areas of our personal lives in which our efforts need to be integrated and balanced- such as inner self, family life, work life, health etc.

Step 7: Goals and Strategies

One needs to develop clear goals and strategies for overcoming the barriers which exist in each Key Result Areas of one's life and give a direction for the next phase of his life. The aim is to develop goals and strategies for the achievement of our vision in the various key result areas of our life as well as for our personal development. Goals should be specific, measurable, achievable, realistic and time-bound. Goals without strategies will remain dreams. Thus strategies are initiatives on how to move forward, realizing time's demand and responding in a proactive manner instead of just reacting. Strategies require implementation. For each goal and accompanying strategy, we need to develop specific action steps.

Step 8: Strategy and Action Plan

The Strategy has to be in alignment with the values and then take each of the strategies and identify which specific tasks we need to perform immediately in order to bring the strategies into life. Our actions don't support our purpose when they are not guided by value.

Step 9: Implementation Process

The implementation process has four aspects- monitoring, timing, response ability and non-violent communication. The aim of monitoring is to introduce a daily self-assessment system to keep on track with action plans and development programmes which show how to maintain my motivation and will power. Timing means one should know the right time to act and learn how to select the time to act when one is at the peak and when one is most vulnerable to defeat. Response-ability provides one with the skills in teamwork and empowerment on the basis of understanding the subtle laws of cause and effect as one applies to his response- ability and practically apply the lessons, one will learn about value-based action. Non- violent communication means recognizing the power available to tap the hidden inner powers and training in the art of nonviolent communication and the keys to effective listening. Our body is mortal and so it seeks security and creates boundaries. But within this body is the immortal Atma that does not seek security and so, does not care for boundaries. Wrapped in mortal flesh, it experiences life and death, again and again. The Atma experiences its childhood, youth and old age before moving on to the next. This body gets attached to the world around it, and so fears death. But the wise, aware of the inner resident's immortality, aware that the flesh goes through cycles of birth and death, do not fear change or death. They know that what matters is the immortal, not the mortal. The idea of rebirth forms the cornerstone of Hindu thought. It is also the mainstay of Buddhist and Jain philosophies. But there are differences. Buddhists do not believe in the existence of the immortal resident (atma), and Jains do not believe in the concept of God (param-atma), but both agree on the concept of rebirth, (punar-janma). In Jainism and Buddhism, the world of rebirth is called samsara, propelled by action (karma) and memories of past actions (sanskaras).

CONCLUSION

Life is larger than one's profession. Life started before we entered our professions and it is naturally assumed that profession occupies only a part of our lifetime. It would be wrong if it engulfs the whole of our time and consumes almost all our physical and mental energy. Our life is not meant for the job, the job is meant to provide us with some of our life's needs. If we cannot sleep because of our job, then we have perhaps, overstepped in our jobs. One must get some time to relax, to know more about other important things in life. Spiritual knowledge guides us to manage our life properly and fulfill all our obligations and enjoy all our rights in a correct way and have the feeling that life is worth living if we have bliss, peace, love and purity and we do service to others. Apart from these, Spirituality helps in developing those qualities in us that enable us to manage our life and by virtue of that experience, we develop a natural ability to manage the organization.

We all live in a life that is filled with different actions, which we perform from the morning to the night. Every action either in the personal, professional, social or financial sphere, is filled with the energy of an intention or a pure desire that I one has to achieve what one aspires for. But things go to wrong when the ambition starts becoming an obsession and it starts affecting our mind or relationships or health or sometimes all of these together.

This causes people to become severely depressive, unenthusiastic and disinterested after ascertain the period of time in their careers and family. Today many people have realized the importance of meditation and relaxation techniques because they have lost the balance in their lives. So the first step on the road to success is revising our purpose that can be achieved at a slower speed than the speed we might see others working at the competition when the competition is mixed with comparisons it becomes negatives or self-harming. So, one should compete without comparison. We need to set smaller goals to be achieved instead of targeting directly at the bigger cause. This is important because this keeps us extremely light in our journey and keeps us on the road to success and does not let us become tired when the going gets tough.

In order to play a leadership role for change within the organization, we must be able to bring about significant changes in our own inner organization. As the external environment changes fast, the importance of self-management increases. It is hardly possible to control the external environment, anymore. The emphasis has accordingly shifted towards managing our inner environment that is to harness our inner resources which we have tended to neglect. The future of our organization rests on the autonomy, maturity and confidence of our people. The skills and abilities that are required now, are how to lead through a never-ending process of change, how to remain calm and confident in the face of upheavals. Change is a continuous process We have to move along with the changing times constantly, moving through rapidly changing times, if we are not able to change and empower ourselves from within, it will become very difficult for us to survive. We need three things to manage any change process. They are knowledge – an understanding of what to change and why to change, desire to change, skills that show us how to change. But if any two are there and one ingredient is missing, change cannot take place in the manner we want. The change adopted in a systematic method according to the need of the hour brings novelty and enthusiasm.

REFERENCES

Development of Self *or Human Resource Development, For Success in Management through Spiritual Wisdom and Meditation*. (n.d.). Brahma Kumari's Ishwariya Vishwa Vidyalaya .

Emet, G., & Tat, M. (2017). Swot Analysis: A Theoretical Review. *Journal of International Social Research*, *51*(10), 995–1005. doi:10.17719/jisr.2017.1832

Levy, D. (1996). *Freud Among the Philosophers: The Psychoanalytic Unconscious and Its Philosophical Critics*. New Haven, CT: Yale University Press.

Neuliep, J. W. (1996). The Influence of Theory X and Y Management Style on the Perception of Ethical Behavior in Organizations. *Journal of Social Behavior and Personality*, (11): 301–311.

Raj-Yoga Meditation. (n.d.). *The Science of Peace and of Social, Economic and over-all Development*. Available from https://www.brahma-kumaris.com/rajyoga-meditation

Ravi Shankar, S. S. (2008). *God Loves Fun*. Bangalore: Sri Sri Publications.

Strachey, J., & Freud, A. (Eds.). (1953-1964). The Standard Edition of the Complete Psychological Works of Sigmund Freud (pp. 1-24). London: Academic Press.

Sujoy, B. K. (2018). We are Spiritual Butterflies Having a Caterpillar Experience. *The World Renewal*, *49*(3), 13–15.

Viral, B. K. (2019). Being Happy Always. *The World Renewal*, *49*(9), 27–29.

Compilation of References

Aaron, R., Joseph, A., Abraham, S., Muliyil, J., George, K., Prasad, J., ... Bose, A. (2005). Suicides in young people in rural southern India. *Lancet*, *363*(9415), 1117–1118. doi:10.1016/S0140-6736(04)15896-0 PMID:15064031

AbdAleati, N. S., Mohd Zaharim, N., & Mydin, Y. O. (2016, December 1). Religiousness and Mental Health: Systematic Review Study. *Journal of Religion and Health*. doi:10.100710943-014-9896-1

Abe, K., Niwa, M., Fujisaki, K., & Suzuki, Y. (2018). EI and empathy have been found to be associated. Empathy is viewed as an ability to understand and share the feelings of another. It is a multi-dimensional construct which includes both cognitive and affective elements. *Bio medical centre*, 2 -9.

Abu-helalah, M., Al-hanaqta, M., Alshraideh, H., & Hijazeen, J. (2014). Quality of life and psychological well-being of breast cancer survivors in Jordan. *Asian Pacific Journal of Cancer Prevention*, *15*(14), 5927–5936. doi:10.7314/APJCP.2014.15.14.5927 PMID:25081724

Acar, C., Tekin-iftar, E., & Yikmis, A. (2016). *Effects of Mother-Delivered Social Stories and Video Modeling in Teaching Social Skills to Children With Autism Spectrum Disorders*. doi:10.1177/0022466916649164

Achmadi, D., Kagohara, D. M., Van Der Meer, L., O'Reilly, M. F., Lancioni, G. E., Sutherland, D., ... Sigafoos, J. (2012). Teaching advanced operation of an iPod-based speech-generating device to two students with autism spectrum disorders. *Research in Autism Spectrum Disorders*, *6*(4), 1258–1264. doi:10.1016/j.rasd.2012.05.005

Addington-Hall, J., & Kalra, L. (2001). Who should measure quality of life? *BMJ (Clinical Research Ed.)*, *322*(7299), 1417–1420. doi:10.1136/bmj.322.7299.1417 PMID:11397754

Aelterman, A., Engels, N., Van Petegem, K., & Verhaeghe, J. P. (2007). The well-being of teachers in Flanders: The importance of a supportive school culture. *Educational Studies*, *33*(3), 285–297. doi:10.1080/03055690701423085

Ae-Ngibise, K. A., Doku, V. C. K., Asante, K. P., & Owusu-Agyei, S. (2015). The experience of caregivers of people living with serious mental disorders: A study from rural Ghana. *Global Health Action*, *8*(1), 10. doi:10.3402/gha.v8.26957 PMID:25967587

Ahmed, A. E., Almuzaini, A. S., Alsadhan, M. A., Alharbi, A. G., Almuzaini, H. S., Ali, Y. Z., & Jazieh, A.-R. (2018). Health-related predictors of quality of life in cancer patients in Saudi Arabia. *Journal of Cancer Education*, *33*(5), 1011–1019. doi:10.100713187-017-1198-3 PMID:28271388

Ahmed, N. Z., Alam, A., Khalid, M., Sheeraz, M., & Qamri, M. A. (2015). An Insight on Malankholia (Melancholia): Unani Perspective. *Medical Journal of Islamic World Academy of Sciences*, *109*(2459), 1–7.

Aktekin, M., Karaman, T., Senol, Y. Y., Erdem, S., Erengin, H., & Akaydin, M. (2001). Anxiety, depression and stressful life events among medical students: A prospective study in Antalya, Turkey. *Medical Education*, *35*(1), 12–17. doi:10.1046/j.1365-2923.2001.00726.x PMID:11123589

Aldridge, D. (1993). Is there evidence for spiritual healing? *Advances*, *9*(4), 4–21.

Al-Dubai, S. A. R., Al-Naggar, R. A., AlShagga, M. A., & Rampal, K. G. (2011). Stress and coping strategies of students in a medical faculty in Malaysia. *The Malaysian Journal of Medical Sciences: MJMS*, *18*(3), 57. PMID:22135602

Al-Faouri, A. H. A. (2011). Investigating the impact of emotional intelligence on technology learning. *IACSIT International Journal of Engineering and Technology*, *11*(3), 58–78.

Al-Gamal, E., & Yorke, J. (2014, March). Perceived breathlessness and psychological distress among patients with chronic obstructive pulmonary disease and their spouses. *Nursing & Health Sciences*, *16*(1), 103–111. doi:10.1111/nhs.12073 PMID:23692348

All About iMood Journal. (n.d.). Retrieved from https://www.imoodjournal.com/

Al-Nawasrah, F. A. (2019). The Relationship between the Mental Health and the Emotional and Social Intelligence among Talented Students in Ajlun Schools. *Brock Journal of Education*, *7*(1), 77–93.

Amenta, M., & Bohnet, N. (1986). *Nursing Care of the Terminally ill*. Boston, MA: Little, Brown, and Company.

Ames, C., & Fletcher-Watson, S. (2010). *A review of methods in the study of attention in autism. Developmental Review*. Elsevier Inc. doi:10.1016/j.dr.2009.12.003

Amir, E., Seruga, B., Niraula, S., Carlsson, L., & Ocaña, A. (2011). Toxicity of adjuvant endocrine therapy in postmenopausal breast cancer patients: A systematic review and meta-analysis. *JNCI: Journal of the National Cancer Institute*, *103*(17), 1299–1309. doi:10.1093/jnci/djr242 PMID:21743022

Amiri, A. M., Peltier, N., Goldberg, C., Sun, Y., Nathan, A., Hiremath, S. V., & Mankodiya, K. (2017). WearSense: Detecting Autism Stereotypic Behaviors through Smartwatches. *Journal of Healthcare*, *5*(11), 2017. PMID:28264474

Anand, B. K., Chhina, G. S., & Singh, B. (2017). Some aspects of Electroencephelographic studies in yogis. In D. Shapiro (Ed.), *Meditation: Classic and Contemporary Perspectives* (pp. 475–476). New York: Routledge. doi:10.4324/9780203785843-50

Andersen, B. L., Yang, H. C., Farrar, W. B., Golden-Kreutz, D. M., Emery, C. F., Thornton, L. M., & Carson, W. E. (2008). Psychologic intervention improves survival for breast cancer patients: A randomized clinical trial. *Cancer, 113*(12), 3450–3458. doi:10.1002/cncr.23969 PMID:19016270

Anderson, W. T., & Golden, L. (1984). Life-style and psychographics: A critical review and recommendation. *Advances in Consumer Research. Association for Consumer Research (U. S.), 11*, 405–411.

Andrich, R., & Caracciolo, A. (2007). Analysing the cost of individual assistive technology programmes. *Disability and Rehabilitation. Assistive Technology, 2*(4), 207–234. doi:10.1080/17483100701325035 PMID:19263539

Andrzejczak, E., Markocka-Mączka, K., & Lewandowski, A. (2013). Partner relationships after mastectomy in women not offered breast reconstruction. *Psycho-Oncology, 22*(7), 1653–1657. doi:10.1002/pon.3197 PMID:23045167

Anzalone, S. M., Xavier, J., Boucenna, S., Billeci, L., Narzisi, A., & Muratori, F. … Chetouani, M. (2018). Quantifying patterns of joint attention during human-robot interactions: An application for autism spectrum disorder assessment. *Pattern Recognition Letters*. doi:10.1016/j.patrec.2018.03.007

Apple, A. C., Schroeder, M. P., Ryals, A. J., Wagner, L. I., Cella, D., Shih, P.-A., ... Wang, L. (2018). Hippocampal functional connectivity is related to self-reported cognitive concerns in breast cancer patients undergoing adjuvant therapy. *NeuroImage. Clinical, 20*(7), 110–118. doi:10.1016/j.nicl.2018.07.010 PMID:30094161

Ardell, D. B. (2002). What is wellness? *The Institute of Rehabilitation and Research*. Retrieved from http://www.ilru.org

Ardell, D. B. (1979). The nature and implications of high level wellness, or why 'normal health' is a rather sorry state of existence. *Health Values, 3*(1), 17–24.

Ardhanareeswarana, K., & Volkmar, F. (2015). Focus: Austism Spectrum Disorders. *Medicine, 88*(1), 3–4. doi:10.1002/ddrr.75

Ardic, C., & Ozturk, G. Z. (2018). The role of stress management and interpersonal communication in preventing violence against family physicians. *International Journal of Research in Medical Sciences, 6*(4), 1094–1100. doi:10.18203/2320-6012.ijrms20181262

Arem, H., Sorkin, M., Cartmel, B., Fiellin, M., Capozza, S., Harrigan, M., ... Irwin, M. L. (2016). Exercise adherence in a randomized trial of exercise on aromatase inhibitor arthralgias in breast cancer survivors: The Hormones and Physical Exercise (HOPE) study. *Journal of Cancer Survivorship: Research and Practice, 10*(4), 654–662. doi:10.100711764-015-0511-6 PMID:26782031

Argyris, C., & Schön, D. A. (1978). *Organizational Learning: A Theory of Action Perspective*. San Francisco, CA: Josse.y-Bass.

Aricò, D., Raggi, A., & Ferri, R. (2016). Cognitive behavioral therapy for insomnia in breast cancer survivors: A review of the literature. *Frontiers in Psychology*, *7*(4), 654–662. doi:10.3389/fpsyg.2016.01162 PMID:27536265

Armstrong, T. (2009). *Multiple intelligences in the classroom*. Ascd.

Arnott, S. (2015). *Reality testing*. The Emotional Intelligence Training Company Inc. Retrieved from https://www.eitrainingcompany.com/2015/12/show-notes-episode-11-reality-testing/

Arslan, N. (2017). Investigating the relationship between educational stress and emotional self-efficacy. *Universal Journal of Educational Research*, *5*(10), 1736–1740. doi:10.13189/ujer.2017.051010

Ashburner, J., Ziviani, J., & Pennington, A. (2012). The Introduction of Keyboarding to Children With Autism Spectrum Disorders With Handwriting Difficulties: A Help or a Hindrance? *Australasian Journal of Special Education*, *36*(01), 32–61. doi:10.1017/jse.2012.6

Ashoka. (n.d.). *Be fearless be kind, empathy toolkit from rules of kindness*. Retrieved from https://befearlessbekind.hasbro.com/wp-content/uploads/pdf/Ashoka_empathytoolkitfromRulesofKindness.pdf

ASL Roma1. (n.d.). *Dipartimento di Salute Mentale* [Mental Health Department]. Retrieved May 14, 2019, from https://www.aslroma1.it/azienda-dipartimentieri/dipartimento-di-salute-mentale

Assagioli, R. (1965). *Psychosynthesis: A manual of principles and techniques*. Oxford, UK: Hobbs, Dorman & Co., Inc.

Assagioli, R. (1974). Jung and psychosynthesis. *Journal of Humanistic Psychology*, *14*(1), 35–55. doi:10.1177/002216787401400104

Astrow, A. B., Puchalski, C. M., & Sulmasy, D. P. (2001). *Religion, spirituality, and health care: Social ethical and practical consideration*. Academic Press.

Aurnhammer-frith, U. T. A. (1969). Emphasis and meaning in recall in normal and autistic children. *Journal of Language and Speech*, *12*(1), 29–38. doi:10.1177/002383096901200103 PMID:5789294

Avis, N. E., Ip, E., & Foley, K. L. (2006). Evaluation of the Quality of Life in Adult Cancer Survivors (QLACS) scale for long-term cancer survivors in a sample of breast cancer survivors. *Health and Quality of Life Outcomes*, *4*(1), 92. doi:10.1186/1477-7525-4-92 PMID:17140438

Avis, N. E., Smith, K. W., McGraw, S., Smith, R. G., Petronis, V. M., & Carver, C. S. (2005). Assessing quality of life in adult cancer survivors (QLACS). *Quality of Life Research: An International Journal of Quality of Life Aspects of Treatment, Care and Rehabilitation*, *14*(4), 1007–1023. doi:10.100711136-004-2147-2 PMID:16041897

Ayres, K. M., Maguire, A., & McClimon, D. (2009). Acquisition and Generalization of Chained Tasks Taught with Computer Based Video Instruction to Children with Autism. *Education and Training in Developmental Disabilities*, *44*(4), 493–508.

Ayyash-Abdo, H., & Sánchez-Ruiz, M. J. (2012). Subjective well-being and its relationship with academic achievement and multilinguality among Lebanese university students. *International Journal of Psychology, 47*(3), 192–202. doi:10.1080/00207594.2011.614616 PMID:22047001

Badea, L., & Panǎ, N. A. (2010). The Role of Empathy in Developing the Leader's Emotional Intelligence. *Theoretical & Applied Economics, 17*(2).

Baetz, M., Larson, D. B., Marcoux, G., Bowen, R., & Griffin, R. (2002). Canadian psychiatric inpatient religious commitment: An association with mental health. *Canadian Journal of Psychiatry, 47*(2), 159–166. doi:10.1177/070674370204700206 PMID:11926078

Bagadia, V. N., Shah, L. P., Pradhan, P. V., & Gada, M. T. (1979). Treatment of mental disorders in India. *Progress in Neuro-Psychopharmacology, 3*(1-3), 109–118. doi:10.1016/0364-7722(79)90075-4 PMID:401334

Baillie, A. J. (2005). Predictive gender and education bias in Kessler's psychological distress Scale (k10). *Social Psychiatry and Psychiatric Epidemiology, 40*(9), 743–748. doi:10.100700127-005-0935-9 PMID:16142511

Baio, J., Wiggins, L., Christensen, D. L., Maenner, M. J., Daniels, J., Warren, Z., … Dowling, N. F. (2018). *Prevalence of Autism Spectrum Disorder Among Children Aged 8 Years* (Vol. 67). Academic Press.

Baird, C. & Calvard, T.S. (2018). Epistemic Vices in Organizations: Knowledge, Truth and Unethical Conduct. *Journal of Buisness Ethics*. doi:10.100710551-018-3897-z

Baker, A. (2001). Crossing the quality chasm: A new health system for the 21st century. *BMJ (Clinical Research Ed.), 323*(7322), 1192. doi:10.1136/bmj.323.7322.1192

Baloch, Q. B., & Kareem, N. (2007). Book Review: *The third wave. Journal of Managerial Sciences, 1*(2), 115–143.

Bambling, M. (2006). Mind, body and heart: Psychotherapy and the relationship between mental and physical health. *Psychotherapy in Australia, 12*(2), 52–59.

Barman, N., & Chakaravorty, P. (2012). A descriptive study to assess the level of stress among family members of selected mentally ill clients attending psychiatry OPD of a tertiary care teaching hospital. *Open Journal of Psychiatry& Allied Sciences., 3*, 65–73.

Bar-On, R. (2013). *The 15 factors of the Bar-On model*. Retrieved from http://www.reuvenbaron.org/wp/the-5-meta-factors-and-15-sub-factors-of-the-bar-on-model

Bar-On, R. (1997). *Bar-On Emotional Quotient Inventory: A Measure of Emotional Intelligence: User's Manualcby Reuven Bar-On*. MHS.

Bar-On, R. (2006). The Bar-On model of emotional social intelligence (ESI). *Psicothema, 18*, 13–25. PMID:17295953

Bar-On, R. (2007). *Description of the EQ-i, EQ-360 and EQ-i: YV*. Retrieved November.

Bartlett, S. J., Moonaz, S. H., Mill, C., Bernatsky, S., & Bingham, C. O. III. (2013). Yoga in rheumatic diseases. *Current Rheumatology Reports*, *15*(12), 387. doi:10.100711926-013-0387-2 PMID:24173693

Barzegar, M., Afzal, E., Maleki, M., & Koochakyazdi, S. (2013). The relationship between Emotional Intelligence and Decision-making Quality in Hospital Managers. *International Journal of Hospital Research*, *2*(2), 64–69.

Baucom, D. H., Porter, L. S., Kirby, J. S., Gremore, T. M., Wiesenthal, N., Aldridge, W., ... Keefe, F. J. (2009). A couple-based intervention for female breast cancer. *Psycho-Oncology*, *18*(3), 276–283. doi:10.1002/pon.1395 PMID:18702064

Baumgartner, R., Baumgartner, K., Irwin, M. L., McTiernan, A., Bernstein, L., Gilliland, F. D., … Ballard-Barbash, R. (2004). Physical activity levels among breast cancer survivors. *Medicine and Science in Sports and Exercise*, *36*(9), 1484-1491. Retrieved from http://www.ncbi.nlm.nih.gov/pmc/articles/PMC3000611/

Bauminger-Zviely, N., Eden, S., Zancanaro, M., Weiss, P. L., & Gal, E. (2013). Increasing social engagement in children with high-functioning autism spectrum disorder using collaborative technologies in the school environment. *Autism*, *17*(3), 317–339. doi:10.1177/1362361312472989 PMID:23614935

Beasley, J. M., Newcomb, P. A., Trentham-Dietz, A., Hampton, J. M., Ceballos, R. M., Titus-Ernstoff, L., ... Holmes, M. D. (2010). Social networks and survival after breast cancer diagnosis. *Journal of Cancer Survivorship: Research and Practice*, *4*(4), 372–380. doi:10.100711764-010-0139-5 PMID:20652435

Beauchemin, J., Gibbs, T., & Granello, P. (2018). Wellness promotion courses in university settings: A review of the outcome research. *Building Healthy Academic Communities Journal*, *2*(1), 36–49. doi:10.18061/bhac.v2i1.6344

Begoli, E., DeFalco, J., & Ogle, C. (2016). The Promise and Relevance of Emerging Technologies in the Education of Children with Autism Spectrum Disorder. In *Advances in Early Childhood and K-12 Education (AECKE)* (pp. 184–203). Hershey, PA: IGI Global. doi:10.4018/978-1-5225-0816-8

Behere, R. V., Muralidharan, K., & Benegal, V. (2009). Complementary and alternative medicine in the treatment of substance use disorders-A review of the evidence. *Drug and Alcohol Review*, *28*(3), 292–300. doi:10.1111/j.1465-3362.2009.00028.x PMID:21462415

Bekele, E., Crittendon, J., Zheng, Z., Swanson, A., Weitlauf, A., Warren, Z., & Sarkar, N. (2014). Assessing the utility of a virtual environment for enhancing facial affect recognition in adolescents with autism. *Journal of Autism and Developmental Disorders*, *44*(7), 1641–1650. doi:10.100710803-014-2035-8 PMID:24419871

Belek, I. (2000). Social class, income, education, area of residence and psychological distress: Does social class have an independent effect on psychological distress in Antalya, Turkey? *Social Psychiatry and Psychiatric Epidemiology*, *35*(2), 94–101. doi:10.1007001270050013 PMID:10784372

Bellah, R. N., Madisen, R., Sullivan, W., Swidler, A., & Tipton, S. (1985). *Habits of the heart: Individualism and commitment in American life*. Berkeley, CA: University of California Press.

Bell, F. (2000). The complex'whole': Exploring homoeopathic and spiritual considerations. *The Australian Journal of Holistic Nursing*, *7*(1), 31. PMID:11898219

Benssassi, E. M., Gomez, J.-C., Boyd, L. E., Hayes, G. R., & Ye, J. (2018). Wearable Assistive Technologies for Autism: Opportunities and Challenges. *IEEE Pervasive Computing*, *17*(2), 11–21. doi:10.1109/MPRV.2018.022511239

Bentenuto, A., De Falco, S., & Venuti, P. (2016). Mother-child play: A comparison of autism spectrum disorder, down syndrome, and typical development. *Frontiers in Psychology*, *7*, 1–9. doi:10.3389/fpsyg.2016.01829 PMID:27920745

Bernard-Opitz, V., Sriram, N., & Nakhoda-Sapuan, S. (2001). Enhancing social problem solving in children with autism and normal children through computer-assisted instruction. *Journal of Autism and Developmental Disorders*, *31*(4), 377–384. doi:10.1023/A:1010660502130 PMID:11569584

Bernstein, A., Bar, J., Ehrman, J. P., Golubic, M., & Roizen, M. (2013). Yoga in management of Overweight and Obesity. *Journal of Lifestyle Medicines*, *8*(1), 33–41. doi:10.1177/1559827613492097

Berryman, C., Ferguson, C. J., & Negy, C. (2018). Social media use and mental health among young adults. *The Psychiatric Quarterly*, *89*(2), 307–314. doi:10.100711126-017-9535-6 PMID:29090428

Bewick, B., Koutsopoulou, G., Miles, J., Slaa, E., & Barkham, M. (2010). Changes in undergraduate students' psychological well-being as they progress through university. *Studies in Higher Education*, *35*(6), 633–645. doi:10.1080/03075070903216643

Bhagavad Gita. (n.d.). Gita Press.

Bharti, R., & Sidana, J. J. (2012). A study of emotional intelligence in relation to academic achievement and academic stress of student-teachers. *Indian Streams Research Journal.*, *2*(9), 1–6.

Bhore Committee Report Government of India. (1946). *Report of the Health Survey and Development Committee* (vol. 2). Delhi: Manager of Publications.

Bhuiyan, P., Khatun, Z., Jahan, S., Morshed, T., Rahman, S., Afsana, N. A., & Rahmatullah, M. (2013). *Use of Quranic verses, amulets, numerology, and medicinal plants for treatment of diseases: a case study of a healer in Narsinghdi district*. Bangladesh: American-Eurasian Journal of Sustainable Agriculture.

Bilodeau, C., & Meissner, J. (2018). The effects of a combined academic and personal counselling initiative for post-secondary student retention. *Canadian Journal of School Psychology, 33*(1), 8–25. doi:10.1177/0829573516644554

Bimbrahw, J., Boger, J., & Mihailidis, A. (2012). Investigating the efficacy of a computerized prompting device to assist children with autism spectrum disorder with activities of daily living. *Assistive Technology, 24*(4), 286–298. doi:10.1080/10400435.2012.680661

Bipolar Disorder Connect - Mobile App. (n.d.). Retrieved from http://ibpf.org/resource/bipolar-disorder-connect-mobile-app

Bisht, D. B. (1985). *Spiritual Dimension of Health*. New Delhi: Directorate General of Health Services.

Bloom, J. R. (2002). Surviving and thriving? *Psycho-Oncology, 11*(2), 89–92. doi:10.1002/pon.606 PMID:11921324

Boniwell, I. (2008). *Positive psychology in a nutshell* (2nd ed.). London: PWBC.

Bonnet-Brilhault, F. (2017). Autism: An early neurodevelopmental disorder. *Archives de Pediatrie, 24*(4), 384–390. doi:10.1016/j.arcped.2017.01.014 PMID:28256376

Booc, C. E. R., San Diego, C. M. D., Tee, M. L., & Caro, J. D. (2016). A mobile application for campus-based psychosocial wellness program. In *Proceedings of the 2016 7th International Conference on Information, Intelligence, Systems & Applications (IISA)* (pp. 1-4). IEEE. 10.1109/IISA.2016.7785426

Bower, P., & Gilbody, S. (2005). Stepped care in psychological therapies: Access, effectiveness and efficiency. *The British Journal of Psychiatry, 186*(1), 11–17. doi:10.1192/bjp.186.1.11 PMID:15630118

Bowles, G. T. (1977). *The People of Asia*. London: Weidenfeld and Nicolson.

Bowling, A. (2003). Current state of the art in quality of life measurement. *Quality of Life, 2003*, 1-8.

Bowling, A., Rowe, G., Adams, S., Sands, P., Samsi, K., Crane, M., ... Manthorpe, J. (2015). Quality of life in dementia: A systematically conducted narrative review of dementia-specific measurement scales. *Aging & Mental Health, 19*(1), 13–31. doi:10.1080/13607863.2014.915923 PMID:24881888

Bowman, E. S. (1989). Understanding and responding to religious material in the therapy of multiple personality disorder. *Dissociation: Progress in the Dissociative Disorders, 2*(4), 231–238.

Bozkurt, F. (2015). *Sağlıklı yaşam ve pazarlama*. İstanbul: Beta Yayınları.

Bozkurt, F., & Ergen, A. (2014). *Promoting healthy lifestyle for sustainable development. In Handbook of Research on Developing Sustainable Value in Economics, Finance, and Marketing*. Hershey, PA: IGI Global.

Brady, M. J., Peterman, A. H., Fitchett, G., Mo, M., & Cella, D. (1999). A case for including spirituality in quality of life measurement in oncology. *Psycho-Oncology*, *8*(5), 417–428. doi:10.1002/(SICI)1099-1611(199909/10)8:5<417::AID-PON398>3.0.CO;2-4 PMID:10559801

Brajša-Žganec, A., & Kaliterna Lipovčan, Lj. (2006). Kvaliteta življenja, životno zadovoljstvo i sreća osoba koje profesionalno pomažu drugima. *Društvena istraživanja*, *4-5*(84-85), 713-728. Retrieved from http://hrcak.srce.hr/10874

Bray, F., Ferlay, J., Soerjomataram, I., Siegel, R. L., Torre, L. A., & Jemal, A. (2018). Global cancer statistics 2018: GLOBOCAN estimates of incidence and mortality worldwide for 36 cancers in 185 countries. *CA: a Cancer Journal for Clinicians*, *68*(6), 394–424. doi:10.3322/caac.21492 PMID:30207593

Brdar, I., & Bakarčić, S. (2006). Suočavanje s neuspjehom u školi: Koliko su važni emocionalna kompetentnost, osobine ličnosti i ciljna orijentacija u učenju? *Psihologijske Teme*, *15*(1), 129–150.

Bressington, D., Mui, J., Yu, C., Leung, S. F., Cheung, K., Wu, C. S. T., ... Chien, W. T. (2019). Feasibility of a group-based Laughter Yoga intervention as an adjunctive treatment for residual symptoms of depression, anxiety and stress in people with depression. *Journal of Affective Disorders*, *248*, 42–51. doi:10.1016/j.jad.2019.01.030 PMID:30711868

Brkić, I., & Rijavec, M. (2011). Izvori stresa, suočavanje sa stresom i životno zadovoljstvo učitelja razredne i predmetne nastave. *Napredak, 152*(2), 211– 225. Retrieved from http://hrcak.srce.hr/file/123100

Bruin, B. (2015). *Ethics and the Global Financial Crisis*. Cambridge University Press. doi:10.1017/CBO9781139237093

Buckingham, M., & Coffman, C. (1999). *First, Break all the Rules: What the world's greatest managers do differently*. New York: Simon & Schuster.

Buckley, M., & Saarni, C. (2009). Emotion regulation: Implications for positive youth development. In R. Gilman, E. S. Huebner, & M. J. Furlong (Eds.), *Handbook of positive psychology in schools* (pp. 107–118). New York, NY: Routledge.

Bullis, R. (1996). *Spirituality in social work practice*. Washington, DC: Taylor & Francis.

Burdak, L. (2016). *Jat Belt: Distribution of Jat Population*. Academic Press.

Cadieux, N., & Marchand, A. (2014). Psychological distress in the workforce: a multilevel and longitudinal analysis of the cases of regulated occupation in Canada. *BMC Public Health*. Retrieved from www.ncbi.nlm.nih.gov/pubmed/25099686

Cale, L. (2018). Young people, social media, physical activity, and health. *Young People, Social Media and Health,* 212-224. doi:10.4324/9781351026987-17

CalmE. (n.d.). Retrieved from https://www.calm.com/

Cameron, K. S., Dutton, J. E., & Quinn, R. E. (2003). *Positive Organizational Scholarship*. San Francisco: Berrett-Koehler.

Campbell-Enns, H., & Woodgate, R. (2015). The psychosocial experiences of women with breast cancer across the lifespan: A systematic review protocol. *JBI Database of Systematic Reviews and Implementation Reports*, *13*(1), 112–121. doi:10.11124/jbisrir-2015-1795 PMID:26447012

Canguilhem, G. (1998). Il normale e il patologico [The Normal and the Pathological] (M. Porro, Trans.). Torino: Einaudi. (Original work published 1966)

Capra, F. (1982). *The Turning Point: Science, Society and the Rising Culture*. London: Fontana Paperbacks.

Carli, R., & Paniccia, R. M. (2003). Analisi della domanda. Teoria e tecnica dell'intervento in psicologia clinica [Analysis of Demand. Theory and technique of intervention in clinical psychology]. Bologna: Il Mulino.

Carli, R., & Paniccia, R. M. (2011). La cultura dei servizi di salute mentale in Italia. Dai malati psichiatrici alla nuova utenza: l'evoluzione della domanda di aiuto e delle dinamiche di rapporto [The culture of Mental Health Services in Italy. From psychiatric patients to new users: The evolution of the aid demand and the dynamics of the relationship]. Milano: FrancoAngeli.

Carli, R., & Paniccia, R. M. (2012). Malattia mentale e senso comune [Mental illness and common sense]. *Rivista di Psicologia Clinica, 2*, 201 - 206. Retrieved from http://www.rivistadipsicologiaclinica.it

Carli, R., Paniccia, R. M., Caputo, A., Dolcetti, F., Finore, E., & Giovagnoli, F. (2016). La relazione che organizza il contesto sanitario: Domanda dell'utenza e risposta dei servizi sanitari, nel territorio e nell'ospedale [The relationship which organizes the healthcare context: Users' demand and response of healthcare services, in the territory and the hospital]. *Rivista di Psicologia Clinica*, *1*, 7–44. doi:10.14645/RPC.2016.1.608

Carlson, D., & Ehrlich, N. (2006). Sources of payment for assistive technology: Findings from a national survey of persons with disabilities. *Assistive Technology*, *18*(1), 77–86. doi:10.1080/10400435.2006.10131908 PMID:16796243

Caron, J., & Liu, A. (2011). Factors associated with psychological distress in the Canadian Population: a comparison of low- income and non-income sub groups. *Community Mental Health Journal, 47*(3), 318-30.

Caronia, L. (1997). Costruire la conoscenza [Building knowledge]. Firenze: La Nuova Italia.

Carr, D., & Felce, J. (2007). The effects of PECS teaching to phase III on the communicative interactions between children with autism and their teachers. *Journal of Autism and Developmental Disorders*, *37*(4), 724–737. doi:10.100710803-006-0203-1 PMID:17006780

Carver, C. S., & Scheier, M. F. (1999). Stress, coping, and self-regulatory processes. In L. A. Pervin & O. P. John (Eds.), *Handbook of personality: Theory and research* (pp. 553–575). New York, NY: Guilford Press.

Census Organisation of India. (2011). *Population Census 2011*. Available at: http://www.census2011.co.in/census/district/102-hazaribagh.html

Čepić, R., & Kalin, J. (2017). *Profesionalni razvoj učitelja: status, ličnost i transverzalne kompetencije*. Rijeka: Učiteljski fakultet Sveučilišta u Rijeci.

Čepić, R., & Pliško-Seferagić, L. (2016). Poticanje razvoja infrastrukture kontinuiranog učenja: izazov za odgajatelje. In N. Tatković, M. Radetić-Paić, & I. Blažević (Eds.), Kompetencijski pristup kvaliteti ranog i predškolskog odgoja i obrazovanja (pp. 281-294). Medulin: Dječji vrtić Medulin i Fakultet za odgojne i obrazovne znanosti Sveučilišta Jurja Dobrile u Puli.

Čepić, R., Tatalović Vorkapić, S., & Ružić, S. (2016). Samovrednovanje kvalitete procesa učenja na individualnoj, timskoj i organizacijskoj razini iz perspektive učitelja. *Školski vjesnik*, *65*, 11-21.

Čepić, R., & Krstović, J. (2011). Through lifelong learning and learning organisations towards sustainable future. *International Journal of Innovation and Learning*, *10*(2), 195–213. doi:10.1504/IJIL.2011.041797

Chadda, R. K. (2014). Caring for the family caregivers of persons with mental illness. *Indian Journal of Psychiatry*, *56*(3), 221. doi:10.4103/0019-5545.140616 PMID:25316932

Chang, E. C., Sanna, L. J., & Yang, K.-M. (2003). Optimism, pessimism, affectivity, and psychological adjustment in US and Korea: A test of a mediation model. *Personality and Individual Differences*, *34*(7), 1195–1208. doi:10.1016/S0191-8869(02)00109-5

Chatterji, S. (2012, January). Government Turns focus on Jat Quota. *Hindustan Times*.

Chattopadhyay, S. (2005). Spiritual and religious themes in psychiatric management: A proposed biopsychosocial model. *The Internet Journal of World Health and Societal Politics*, *2*(1).

Chen, C. (2016). The role of resilience and coping styles in subjective well-being among Chinese university students. *The Asia-Pacific Education Researcher*, *25*(3), 377–387. doi:10.100740299-016-0274-5

Cheng, Y., Huang, C.-L., & Yang, C.-S. (2015). Using a 3D Immersive Virtual Environment System to Enhance Social Understanding and Social Skills for Children With Autism Spectrum Disorders. *Focus on Autism and Other Developmental Disabilities*, *30*(4), 222–236. doi:10.1177/1088357615583473

Chen, K. H. (2018). Effects of multimedia teaching integrated social story on autistic children ' s social interaction. *Quality & Quantity*, *52*(S2), 1399–1408. doi:10.100711135-018-0731-8

Chen, M. (2009). Attitude toward organic foods among taiwanese as related to health consciousness, environmental attitudes, and the mediating effects of a healthy lifestyle. *British Food Journal*, *111*(2), 165–178. doi:10.1108/00070700910931986

Cheung, Y. B., Luo, N., Ng, R., & Lee, C. F. (2014). Mapping the functional assessment of cancer therapy - Breast (FACT-B) to the 5-level EuroQoL group's 5-dimension questionnaire (EQ-5D-5L) utility index in a multi-ethnic Asian population. *Health and Quality of Life Outcomes*, *12*(1), 180. doi:10.118612955-014-0180-6 PMID:25495840

Chien, W. T., Chan, S. W., & Thompson, D. R. (2006). Effects of a mutual support group for families of Chinese people with schizophrenia: 18- month follow-up. *The British Journal of Psychiatry*, *189*(1), 41–49. doi:10.1192/bjp.bp.105.008375 PMID:16816305

Chopik, W. J., Newton, N. J., Ryan, L. H., Kashdan, T. B., & Jarden, A. J. (2019). Gratitude across the life span: Age differences and links to subjective well-being. *The Journal of Positive Psychology*, *14*(3), 292–302. doi:10.1080/17439760.2017.1414296 PMID:31105762

Chowdhry, P. (1994). *The Veiled Women: Shifting Gender Equations in Rural Haryana 1880–1990*. New Delhi: Oxfor University Press.

Ciarrochi, J., Heaven, P. C. L., & Davies, F. (2007). The impact of hope, self-esteem, and attributional style on adolescents' school grades and emotional well-being: A longitudinal study. *Journal of Research in Personality*, *41*(6), 1161–1178. doi:10.1016/j.jrp.2007.02.001

Cihak, D. F. (2007). Teaching students with autism to read pictures. *Research in Autism Spectrum Disorders*, *1*(4), 318–329. doi:10.1016/j.rasd.2006.12.002

Cihak, D., Fahrenkrog, C., Ayres, K. M., & Smith, C. (2010). The Use of Video Modeling via a Video iPod and a System of Least Prompts to Improve Transitional Behaviors for Students with Autism Spectrum Disorders in the General Education Classroom. *Journal of Positive Behavior Interventions*, *12*(2), 103–115. doi:10.1177/1098300709332346

Clark, M. L. E., Austin, D. W., & Craike, M. J. (2014). Professional and Parental Attitudes Toward iPad Application Use in Autism Spectrum Disorder. *Focus on Autism and Other Developmental Disabilities*. doi:10.1177/1088357614537353

Clifford, T., & Minnes, P. (2013). Logging on: Evaluating an online support group for parents of children with autism spectrum disorders. *Journal of Autism and Developmental Disorders*, *43*(7), 1662–1675. doi:10.100710803-012-1714-6 PMID:23143075

Clyburn, L. D., Stones, M. J., Hadjistavropoulos, T., & Tuokko, H. (2000). Predicting caregiver burden and depression in Alzheimer's disease. *The Journals of Gerontology. Series B, Psychological Sciences and Social Sciences*, *55*(1), S2–S13. doi:10.1093/geronb/55.1.S2 PMID:10728125

Coggi, C., & Ricchiardi, P. (2005). Progettare la ricerca empirica in educazione [Planning empirical research in education]. Roma: Carocci Editore.

Cohen, M. (2010). Wellness and the thermodynamics of a healthy lifestyle. *Asia-Pacific Journal of Health, Sport and Physical Education*, *1*(2), 5–12. doi:10.1080/18377122.2010.9730326

Colby, K. M. (1967). Computer simulation of change in personal belief systems. *Journal of Systems Research and Behavioral Science*, *12*(3), 248–253. PMID:6059766

Coleman, S. B., Kaplan, J. D., & Downing, R. W. (1986). Life Cycle and Loss— The Spiritual Vacuum of Heroin Addiction. *Family Process*, *25*(1), 5–23. doi:10.1111/j.1545-5300.1986.00005.x PMID:3956709

Collie, R. J., & Martin, A. J. (2017). Students' adaptability in mathematics: Examining self-reports and teachers' reports and links with engagement and achievement outcomes. *Contemporary Educational Psychology*, *49*, 355–366. doi:10.1016/j.cedpsych.2017.04.001

Collings, R., Swanson, V., & Watkins, R. (2014). The impact of peer mentoring on levels of student wellbeing, integration and retention: A controlled comparative evaluation of residential students in UK higher education. *Higher Education*, *68*(6), 927–942. doi:10.100710734-014-9752-y

Collon, D. (1987). *First impressions: cylinder seals in the ancient Near East*. London: British Museum Publications.

Colucci, E., & Martin, G. (2008). Religion and Spirituality Along the Suicidal Path. *Suicide & Life-Threatening Behavior*, *38*(2), 229–244. doi:10.1521uli.2008.38.2.229 PMID:18444780

Conley, C. S., Travers, L. V., & Bryant, F. B. (2013). Promoting psychosocial adjustment and stress management in first-year college students: The benefits of engagement in a psychosocial wellness seminar. *Journal of American College Health*, *61*(2), 75–86. doi:10.1080/07448481.2012.754757 PMID:23409857

Constantin, A., Johnson, H., Smith, E., Lengyel, D., & Brosnan, M. (2017). Designing computer-based rewards with and for children with Autism Spectrum Disorder and/or Intellectual Disability. *Computers in Human Behavior*, *75*, 404–414. doi:10.1016/j.chb.2017.05.030

Copley, J., & Ziviani, J. (2004). Barriers to the use of assistive technology for children with multiple disabilities. *Occupational Therapy International*, *11*(4), 229–243. doi:10.1002/oti.213 PMID:15771212

Corbett, B. A. (2003). Video modeling: A window into the world of autism. *The Behavior Analyst Today*, *4*(3), 88–96. doi:10.1037/h0100025

Corbin, C. B., & Pangrazi, R. P. (2001). Towards a uniform definition of wellness: A commentary. *President's Council on Physical Fitness and Sports Research Digest*, *3*(15), 1–8.

Corbin, C. B., Welk, G. J., Corbin, W. R., & Welk, K. A. (2008). *Concepts of physical fitness: active lifestyles for wellness*. Boston: McGraw Hill.

Cory, D. (2015). *Healthy self-regard in effective leaders*. The Emotional Intelligence Training Company Inc. retrieved from https://www.eitrainingcompany.com/2015/02/healthy-self-regard-in-effective-leaders/

Cowen, V., & Adams, T. (2005). Physical and Perceptual Benefits of Yoga Asana Practice: Results of a Pilot Study. *Journal of Bodywork and Movement Therapies*, *9*(3), 211–219. doi:10.1016/j.jbmt.2004.08.001

Cozy Apps, L. (2014, August 27). *Quit That! - Habit Tracker*. Retrieved from https://apps.apple.com/us/app/quit-that-habit-tracker/id909400800

Creighton, C. (2018, March 22). *Validity of the Blue Whale Challenge is Disputed, but Social Media's Impact on Young People's Mental Health is Real*. Retrieved from https://www.einpresswire.com/article/393609296/validity-of-the-blue-whale-challenge-is-disputed-but-social-media-s-impact-on-young-people-s-mental-health-is-real

Cressy, J. (2011). The roles of physical activity and health in enhancing student engagement: Implications for leadership in post-secondary education. *The College Quarterly*, *14*(4), n4. Retrieved from https://search-ebscohost-com.ezp.waldenulibrary.org/login.aspx?direct=true&db=eric&AN=EJ967640&site=eds-live&scope=site

Crompton, M. (2010). *Improving self-awareness increases your emotional intelligence. inter business issues.* Retrieved from https://peoriamagazines.com/ibi/2010/apr/improving-self-awareness-increases-your-emotional-intelligence

Crowley, C., & Munk, D. (2017). An examination of the impact of a college level meditation course on college student well-being. *College Student Journal*, *91*(1). Retrieved from https://search-ebscohost-com.ezp.waldenulibrary.org/login.aspx?direct=true&db=edsgea&AN=edsgcl.487602756&site=eds-live&scope=site

Csikszentmihalyi, M. (1975). *Beyond boredom and anxiety*. San Francisco: Jossey Bass. Row.

Csikszentmihalyi, M. (1978). Attention and the holistic aproach to behavior. In K. S. Pope & J. L. Singer (Eds.), *The stream of consciousness* (pp. 335–358). New York: Plenum. doi:10.1007/978-1-4684-2466-9_13

Csikszentmihalyi, M. (1997). *Finding Flow*. New York: Basic Books.

Csikszentmihalyi, M. (2000). *Beyond boredom and anxiety. Experiencing flow in work and play*. San Francisco: Jossey-Bass. (Original work published 1975)

Csikszentmihalyi, M. (2006). *Zanesenost [Flow]*. Zagreb: Naklada Slap. (in Croatian)

Csikszentmihalyi, M., & Csikszentmihalyi, I. S. (1988). *Optimal Experience: Psychological studies of flow in consciousness*. Cambridge, UK: Cambridge University Press. doi:10.1017/CBO9780511621956

Da Silva, T. L., Ravindran, L. N., & Ravindran, A. V. (2009). Yoga in the treatment of mood and anxiety disorders: A review. *Asian Journal of Psychiatry*, *2*(1), 6–16. doi:10.1016/j.ajp.2008.12.002 PMID:23051013

Dabas, P & Sing, A. (2018). Bhagavad Gita teachings and positive psychology: Efficacy for semi-urban Indian students of NCR. *Cogent Psychology, 5*(1).

Dalal, A. K. (2016). *Cultural Psychology of Health in India: Well-being, Medicine and Traditional Health Care*. New Delhi: Sage Publication.

Das, S. (2017). Suicide among the elderly: A psychological perspective. *International Journal of Social Work and Human Services Practice*, *5*(1), 35–42.

Dastan, N. B., & Buzlu, S. (2012). Psychoeducation intervention to improve adjustment to cancer among Turkish stage I-II breast cancer patients: A randomized controlled trial. *Asian Pacific Journal of Cancer Prevention*, *13*(10), 5313–5318. doi:10.7314/APJCP.2012.13.10.5313 PMID:23244155

Data & Statistics on Autism Spectrum Disorder. (2019). Retrieved from https://www.cdc.gov/ncbddd/autism/data.html

Data Blog. (2018, June 19). Retrieved from https://health-infobase.canada.ca/datalab/blog.html

Datta, N. (1999a). *Forming an Identity: A Social History of the Jats*. New Delhi: Oxfor University Press.

Datta, N. (1999b). Jats: Trading Caste Status for Empowerment. *Economic and Political Weekly*, *34*(45), 6–12.

Dawson, G., Meltzoff, A. N., Osterling, J., & Rinaldi, J. (2006). Neuropsychological Correlates of Early Symptoms of Autism. *Child Development*, *69*(5), 1276–1285. doi:10.1111/j.1467-8624.1998.tb06211.x PMID:9839415

Day, J., Woolrich, W., & Strong, H. (2001). The stability of impact of assistive devices. *Disability and Rehabilitation*, *23*(9), 400–404. doi:10.1080/09638280010008906 PMID:11394591

Dayalan, H., Subramanian, S., & Elango, T. (2010). Psychological well-being in medical students during exam stress: Influence of short-term practice of mind sound technology. *Indian Journal of Medical Sciences*, *64*(11), 501. doi:10.4103/0019-5359.102122 PMID:23051942

De Villiers, R. (2010). The incorporation of soft skills into accounting curricula: Preparing accounting graduates for their unpredictable futures. *Meditari Accountancy Research*, *18*(2), 1–22. doi:10.1108/10222529201000007

Delle Fave, A., & Massimini, F. (2004). Bringing subjectivity into focus: optimal experiances, life themes and person-centred rehabilitation. In P. A. Linley & S. Joseph (Eds.), *Positive Psyhology in Practice* (pp. 581–597). London: Wiley & Sons.

Demetrio, D. (1992). Micropedagogia. La ricerca qualitativa in educazione [Micropedagogy. Qualitative research in education]. Firenze: La Nuova Italia.

Deniz, S. (2013). The relationship between emotional intelligence and problem solving skills in prospective teachers. *Educational Research Review*, *8*(24), 2339–2345.

Denovan, A., & Macaskill, A. (2017). Stress and subjective well-being among first year UK undergraduate students. *Journal of Happiness Studies*, *18*(2), 505–525. doi:10.100710902-016-9736-y

DeNysschen, C. A., Burton, H., Ademuyiwa, F., Levine, E., Tetewsky, S., & O'Connor, T. (2014). Exercise intervention in breast cancer patients with aromatase inhibitor-associated arthralgia: A pilot study. *European Journal of Cancer Care, 23*(4), 493–501. doi:10.1111/ecc.12155 PMID:24289215

Derry, H., Jaremka, L., Bennett, J., Peng, J., Andridge, R., Shapiro, C., ... Keicol-Glaser, J. (2014). (2014). Yoga and self-reported cognitive problems in breast cancer survivors: A randomized controlled trial. *Journal of Psychological. Social and Behavioural Dimensions of Cancer, 24*(8), 958–966. PMID:25336068

DeSantis, C. E., Ma, J., Goding Sauer, A., Newman, L. A., & Jemal, A. (2017). Breast cancer statistics, 2017, racial disparity in mortality by state. *CA: a Cancer Journal for Clinicians, 67*(6), 439–448. doi:10.3322/caac.21412 PMID:28972651

DeSteno, D. A., & Salovey, P. (1997). The effects of mood on the structure of the self-concept. *Cognition and Emotion, 11*(4), 351–372. doi:10.1080/026999397379836

Development of Self *or Human Resource Development, For Success in Management through Spiritual Wisdom and Meditation.* (n.d.). Brahma Kumari's Ishwariya Vishwa Vidyalaya .

Di Bella, O., Cocchiara, R. A., De Luca, A., Frusone, F., Aceti, V., Sestili, C., D'Egidio, V., Mannocci, … Torre, G.L (2018). Functional Assessment of Cancer Therapy Questionnaire for Breast Cancer (FACT-B+4): Italianversion validation. *Clin. Ter., 169*(4), e151-e154. doi:10.7417/T.2018.2071

Diagnostic and Statistical Manual of Mental Disorders. (1994). (4th ed.). Washington, DC: American Psychiatric Association.

Dieli-Conwright, C. M., Mortimer, J. E., Schroeder, E. T., Courneya, K., Demark-Wahnefried, W., Buchanan, T. A., ... Bernstein, L. (2014). Randomized controlled trial to evaluate the effects of combined progressive exercise on metabolic syndrome in breast cancer survivors: Rationale, design, and methods. *BMC Cancer, 14*(1), 238. doi:10.1186/1471-2407-14-238 PMID:24708832

Diener, E., Lukas, R.E. & Oishi, S. (2002). Subjective Well-Being. The Science of Happiness and the Satisfaction. Part III. *Emotional-Focused Approaches*, 63-73.

Diener, E., Wirtz, D., Tov, W., Kim-Prieto, C., Choi, D. W., Oishi, S., & Biswas-Diener, R. (2010). New well-being measures: Short scales to assess flourishing and positive and negative feelings. *Social Indicators Research, 97*(2), 143–156. doi:10.100711205-009-9493-y

Diener, E. D., Emmons, R. A., Larsen, R. J., & Griffin, S. (1985). The satisfaction with life scale. *Journal of Personality Assessment, 49*(1), 71–75. doi:10.120715327752jpa4901_13 PMID:16367493

Diener, E., & Suh, M. E. (1998). Subjective Well-Being and Age: An International Analysis. In K. W. Schaie & M. P. Lawton (Eds.), *Annual Review of Gerontology and Geriatrics: Focus on Emotion and Adult Development*. New York, NY: Springer Publishing Company.

Dilip, V., Jeste, M. D., Ipsit, V., & Vahia, M. D. (2014). Comparison of the conceptualization of wisdom in ancient Indian literature with modern views: Focus on the Bhagavad Gita. *Psychiatry*, *71*, 197–209. PMID:18834271

Diwakar, N., & Ahamad, T. (2015). Skill development of women through vocational training. *International Journal of Applied Research.*, *1*(6), 79–83.

Dominic Claeys-Jackson. (2017). *5 ways to manage student stress*. Retrieved from https://www.prospects.ac.uk/applying-for-university/university-life/5-ways-to-manage-student-stress

Domović, V. (2003). *Školsko ozračje i učinkovitost škole*. Jastrebarsko: Naklada Slap.

Draper, B. (2004). *Dealing with Dementia: A guide to Alzheimer's Disease and Depression in Caregivers of Patients with Dementia*. Academic Press.

Drescher, K. D., & Foy, D. W. (1995). *Spirituality and Trauma Treatment: Suggestions for Including Spirituality as a Coping Resource - the National Center for Post Traumatic Stress Disorder Napa County, California*. Retrieved November 5, 2019, from http://napa.networkofcare.org/veterans/library/article.aspx?id=384&cat=473

Dvořáková, K., Kishida, M., Li, J., Elavsky, S., Broderick, P. C., Agrusti, M. R., & Greenberg, M. T. (2017). Promoting healthy transition to college through mindfulness training with first-year college students: Pilot randomized controlled trial. *Journal of American College Health*, *65*(4), 259–267. doi:10.1080/07448481.2017.1278605 PMID:28076182

Edwards, E., & Maxwell, M. (2002). Psychological interventions for women with metastatic breast cancer. Cochrane Database of Systematic Reviews, 44, 3137-3150. doi:10.1002/14651858.CD004253

Ehman, J. W., Ott, B. B., Short, T. H., Ciampa, R. C., & Hansen-Flaschen, J. (1999). Do patients want physicians to inquire about their spiritual or religious beliefs if they become gravely ill? *Archives of Internal Medicine*, *159*(15), 1803–1806. doi:10.1001/archinte.159.15.1803 PMID:10448785

Eikemo, T. E., Bambra, C., Huijts, T., & Fitzgerald, R. (2016). The First Pan-European Sociological Health Inequalities Survey of the General Population: The European Social Survey Rotating Module on the Social Determinants of Health. *European Sociological Review*, *33*(1), 137–153. Retrieved from https://watermark.silverchair.com/jcw019.pdf

El Ansari, W., Stock, C., John, J., Deeny, P., Phillips, C., Snelgrove, S., ... Mabhala, A. (2011). Health promoting behaviours and lifestyle characteristics of students at seven universities in the UK. *Central European Journal of Public Health*, *19*(4), 197–204. doi:10.21101/cejph.a3684 PMID:22432394

Election Commission of India. (2014). *Systematic Voters' Education and Electoral Participation*. State Sveep Plan 2014, Jharkhand, Office of the Chief Electoral Officer, Jharkhand. Available at: http://eci.nic.in/eci_main1/SVEEP/statesweepplan2014/JHARKHAND.pdf

El-Hashimi, D., & Gorey, K. M. (2019). Yoga-Specific Enhancement of Quality of Life Among Women With Breast Cancer: Systematic Review and Exploratory Meta-Analysis of Randomized Controlled Trials. *Journal of Evidence-Based Integrative Medicine, 24.*

El-Hashimi, D., & Gorey, K. M. (2019). Yoga-specific enhancement of quality of life among women with breast cancer: Systematic review and exploratory meta-analysis of randomized controlled trials. *Journal of Evidence-Based Integrative Medicine, 24*(6). doi:10.1177/2515690X19828325 PMID:30791697

Emaus, A., Veierod, M. B., Tretli, S., Finstad, S. E., Selmer, R., Furberg, A.-S., ... Thune, I. (2010). Metabolic profile, physical activity, and mortality in breast cancer patients. *Breast Cancer Research and Treatment, 121*(3), 651–660. doi:10.100710549-009-0603-y PMID:19882245

Emet, G., & Tat, M. (2017). Swot Analysis: A Theoretical Review. *Journal of International Social Research, 51*(10), 995–1005. doi:10.17719/jisr.2017.1832

Enea, H., & Colby, K. M. (1973). Idiolectic language-analysis for understanding doctor-patient dialogues. In *3rd International Joint Conference on Artificial Intelligence* (pp. 278–290). Academic Press.

Erickson, E. H., Erickson, J. M., & Kivnick, H. W. (1986). *Vital involvement in old age*. New York: Norton.

Erikson, J. M. (1988). *Wisdom and the senses*. New York: W.W. Norton.

Escobar, A., Trujillo-Martín Mdel, M., Rueda, A., Pérez-Ruiz, E., Avis, N. E., & Bilbao, A. (2015). Cross-cultural adaptation, reliability and validity of the Spanish version of the Quality of Life in Adult Cancer Survivors (QLACS) questionnaire: application in a sample of short-term survivors. *Health Qual Life Outcomes, 13,* 182. doi:10.118612955-015-0378-2

Esmaeili, N., & Jamkhaneh, E. B. (2013). The relationship between emotional intelligence and mental health in humanism college students at IAU, Qaemshahr Branch, Iran. *Journal of Basic and Applied Scientific Research, 3*(2), 68–76.

Esmaeily, M., Ahadi, H., Delavar, A., & Shafiabadi, A. (2007). Effects of emotional intelligence training on enhancing mental health. *Majallah-i Ravanpizishki va Ravanshinasi-i Balini-i Iran, 13*, 158–165.

Everyday Health. (2018, October 25). *Trusted Medical Information, Expert Health Advice, News, Tools, and Resources*. Retrieved from https://www.everydayhealth.com/

Eyre, H., Siddarth, P., Acevedo, B., & Dyk, K. (2017). A Randomized controlled trial of Kundalini Yoga in mild cognitive impairment. *International Psychogeriatrics, 29*(4), 557–567. doi:10.1017/S1041610216002155 PMID:28088925

Falb, M. D., & Pargament, K. I. (2014). Religion, Spirituality, and Positive Psychology: Strengthening Well-Being. In Perspectives on the Intersection of Multiculturalism and Positive Psychology. Cross-Cultural Advancements in Positive Psychology (7th ed.). Dordrecht: Springer.

Falsetti, S. A., Resick, P. A., & Davis, J. L. (2003). Changes in religious beliefs following trauma. *Journal of Traumatic Stress*, *16*(4), 391–398. doi:10.1023/A:1024422220163 PMID:12895022

Farina, A. (1982). The stigma of mental disorders. In A. Miller (Ed.), *The Eye of the Beholder* (pp. 305–363). New York: Praeger.

Febrilia, I., & Warokka, A. (2014). *The effects of positive and negative mood on university students' learning and academic performance: Evidence from Indonesia*. Academic Press.

Fekih-Romdhane, F., Henchiri, H., Ridha, R., Labbane, R., & Cheour, M. (2019). Niveau de détresse psychologique et de fardeau perçu chez les conjoints de femmes atteintes d'un cancer du sein. *L'Encéphale*, *45*(2), 190–192. doi:10.1016/j.encep.2018.09.003 PMID:30428997

Feldman, D. B., & Dreher, D. E. (2012). Can hope be changed in 90 minutes? Testing the efficacy of a single-session goal-pursuit intervention for college students. *Journal of Happiness Studies*, *13*(4), 745–759. doi:10.100710902-011-9292-4

Ferrer, R. A., Huedo-Medina, T. B., Johnson, B. T., Ryan, S., & Pescatello, L. S. (2011). Exercise interventions for cancer survivors: A meta-analysis of quality of life outcomes. *Annals of Behavioral Medicine*, *41*(1), 32–47. doi:10.100712160-010-9225-1 PMID:20931309

Ferster, C. B., & Demyer, M. K. (1961). The development of performances in autistic children in an automatically controlled environment. *Journal of Chronic Diseases*, *13*(4), 312–345. doi:10.1016/0021-9681(61)90059-5 PMID:13699188

Firman, J., & Gila, A. (2012). *Psychotherapy of Love, A: Psychosynthesis in Practice*. Albany, NY: State University of New York Press.

Fishbach, A., & Labroo, A. A. (2007). Be better or be merry: How mood affects self-control. *Journal of Personality and Social Psychology*, *93*(2), 158–173. doi:10.1037/0022-3514.93.2.158 PMID:17645393

Fisher, J. W. (2009). Investigating Australian education students' views about spiritual well-being, as compared with teachers in schools. *International Journal of Children's Spirituality*, *14*(2), 151–167. doi:10.1080/13644360902830358

Fisher, J. W., & Wong, P. H. (2013). Comparing levels of spiritual well-being and support among pre-service teachers in Hong Kong and Australia. *Religious Education Journal of Australia*, *29*(1), 34.

Fitzpatrick, R. B. (2010). AbleData: A resource of assistive technology information. *Medical Reference Services Quarterly*, *29*(3), 260–268. doi:10.1080/02763869.2010.494510 PMID:20677066

Foster, R. M. P. (2016). *The power of emotional intelligence for facilitating psychologically flexible thinking: a contextual perspective in decision making and workplace flourishing*. Academic Press.

Fowler, J. W. (1981). *Stages of faith: The psychology of human development and the quest for meaning*. San Francisco: Harper and Row.

Fredrickson, B. L. (1998). What good are positive emotions? *Review of General Psychology*, *2*(3), 300–319. doi:10.1037/1089-2680.2.3.300 PMID:21850154

Fredrickson, B. L. (2001). The role of positive emotions in positive psychology: The broaden-and-build theory of positive emotions. *The American Psychologist*, *56*(3), 218–226. doi:10.1037/0003-066X.56.3.218 PMID:11315248

Freed, R. S., & Freed, S. A. (1990). Ghost Illness in a North Indian village. *Social Science & Medicine, 30*(5), 617–623.

Freed, R. S., & Freed, S. A. (1993). Ghost: Life and Death in North India (No. 72). New York: Academic Press.

Freedman, J., & Jensen, A. (2008). A case for emotional intelligence in our schools. *Six seconds: The Emotional Intelligence Network*.

Friedenreich, C. M., & Cust, A. E. (2008). Physical activity and breast cancer risk: Impact of timing, type and dose of activity and population subgroup effects. *British Journal of Sports Medicine*, *42*(8), 636–647. doi:10.1136/bjsm.2006.029132 PMID:18487249

Frijns, M. (2010). *Determinants of life satisfaction: a cross-regional comparison* (Unpublished final thesis). Maastricht University, School of Business and Economics, Master of Science in International Business Concentration.

Frost, R. E. (1981). An interactive computer environment for autistic children. In *The Johns Hopkins First National Search for Applications of Personal Computing to Aid the Handicapped* (p. 1981). Los Angeles, CA: IEEE Computer Society.

Frutos, M., Bustos, I., Zapirain, B. G., & Zorrilla, A. M. (2011). Computer game to learn and enhance speech problems for children with autism. *Proceedings of CGAMES'2011 USA - 16th International Conference on Computer Games: AI, Animation, Mobile, Interactive Multimedia, Educational and Serious Games*, 209–216. 10.1109/CGAMES.2011.6000340

Fuchs, S. (1974). *The Aboriginal Tribes of India*. Delhi: Macmillan.

Furnham, A., & Petrides, K. V. (2003). Trait emotional intelligence and happiness. *Social Behavior and Personality*, *31*(8), 815–823. doi:10.2224bp.2003.31.8.815

Galalae, R. M., Michel, J., Siebmann, J. U., Küchler, T., Eilf, K., & Kimmig, B. (2005). Significant negative impact of adjuvant chemotherapy on health-related quality of life (HR-QoL) in women with breast cancer treated by conserving surgery and postoperative 3-D radiotherapy. *Strahlentherapie und Onkologie*, *181*(10), 645–651. doi:10.100700066-005-1403-x PMID:16220403

Galante, J., Dufour, G., Benton, A., Howarth, E., Vainre, M., Croudace, T. J., ... Jones, P. B. (2016). Protocol for the Mindful Student Study: A randomised controlled trial of the provision of a mindfulness intervention to support university students' well-being and resilience to stress. *BMJ (Clinical Research Ed.)*, *6*(11), 1–8. doi:10.1136/bmjopen-2016-012300 PMID:28186934

Galderisi, S., Heinz, A., Kastrup, M., Beezhold, J., & Sartorius, N. (2015, June). *Toward a new definition of mental health*. Retrieved from https://www.ncbi.nlm.nih.gov/pmc/articles/PMC4471980/

Galway, K., Black, A., Cantwell, M., Cardwell, C. R., Mills, M., & Donnelly, M. (2012). Psychosocial interventions to improve quality of life and emotional wellbeing for recently diagnosed cancer patients. *Cochrane Database of Systematic Reviews*, *181*(10), 645–651. doi:10.1002/14651858.CD007064.pub2 PMID:23152241

Ganesh, S., Lye, M.-S., & Lau, F. N. (2016). Quality of life among breast cancer patients in Malaysia. *Asian Pacific Journal of Cancer Prevention*, *17*(4), 1677–1684. doi:10.7314/APJCP.2016.17.4.1677 PMID:27221837

Ganz, J. B., Boles, M. B., Goodwyn, F. D., & Flores, M. M. (2014). Efficacy of Handheld Electronic Visual Supports to Enhance Vocabulary in Children With ASD. *Focus on Autism and Other Developmental Disabilities*, *29*(1), 3–12. doi:10.1177/1088357613504991

Ganz, J. B., & Simpson, R. L. (2004). Effects on communicative requesting and speech development of the picture exchange communication system in children with characteristics of autism. *Journal of Autism and Developmental Disorders*, *34*(4), 395–409. doi:10.1023/B:JADD.0000037416.59095.d7 PMID:15449515

Ganz, P. (2002). Quality of life in long-term, disease-free survivors of breast cancer: A follow-up study. *CancerSpectrum Knowledge Environment*, *94*(1), 39–49. PMID:11773281

Garg, P., & Rastogi, R. (2009). Emotional intelligence and stress resiliency: A relationship study. *International Journal of Educational Advancement*, *1*(1), 1–16.

Garrison, K., Zeffiro, T., Scheinost, D., Constable, R., & Brewer, J. (2015). Meditation leads to reduced default mode network activity beyond an active task. *Cognitive, Affective & Behavioral Neuroscience*, *15*(3), 712–720. doi:10.375813415-015-0358-3 PMID:25904238

Garzotto, F., Messina, N., Matarazzo, V., Moskwa, L., Oliva, G., & Facchini, R. (2018). Empowering Interventions for Persons with Neurodevelopmental Disorders through Wearable Virtual Reality and Bio-sensors. *Conference on Human Factors in Computing Systems - CHI '18*, 1–6. 10.1145/3170427.3188636

Geertz, C. (1973). *The Interpretation of Cultures: Selected essays*. New York: Basic Books Inc. Publishers.

George, J. M. (2000). Emotions and leadership: The role of emotional intelligence. *Human Relations*, *53*(8), 1027–1055. doi:10.1177/0018726700538001

Get the Headspace App. (n.d.). Retrieved from https://www.headspace.com/headspace-meditation-app

Gieck, D. J., & Olsen, S. (2007). Holistic wellness as a means to developing a lifestyle approach to health behavior among college students. *Journal of American College Health*, *56*(1), 29–36. doi:10.3200/JACH.56.1.29-36 PMID:17711823

Gil, J. M., Gracia, A., & Sanchez, M. (2000). Market segmentation and willingness to pay for organic products in Spain. *The International Food and Agribusiness Management Review*, *3*(2), 207–226. doi:10.1016/S1096-7508(01)00040-4

Gillespie-Lynch, K., Kapp, S. K., Shane-Simpson, C., Smith, D. S., & Hutman, T. (2014). Intersections between the autism spectrum and the internet: Perceived benefits and preferred functions of computer-mediated communication. *Intellectual and Developmental Disabilities*, *52*(6), 456–469. doi:10.1352/1934-9556-52.6.456 PMID:25409132

Ginzburg, C. (1986). Miti, emblemi e spie [Myths, emblems and clues]. Torino: Einaudi.

Gleason, M. E. (2011). Intrapersonal intelligence strategies in the developmental writing classroom. *Inquiry*, *16*(1), 95–105.

Gockel, A. (2011). Client perspectives on spirituality in the therapeutic relationship. *The Humanistic Psychologist*, *39*(2), 154–168. doi:10.1080/08873267.2011.564959

Goldenberg, E. P. (1979). *Special technology for special children.* Academic Press.

Goldenberg, E. P. (1987). *Exploring Language with Logo.* The MIT Press.

Goldman, R. (1968). *Religious thinking from childhood to adolescence.* New York: Seabury.

Goleman, D. (1995). *Emotional intelligence: why it can matter more than IQ?* New York: Bantam.

Goleman, D. (1998). *Working with Emotional Intelligence.* New York: Bantam Books.

Gonsiorek, J. C., Richards, P. S., Pargament, K. I., & McMinn, M. R. (2009). Ethical challenges and opportunities at the edge: Incorporating spirituality and religion into psychotherapy. *Professional Psychology, Research and Practice*, *40*(4), 385–395. doi:10.1037/a0016488

Goodwin, J., Behan, L., Kelly, P., McCarthy, K., & Horgan, A. (2016). Help-seeking behaviors and mental well-being of first year undergraduate university students. *Psychiatry Research*, *246*, 129–135. doi:10.1016/j.psychres.2016.09.015 PMID:27693865

Gordon, N. H., & Siminoff, L. A. (2010). Measuring quality of life of long-term breast cancer survivors: The long term quality of life - breast cancer (LTQOL-BC) scale. *Journal of Psychosocial Oncology*, *28*(6), 589–609. doi:10.1080/07347332.2010.516806 PMID:21058158

Gosh, S. (2014). Equity in the utilization of healthcare services in India: Evidence from National Sample Survey. *International Journal of Health Policy and Management*, *2*(1), 29–38. doi:10.15171/ijhpm.2014.06 PMID:24596902

Government of India. (n.d.). *National Rural Health Mission e meeting people's health needs in rural areas: framework for implementation. 2005-2012.* Ministry of Health and Family Welfare. Available from: http://www.nrhm.gov.in/images/pdf/about-nrhm/nrhm-framework-implementation/nrhmframework-latest.pdf

Goyal, N. G., Levine, B. J., Van Zee, K. J., Naftalis, E., & Avis, N. E. (2018). Trajectories of quality of life following breast cancer diagnosis. *Breast Cancer Res Treat., 169*(1), 163-173. doi:10.100710549-018-4677-2

Grainger, C., Williams, D. M., & Lind, S. E. (2014). Online action monitoring and memory for self-performed actions in autism spectrum disorder. *Journal of Autism and Developmental Disorders, 44*(5), 1193–1206. doi:10.100710803-013-1987-4 PMID:24193578

Green, J., & Shellenberger, R. (1991). *The Dynamics of Health and Wellness: A Biopsychosocial Approach*. Chicago: Holt, Rinehart & Winston.

Greysen, H. M., Hong, O. S., & Katz, P. (2019). The Association Between Yoga Use, Physical Function, and Employment in Adults With Rheumatoid Arthritis. *Holistic Nursing Practice, 33*(2), 71–79. doi:10.1097/HNP.0000000000000296 PMID:30747775

Grimison, P. S., & Stockler, M. R. (2007). Quality of life and adjuvant systemic therapy for early-stage breast cancer. *Expert Review of Anticancer Therapy, 7*(8), 1123–1134. doi:10.1586/14737140.7.8.1123 PMID:18028021

Grossard, C., Grynspan, O., Serret, S., Jouen, A. L., Bailly, K., & Cohen, D. (2017). Serious games to teach social interactions and emotions to individuals with autism spectrum disorders (ASD). *Computers & Education, 113*, 195–211. doi:10.1016/j.compedu.2017.05.002

Gruetzner, H. (2001). *Alzheimer's: A caregiver's guide and sourcebook*. New York: John Wiley.

Gujral, D. H. K. (2013). Emotional intelligence buffers stress: A study on emotional intelligence and coping styles. *EXCEL International Journal of Multidisciplinary Management Studies, 3*(11), 76–82.

Gupta, G., & Kumar, S. (2010). Mental health in relation to emotional intelligence and self-efficacy among college students. *Journal of the Indian Academy of Applied Psychology, 36*(1), 61–67.

Guthrie, C. (2010). *Befriending the Body: Find Peace and Relief from Autoimmune Disorders through Yoga*. Retrieved from https://www.yogajournal.com/lifestyle/befriend-the-body

Hahn, E. A., Segawa, E., Kaiser, K., Cella, D., & Smith, B. D. (2015). Validation of the Functional Assessment of Cancer Therapy-Breast (FACT-B) quality of life instrument. *Journal of Clinical Oncology, 33*(15suppl), e17753–e17753. doi:10.1200/jco.2015.33.15_suppl.e17753

Halama, P. (2010). Hope as a mediator between personality traits and life satisfaction. *Studia Psychologica, 52*(4), 309–314.

Han, L., & Li, X. (2014). The appliance of affective computing in man-machine dialogue: Assisting therapy of having autism. In *4th International Conference on Communication Systems and Network Technologies, CSNT 2014* (pp. 1093–1096). 10.1109/CSNT.2014.223

Harding, R., Powell, R. A., Kiyange, F., Downing, J., & Mwangi-Powell, F. (2010). Provision of Pain- and Symptom-Relieving Drugs for HIV/AIDS in Sub-Saharan Africa. *Journal of Pain and Symptom Management, 40*(3), 405–415. doi:10.1016/j.jpainsymman.2009.12.025 PMID:20685071

Hardy, J. (2016). *A psychology with a soul: Psychosynthesis in evolutionary context*. Routledge. doi:10.4324/9781315562124

Harter, J. K., & Creglow, A. (1999). A meta-analysis and utility analysis of the relationship between core employee opinions and business outcomes. In M. Buckingham & C. Coffman (Eds.), First, break all the rules (pp. 255-267). New York: Simon & Schuster.

Hartman, C. L., Evans, K. E., & Anderson, D. M. (2017). Promoting adaptive coping skills and subjective well-being through credit-based leisure education courses. *Journal of Student Affairs Research and Practice*, *54*(3), 303–315. doi:10.1080/19496591.2017.1331852

Hazen, E. P., Stornelli, J. L., O'Rourke, J. A., Koesterer, K., & McDougle, C. J. (2014). Sensory symptoms in autism spectrum disorders. *Harvard Review of Psychiatry*, *22*(2), 112–124. doi:10.1097/01.HRP.0000445143.08773.58 PMID:24614766

Heinl, D., Prinsen, C. A. C., Deckert, S., Chalmers, J. R., Drucker, A. M., Ofenloch, R., ... Apfelbacher, C. (2016). Measurement properties of adult quality-of-life measurement instruments for eczema: A systematic review. *Allergy*, *71*(3), 358–370. doi:10.1111/all.12806 PMID:26564008

Heinl, D., Prinsen, C. A. C., Sach, T., Drucker, A. M., Ofenloch, R., Flohr, C., & Apfelbacher, C. (2017). Measurement properties of quality-of-life measurement instruments for infants, children and adolescents with eczema: A systematic review. *British Journal of Dermatology*, *176*(4), 878–889. doi:10.1111/bjd.14966 PMID:27543747

Heinonen, K., Räikkönen, K., & Keltikangas-Järvinen, L. (2005). Dispositional optimism: Development over 21 years from the perspectives of perceived temperament and mothering. *Personality and Individual Differences*, *38*(2), 425–435. doi:10.1016/j.paid.2004.04.020

Hellman, M. (2017). *Promoting Vices- An Introduction to Research on the Advertising of Coercive Products*. University of Helsinki.

Hetzroni, O. E., & Tannous, J. (2004). Effects of a computer-based intervention program on the communicative functions of children with autism. *Journal of Autism and Developmental Disorders*, *34*(2), 95–113. doi:10.1023/B:JADD.0000022602.40506.bf PMID:15162930

Higgins, K., & Boone, R. (1996). Creating individualized computer-assisted instruction for students with autism using multimedia. *Focus on Autism and Other Developmental Disabilities*, *11*(2), 69–78. doi:10.1177/108835769601100202

Hills, P., & Argyle, M. (2001). Happiness, introversion-extraversion and happy introverts. *Personality and Individual Differences*, *30*(4), 595–608. doi:10.1016/S0191-8869(00)00058-1

Hilton, L., Maher, A. R., Colaiaco, B., Apaydin, E., Sorbero, M. E., Booth, M., ... Hempel, S. (2017). Meditation for posttraumatic stress: Systematic review and meta-analysis. *Psychological Trauma: Theory, Research, Practice, and Policy*, *9*(4), 453–460. doi:10.1037/tra0000180 PMID:27537781

Hochmair, I. (2013). The importance of being flexible. *Nature Medicine*, *19*(10), 1240–1244. doi:10.1038/nm.3341 PMID:24100995

Hocking, C. (1999). Function or feelings: factors in abandonment of assistive devices. *Technology and Disability, 11*(1, 2), 3-11.

Hoeing, J., & Hamilton, M. W. (1966). The schizophrenia patients in the community and is effect on the household. *The International Journal of Social Psychiatry, 12*(3), 165–176. doi:10.1177/002076406601200301 PMID:5964677

Hojan, K., Molińska-Glura, M., & Milecki, P. (2013). Physical activity and body composition, body physique, and quality of life in premenopausal breast cancer patients during endocrine therapy: A feasibility study. *Acta Oncologica, 52*(2), 319–326. doi:10.3109/0284186X.2012.744468 PMID:23193959

Holm, M. B. (2000). Our mandate for the new millennium: Evidence-based practice. *The American Journal of Occupational Therapy, 54*(6), 575–585. doi:10.5014/ajot.54.6.575 PMID:11100239

Home Page. (n.d.). Retrieved from https://www.treatmyocd.com/

Home. (n.d.). Retrieved from https://www.mentalhealth.org.uk/

Home. (n.d.). Retrieved from https://www.mind.org.uk/

Hopkins, I. M., Gower, M. W., Perez, T. A., Smith, D. S., Amthor, F. R., Casey Wimsatt, F., & Biasini, F. J. (2011). Avatar assistant: Improving social skills in students with an asd through a computer-based intervention. *Journal of Autism and Developmental Disorders, 41*(11), 1543–1555. doi:10.100710803-011-1179-z PMID:21287255

Hopwood, P., Haviland, J., Mills, J., Sumo, G., & Bliss, J. (2007). The impact of age and clinical factors on quality of life in early breast cancer: An analysis of 2208 women recruited to the UK START Trial (Standardisation of Breast Radiotherapy Trial). *The Breast, 16*(3), 241–251. doi:10.1016/j.breast.2006.11.003 PMID:17236771

Hosotani, R., & Imai-Matsumura, K. (2011). Emotional experience, expression, and regulation of high-quality Japanese elementary school teachers. *Teaching and Teacher Education, 27*(6), 1039–1048. doi:10.1016/j.tate.2011.03.010

Hosseini, H. S. (2007, September). *Problem solving by intelligent water drops. In 2007 IEEE congress on evolutionary computation* (pp. 3226–3231). IEEE. doi:10.1109/CEC.2007.4424885

House, J. S., Landis, K. R., & Umberson, D. (1988). Social relationships and health. *Science, 241*(4865), 540–545. doi:10.1126cience.3399889 PMID:3399889

Hou, Y., Feng, X., Yang, X., Yang, Z., Zhang, X., & Koenig, H. G. (2018). Religion and subjective well-being in Chinese college students: Does meaningfulness matter? *Archiv Für Religionspsychologie. Archiv für Religionspsychologie, 40*(1), 60–79. doi:10.1163/15736121-12341351

Howlett, N., Pine, K., Orakçıoğlu, I., & Fletcher, B. (2013). The influence of clothing on first impressions: Rapid and positive responses to minor changes in male attire. *Journal of Fashion Marketing and Management: An International Journal*, *17*(1), 38–48. doi:10.1108/13612021311305128

Hsieh, M. C., Wang, T. S., Fan, C. P., & Huang, C. I. (2014). A study of the emotional intelligence and interpersonal relationships of college students in Southern Taiwan. *Universal Journal of Management*, *2*(8), 133–138.

Hwang, S. Y., Chang, S. J., & Park, B.-W. (2013). Does chemotherapy really affect the quality of life of women with breast cancer? *Journal of Breast Cancer*, *16*(2), 229. doi:10.4048/jbc.2013.16.2.229 PMID:23843858

Iarocci, G., Burack, J. A., Shore, D. I., Mottron, L., & Enns, J. T. (2006). Global-local visual processing in high functioning children with autism: Structural vs. implicit task biases. *Journal of Autism and Developmental Disorders*, *36*(1), 117–129. doi:10.100710803-005-0045-2 PMID:16397823

Ibbetson, D. (1916). *Punjab Castes*. Lahore: Indian Press.

Ibrahim, E. M., & Al-Homaidh, A. (2011). Physical activity and survival after breast cancer diagnosis: Meta-analysis of published studies. *Medical Oncology (Northwood, London, England)*, *28*(3), 753–765. doi:10.100712032-010-9536-x PMID:20411366

IDeaSS Italy. (n.d.). *From the asylum to territorial services for mental health*. Retrieved May 14, 2019, from http://www.triestesalutementale.it/english/doc/BrochureTriesteENG.pdf

Igbinovia, M. O. (2016). *Emotional Self Awareness and Information Literacy Competence as Correlates of Task Performance of Academic Library Personnel*. Academic Press.

Ilies, R., Yao, J., Curseu, P. L., & Liang, A. X. (2019). Educated and Happy: A Four-Year Study Explaining the Links Between Education, Job Fit, and Life Satisfaction. *Applied Psychology*, *68*(1), 150–176. doi:10.1111/apps.12158

Inagaki, M., Yoshikawa, E., Matsuoka, Y., Sugawara, Y., Nakano, T., Akechi, T., ... Uchitomi, Y. (2006). Smaller regional volumes of brain gray and white matter demonstrated in breast cancer survivors exposed to adjuvant chemotherapy. *Cancer*, *109*(1), 146–156. doi:10.1002/cncr.22368 PMID:17131349

Inan, F. S., & Ustun, B. (2019). After the pychoeducational intervention: Turkish breast cancer survivors' experiences. *European Journal of Breast Health*, *15*(1), 37–42. doi:10.5152/ejbh.2018.4255 PMID:30816352

Individual. (n.d.). In *Merriam-Webster's dictionary*. Retrieved from https://www.merriam-webster.com/dictionary/individual

Ingram, P. B., Warlick, C. A., Ternes, M. S., & Krieshok, T. S. (2018). Examining the feasibility of the integrated hope scale in American college students. *Counselling Psychology Quarterly*, *31*(3), 336–352. doi:10.1080/09515070.2017.1318111

Institute of Medicine (US) Committee on Health and Behavior, Research, Practice, and Policy. (2001). *Health and Behavior: The Interplay of Biological, Behavioral, and Societal Influences.* Washington, DC: National Academies Press. Retrieved from https://www.ncbi.nlm.nih.gov/books/NBK43743/doi:10.17226/9838

Ioannidou & Konstantikaki. (2008). Empathy and emotional intelligence: What is it really about? *International. Journal of Caring Sciences, 1*(3), 118.

Irwin, M. L., Crumley, D., McTiernan, A., Bernstein, L., Baumgartner, R., Gilliland, F. D., ... Ballard-Barbash, R. (2003). Physical activity levels before and after a diagnosis of breast carcinoma. *Cancer, 97*(7), 1746–1757. doi:10.1002/cncr.11227 PMID:12655532

Isen, A. M. (2002). A role of neuropsychology in understanding the facilitating influence of positive affect on social behavior and cognitive process. In C. R. Snyder & S. J. Lopez (Eds.), *Handbook of positive psychology* (pp. 528–540). New York: Oxford University Press.

Iseselo, M. K., Kajula, L., & Yahya-Malima, K. I. (2016). The psychosocial problems of families caring for relatives with mental illnesses and their coping strategies: A qualitative urban based study in Dar es Salaam, Tanzania. *BMC Psychiatry, 16*(1), 146. doi:10.118612888-016-0857-y PMID:27177934

Italian Civil Code. (1942). Retrieved May 14, 2019, from https://www.brocardi.it/codice-civile/libro-quinto/titolo-iii/capo-ii/art2229.html

Jafari, N., Farajzadegan, Z., Zamani, A., Bahrami, F., Emami, H., & Loghmani, A. (2013). Spiritual well-being and quality of life in Iranian women with breast cancer undergoing radiation therapy. *Support Care Cancer, 21*(5), 1219-1225. doi:10.100700520-012-1650-1

Janelsins, M. C., Davis, P. G., Wideman, L., Katula, J. A., Sprod, L. K., Peppone, L. J., ... Mustian, K. M. (2011). Effects of tai chi chuan on insulin and cytokine levels in a randomized controlled pilot study on breast cancer survivors. *Clinical Breast Cancer, 11*(3), 161–170. doi:10.1016/j.clbc.2011.03.013 PMID:21665136

Jeffery, R., & Jeffery, P. (1997). *Population, Gender and Politics: Demographic change in rural North India.* Cambridge, UK: Cambridge University Press. doi:10.1017/CBO9780511621550

Jeleč Kaker, D. (2009). Zadovoljstvo poslom i sagorijevanje na poslu socijalnih radnika u zdravstvu u Republici Sloveniji. *Ljetopis Socijalnog Rada, 16*(3), 537–549. http://hrcak.srce.hr/47814

Jeong, Y., Kim, J. Y., Ryu, J. S., Lee, K. E., Ha, E. H., & Park, H. (2010). The associations between social support, health-related behaviors, socioeconomic status and depression in medical students. *Epidemiology and Health, 32*, e2010009. doi:10.4178/epih/e2010009 PMID:21191462

Johannsen, M., O'Connor, M., O'Toole, M. S., Jensen, A. B., Hojris, I., & Zachariae, R. (2016). Efficacy of mindfulness-based cognitive therapy on late post-treatment pain in women treated for primary breast cancer: A randomized controlled trial. *Journal of Clinical Oncology, 34*(28), 3390–3399. doi:10.1200/JCO.2015.65.0770 PMID:27325850

Johnson, K. K., Schofield, N. A., & Yurchisin, J. (2002). Appearance and dress as a source of information: A qualitative approach to data collection. *Clothing & Textiles Research Journal, 20*(3), 125–137. doi:10.1177/0887302X0202000301

Jones, N. B. (2017). An Ethological Study of Some Aspects of Social Behaviour of Children in. *Primate Ethology*, 347.

Jong, M. C., Boers, I., Schouten van der Velden, A. P., van der Meij, S., Göker, E., Timmer-Bonte, A. N. J. H., & van Wietmarschen, H. A. (2018). A randomized study of yoga for fatigue and quality of life in women with breast cancer undergoing (neo) adjuvant chemotherapy. *Journal of Alternative and Complementary Medicine (New York, N.Y.), 24*(9-10), 942–953. doi:10.1089/acm.2018.0191 PMID:30247961

Jordan, J. A., McRorie, M., & Ewing, C. (2010). Gender differences in the role of emotional intelligence during the primary–secondary school transition. *Emotional & Behavioural Difficulties, 15*(1), 37–47. doi:10.1080/13632750903512415

Jorfi, H., Jorfi, S., Yaccob, H. F. B., & Shah, I. M. (2010). Emotional intelligence: The relationship between self-regard and communication effectiveness. *World Academy of Science, Engineering and Technology, International Journal of Social, Behavioral, Educational, Economic. Business and Industrial Engineering, 4*(9), 1989–1995.

Josephson, A. M. (1993). The Interactional problems of Christian families and their relationship to developmental psychopathology: Implications for treatment. *Journal of Psychology and Christianity, 12*(4), 312–328.

Jungbauer, J., Wittmund, B., Dietrich, S., & Angermeyer, M. C. (2004). The disregarded caregivers: Subjective burden in spouses of schizophrenia patients. *Schizophrenia Bulletin, 30*(3), 665–675. doi:10.1093/oxfordjournals.schbul.a007114 PMID:15631259

Jutai, J. W., Fuhrer, M. J., Demers, L., Scherer, M. J., & DeRuyter, F. (2005). Toward a taxonomy of assistive technology device outcomes. *American Journal of Physical Medicine & Rehabilitation, 84*(4), 294–302. doi:10.1097/01.PHM.0000157313.88732.DC PMID:15785265

Juvet, L. K., Elvsaas, I.-K. Ø., Leivseth, G., Anker, G., Bertheussen, G. F., Falkmer, U., … Norderhaug, I. N. (2009). Rehabilitation of breast cancer patients. *Rehabilitation of Breast Cancer Patients*. Retrieved from http://www.ncbi.nlm.nih.gov/pubmed/29319956

Kahneman, D. (1999). Objective happiness. *Well-Being: The Foundations of Hedonic Psychology, 3*(25), 1-23.

Kahn, S. R., Akaberi, A., Granton, J. T., Anderson, D. R., Wells, P. S., Rodger, M. A., ... Dennie, C. (2017). Quality of life, dyspnea, and functional exercise capacity following a first episode of pulmonary embolism: Results of the ELOPE cohort study. *The American Journal of Medicine, 130*(8), 990–e9. doi:10.1016/j.amjmed.2017.03.033 PMID:28400247

Kalanjiam, V., & Manoharan, M. G. (2016). A study of the relationship between stress, adaptability and temporomandibular disordersy. *International Journal of Current Research and Review, 8*(4), 1.

Kammath, R., Robin, S., & Chandrasekaran, V. (2014). Common mental disorder: A challenge among people living with Human Immuno Deficiency virus infection/ acquired immunodeficiency syndrome in Udupi, India. *Annals of Medical and Health Sciences Research*, *4*(2), 242–247. doi:10.4103/2141-9248.129051 PMID:24761246

Kang, Y., & Chang, Y. (2018). Using game technology to teach six elementary school children with autism to take a shower independently. *Developmental Neurorehabilitation*, *00*(00), 1–9. doi:10.1080/17518423.2018.1501778 PMID:30060690

Kanner, L. (1943). *Autistic Disturbances of Affective Contact*. Academic Press.

Kara, B., & Kaya, G. (2017). Functional status and associated factors in patients with colon cancer receiving chemotherapy. *Journal of Archives in Military Medicine*, 372-380. doi:10.5812/jamm.11882

Kashdan, T. B., & Rottenberg, J. (2010). Psychological flexibility as a fundamental aspect of health. *Clinical Psychology Review*, *30*(7), 865–878. doi:10.1016/j.cpr.2010.03.001 PMID:21151705

Kaur, R., & Pathak, R. K. (2017). Treatment Gap in Mental Healthcare Reflections from Policy and Research. *Economic and Political Weekly*, *52*(31).

Kauric-Klein, Z. (2018). Effect of yoga on physical and psychological outcomes in patients on chronic hemodialysis. *Complementary Therapies in Clinical Practice*. PMID:30712744

Kaur, M., & Kochar, G. K. (2017). Impact of Anaemia on Morpho-physiological Variables of Rural Jat Women. *Journal of Life Science*, *2*(1), 17–20. doi:10.1080/09751270.2010.11885148

Kaur, S. (2018). Emotional intelligence in relation to mental health and adjustment among students. *International Journal of Advanced Research and Development.*, *3*(1), 304–308.

Kaushik, P., & Bhatia, M. S. (2013). Burden and quality of life in spouses of patients with schizophrenia and bipolar disorders. *Delhi Psychiatry Journal.*, *16*, 83–88.

Kauts, D. S. (2016). Emotional Intelligence and Academic Stress among College Students. *Educational Quest*, *7*(3), 149.

Kemp, B. J. (1999). Quality of life while aging with a disability. *Assistive Technology*, *11*(2), 158–163. doi:10.1080/10400435.1999.10131999 PMID:11010065

Kern, M. L., Waters, L. E., Adler, A., & White, M. A. (2015). A multidimensional approach to measuring well-being in students: Application of the PERMA framework. *The Journal of Positive Psychology*, *10*(3), 262–271. doi:10.1080/17439760.2014.936962 PMID:25745508

Kessler, R. C., Barker, P. R., Colpe, L. J., Epstein, J. F., Gfroerer, J. C., Hiripi, E., & Zaslavaky, A. M. (2003). Screening for serious mental illness in the general population. *Archives of General Psychiatry*, *60*(2), 184–189. doi:10.1001/archpsyc.60.2.184 PMID:12578436

Khanna, S. K. (2003). Jat. In Encyclopedia of Medical Anthropology: Health and Illness in the World's Cultures Topics - Volume 1; Cultures (pp. 777–783). Springer International Publishing.

Khanna, S. K. (1995). *Gender Discrimination, Maternal Health, and Pregnancy Outcomes in North India*. Syracuse University.

Khanna, S. K. (1997). Traditions and Reproductive Technology in an Urbanizing North Indian Village. *Social Science & Medicine*, *44*(2), 171–180. doi:10.1016/S0277-9536(96)00144-X PMID:9015870

Khanna, S. K. (2001). Shahri Jat and dehati Jatni: The Indian peasant community in transition. *Contemporary South Asia*, *10*(1), 37–53. doi:10.1080/09584930120062029

Khona, N., Kima, A., & Aidossovaa, Z. (2016). *Problem Solving Design for Emotional Intelligence Training of Middle Managers*. Academic Press.

Khosla, M., & Dokania, V. (2010). Does happiness promote emotional intelligence. *Journal of the Indian Academy of Applied Psychology*, *36*(1), 45–54.

Khullar, V., Singh, H. P., & Bala, M. (2017). ASD Faces are Less Explainable. *Autism - Open Access Research*, *7*(3), 3–7. doi:10.4172/2165-7890.1000210

Kickbusch, I. (2012). 21st century determinants of health and wellbeing: A new challenge for health promotion. *Global Health Promotion*, *19*(3), 5–7. doi:10.1177/1757975912454783 PMID:24802779

Kidd, I. J. (2016). Charging Others with Epistemic Vices. *The Monist*, *99*(2), 181–197. doi:10.1093/monist/onv035

Kim, I. & Loadman, W. E. (1994). *Predicting teacher job satisfaction*. ERIC Document Reproduction Service No. ED 383707.

Kim, B., & Kim, Y. (2017). College students' social media use and communication network heterogeneity: Implications for social capital and subjective well-being. *Computers in Human Behavior*, *73*, 620–628. doi:10.1016/j.chb.2017.03.033

Kim, E. S., Berkovits, L. D., Bernier, E. P., Leyzberg, D., Shic, F., Paul, R., & Scassellati, B. (2013). Social robots as embedded reinforcers of social behavior in children with autism. *Journal of Autism and Developmental Disorders*, *43*(5), 1038–1049. doi:10.100710803-012-1645-2 PMID:23111617

Kingston, D., McDonald, S., Austin, M. P., & Tough, S. (2015). *Association between Prenatal and Postnatal Psychological Distress and Toddler Cognitive Development: A Systematic Review*. Released on 21/5/015. Retrieved from www.ncbi.nlm.nih.gov/pubmed/?term=maternal+psychological+distress+and+todler+cognitive+development

Kinney, E. M., Vedora, J., & Stromer, R. (2003). Computer-Presented Video Models to Teach Generative Spelling to a Child with an Autism Spectrum Disorder. *Journal of Positive Behavior Interventions*, *5*(1), 22–29. doi:10.1177/10983007030050010301

Kirmayer, L. J. (1989). Cultural variations in the response to psychiatric disorders and psychological distress. *Social Science & Medicine*, *29*(3), 327–339. doi:10.1016/0277-9536(89)90281-5 PMID:2669146

Kirsten, T. G. J. C., van der Walt, H. J. L., & Viljoen, C. T. (2009). Health, Well-being and Wellness: An Anthropological Eco-systemic Approach. *Health SA Gesondheid*, *14*(1), 1–7. doi:10.4102/hsag.v14i1.407

Kleinman, A. (1991). *Rethinking Psychiatry. From Cultural Category to Personal Experience*. New York: The Free Press.

Klin, A., Jones, W., Schultz, R., & Volkmar, F. (2003). The enactive mind, or from actions to cognition : Lessons from autism. *Philosophical Transactions of the Royal Society*, *358*(1430), 345–360. doi:10.1098/rstb.2002.1202 PMID:12639332

Knight, V. F., Wood, C. L., Spooner, F., Browder, D. M., & O'Brien, C. P. (2015). An Exploratory Study Using Science eTexts With Students With Autism Spectrum Disorder. *Focus on Autism and Other Developmental Disabilities*, *30*(2), 86–99. doi:10.1177/1088357614559214

Knobf, M. T., Thompson, A. S., Fennie, K., & Erdos, D. (2014). The effect of a community-based exercise intervention on symptoms and quality of life. *Cancer Nursing*, *37*(2), E43–E50. doi:10.1097/NCC.0b013e318288d40e PMID:23519041

Koenig, H. G. (1998). Religious attitudes and practices of hospitalized medically ill older adults. *International Journal of Geriatric Psychiatry*, *13*(4), 213–224. doi:10.1002/(SICI)1099-1166(199804)13:4<213::AID-GPS755>3.0.CO;2-5 PMID:9646148

Koenig, H. G. (2015). Religion, spirituality, and health: A review and update. *Advances in Mind-Body Medicine*, *29*(3), 19–26. PMID:26026153

Koenig, H. G., George, L. K., Meador, K. G., Blazer, D. G., & Dyck, P. B. (1994). Religious affiliation and psychiatric disorder among protestant baby boomers. *Hospital & Community Psychiatry*, *45*(6), 586–596. doi:10.1176/ps.45.6.586 PMID:8088740

Kolenda, P. (1987). *Regional Differences in Family Structure in India*. Jaipur: Rawat Publications.

Koller-Trbović, N., Žižak, A., & Tasić, D. (1996). Zadovoljstvo odgajatelja osobnim životom u promijenjenim okolnostima. *Kriminologija & Socijalna Integracija*, *4*(2), 120–126.

Koo, S. H., Gaul, K., Rivera, S., Pan, T., & Fong, D. (2018). Wearable Technology Design for Autism Spectrum Disorders. *Archives of Design Research*, *31*(1), 37–55. doi:10.15187/adr.2018.02.31.1.37

Korkut-Owen & Owen, D.W. (2012). İyilik hali yıldızı modeli, uygulanması ve değerlendirilmesi. *Uluslararası Avrasya Sosyal Bilimler Dergisi*, *3*(9), 24–33.

Korkut-Owen, F., & Demirbaş Çelik, N. (2018). Lifelong healthy lifestyle and wellness. *Psikiyatride Güncel Yaklasimlar*, *10*(4), 440–453.

Koydemir, S., & Sun-Selışık, Z. E. (2016). Well-being on campus: Testing the effectiveness of an online strengths-based intervention for first year college students. *British Journal of Guidance & Counselling*, *44*(4), 434–446. doi:10.1080/03069885.2015.1110562

Krishnamurthy, S., & Chetlapalli, S. K. (2015). Internet addiction: Prevalence and risk factors: A cross-sectional study among college students in Bengaluru, the Silicon Valley of India. *Indian Journal of Public Health*, *59*(2), 115. doi:10.4103/0019-557X.157531 PMID:26021648

Kroenke, C. H., Kubzansky, L. D., Schernhammer, E. S., Holmes, M. D., & Kawachi, I. (2006). Social networks, social support, and survival after breast cancer diagnosis. *Journal of Clinical Oncology*, *24*(7), 1105–1111. doi:10.1200/JCO.2005.04.2846 PMID:16505430

Kroenke, C. H., Quesenberry, C., Kwan, M. L., Sweeney, C., Castillo, A., & Caan, B. J. (2013). Social networks, social support, and burden in relationships, and mortality after breast cancer diagnosis in the Life After Breast Cancer Epidemiology (LACE) study. *Breast Cancer Research and Treatment*, *137*(1), 261–271. doi:10.100710549-012-2253-8 PMID:23143212

Krumeich, A., Weijts, W., Reddy, P., & Meijer-Weitz, A. (2016). The Benefits of Anthropological Approaches for Health Promotion Research and Practice. *Health Education Research*, *16*(2), 121–130. doi:10.1093/her/16.2.121 PMID:11345657

Küçükemiroğlu, O. (1997). Market segmentation by using consumer lifestyle dimensions and ethnocentrism: An empirical study. *European Journal of Marketing*, *33*(5/6), 470–487. doi:10.1108/03090569910262053

Kuhn, T. S. (1970). Logic of Discovery or Psychology of Research? In I. Lakatos & A. Musgrave (Eds.), *Criticism and the Growth of Knowledge* (pp. 1–22). Cambridge, UK: Cambridge University Press. doi:10.1017/CBO9781139171434.003

Kukreja, R. (2018). Caste and Cross-region Marriages in Haryana, India: Experience of Dalit cross-region brides in Jat households. *Modern Asian Studies*, *52*(2), 492–531. doi:10.1017/S0026749X16000391

Kumar, D. (2018). Changing Agricultural Practices and their Impact on Rural Social Institutions in Uttar Pradesh, India. National Institute of Technology, Rourkela.

Kumar, A. (2011). Mental health services in rural India: Challenges and prospects. *Health*, *3*(12), 757–761. doi:10.4236/health.2011.312126

Kumar, D., Kumar, P., Singh, A. R., & Bhandari, S. S. (2012). Knowledge and attitude towards mental illness of key informants and general population: A comparative study. *Dysphrenia*, *3*(1), 57–64.

Kumar, D., & Mishra, N. R. (2017). Caste Hierarchy and New Agro-technological Practices : Some Anthropological thoughts on Western Uttar Pradesh. *Man in India*, *97*(11), 285–300.

Kumar, S., Dagli, R. J., Mathur, A., Jain, M., Prabu, D., & Kulkarni, S. (2009). Perceived sources of stress amongst Indian dental students. *European Journal of Dental Education*, *13*(1), 39–45. doi:10.1111/j.1600-0579.2008.00535.x PMID:19196292

Kumar, S., & Mohanty, S. (2007). Spousal burden of care in schizophrenia. *Journal of the Indian Academy of Applied Psychology*, *33*, 189–194.

Kumar, S., Singh, A. R., Verma, A. N., Verma, P. K., & Chaudhary, S. (2009). Subjective burden on spouses of schizophrenia patients. *Industrial Psychiatry Journal*, *18*(2), 97–100. doi:10.4103/0972-6748.62268 PMID:21180485

Kundi, G. (2016). *Why Indian Students are more stressed than ever?* Retrieved October 18, 2016, from http://www.studyin-uk.in/blog/why-indianstudents-are-more-stressed-than-ever/

Kuppuswamy, M., Kamaldeen, D., Pitani, R., Amaldas, J., & Shanmugam, P. (2017). Effects of Bhramari Pranayam on Health - A Systematic Review. *Journal of Traditional and Complementary Medicine*, *8*(1), 11–16. doi:10.1016/j.jtcme.2017.02.003 PMID:29321984

Kuriakose, S., & Lahiri, U. (2015). Understanding the Psycho-Physiological Implications of Interaction with a Virtual Reality-Based System in Adolescents with Autism: A Feasibility Study. *IEEE Transactions on Neural Systems and Rehabilitation Engineering*, *23*(4), 665–675. doi:10.1109/TNSRE.2015.2393891 PMID:25643409

Kushi, L. H., Doyle, C., McCullough, M., Rock, C. L., Demark-Wahnefried, W., Bandera, E. V., ... Gansler, T. (2012). American Cancer Society guidelines on nutrition and physical activity for cancer prevention. *CA: a Cancer Journal for Clinicians*, *62*(1), 30–67. doi:10.3322/caac.20140 PMID:22237782

Kuzeff, R. M. (1998). Homeopathy, sensation of well-being and CD4 levels: A placebo-controlled, randomized trial. *Complementary Therapies in Medicine*, *6*(1), 4–9. doi:10.1016/S0965-2299(98)80050-2

Kwon, Y.-H. (1994). Feeling toward one's clothing and self-perception of emotion, sociability, and work competency. *Journal of Social Behavior and Personality*, *9*(1), 129–139.

Lahart, I. M., Metsios, G. S., Nevill, A. M., & Carmichael, A. R. (2015). Physical activity, risk of death and recurrence in breast cancer survivors: A systematic review and meta-analysis of epidemiological studies. *Acta Oncologica*, *54*(5), 635–654. doi:10.3109/0284186X.2014.998275 PMID:25752971

Lahart, I. M., Metsios, G. S., Nevill, A. M., & Carmichael, A. R. (2018). Physical activity for women with breast cancer after adjuvant therapy. *Cochrane Database of Systematic Reviews*, *1*(1), CD011292. doi:10.1002/14651858.CD011292.pub2 PMID:29376559

Lambert, L., Passmore, H. A., & Holder, M. D. (2015). Foundational frameworks of positive psychology: Mapping well-being orientations. *Canadian Psychology*, *56*(3), 311–321. doi:10.1037/cap0000033

Lang, C. (2018). Translation and purification: Ayurvedic psychiatry, allopathic psychiatry, spirits and occult violence in Kerala, South India. *Anthropology & Medicine*, *25*(2), 141–161. doi:10.1080/13648470.2017.1285001 PMID:28480739

Larson, D. B., Larson, S. S., & Koenig, H. G. (2001). The patient's spiritual/religious dimension: A forgotten factor in mental health. *Directions in Psychiatry*, *21*(4), 10–15.

Larson, D. B., Swyers, J. P., & McCullough, M. E. (1998). *Scientific research on spirituality and health: A consensus report*. Rockville, MD: National Institute for Healthcare Research.

Lash, T. L., & Silliman, R. A. (2002). Long-term follow-up of upper-body function among breast cancer survivors. *The Breast Journal*, *8*(1), 28–33. doi:10.1046/j.1524-4741.2002.08006.x PMID:11856158

Law, M. (2002). Participation in the occupations of everyday life. *The American Journal of Occupational Therapy*, *56*(6), 640–649. doi:10.5014/ajot.56.6.640 PMID:12458856

Lazarus, R. S. (1999). *Stress and emotion: A new synthesis*. New York: Springer.

Lazzarino, A. L., Yiengpruqsawan, V., Seubsman, S. A., Steptoe, A., & Sleigh, A. C. (2014). The association between unhealthy behaviors, mental stress and low socio economic status in an international comparison of representative samples from Thailand and England. *Globalization and Health*, *10*(10).

Leary, K. A., & DeRosier, M. E. (2012). Factors promoting positive adaptation and resilience during the transition to college. *Psychology (Irvine, Calif.)*, *3*(12), 1215–1222. doi:10.4236/psych.2012.312A180

LeBlanc, L. A., Coates, A. M., Daneshvar, S., Charlop-Christy, M. H., Morris, C., & Lancaster, B. M. (2003). Using video modeling and reinforcement to teach perspective-taking skills to children with autism. *Journal of Applied Behavior Analysis*, *36*(2), 253–257. doi:10.1901/jaba.2003.36-253 PMID:12858990

Lee, A., Lang, R., Davenport, K., Moore, M., Rispoli, M., Van Der Meer, L., ... Chung, C. (2015). Comparison of therapist implemented and iPad-assisted interventions for children with autism. *Developmental Neurorehabilitation*, *18*(2), 97–103. doi:10.3109/17518423.2013.830231 PMID:24088050

Leung, J., Pachana, N. A., & McLaughlin, D. (2014). Social support and health-related quality of life in women with breast cancer: A longitudinal study. *Psycho-Oncology*, *23*(9), 1014–1020. doi:10.1002/pon.3523 PMID:24700668

Levus, N. (2012). Self-regard in the structure of personality behavioural manifestations. *Journal of Education Culture and Society*, (2).

Levy, D. (1996). *Freud Among the Philosophers: The Psychoanalytic Unconscious and Its Philosophical Critics*. New Haven, CT: Yale University Press.

Lewis, L., Charron, N., Clamp, C., & Craig, M. (2016). Soft systems methodology as a tool to aid a pilot study in robot-assisted therapy. *ACM/IEEE International Conference on Human-Robot Interaction*, 467–468. 10.1109/HRI.2016.7451809

Lewis, O. (1958). *Village Life in Northern India: Studies in a Delhi Village*. New York: Vintage Books.

Liebana-Pressa, C., Fernandez-Martinez, M. E., Gandara, A. R., Muñoz-Villanueva, M. C., Vázquez-Casares, A. M., & Rodríguez-Borrego, M. A. (2014). Psychological distress in health science college students and its relationship with academic engagement. [PubMed]. *Revista da Escola de Enfermagem da U S P., 48*(4), 715–722.

Link, B., & Phelan, J. (2001). Conceptualizing stigma. *Annual Review of Sociology, 27*(1), 363–385. doi:10.1146/annurev.soc.27.1.363

Liu, H., Peng, F., Zeng, X., Zhao, J., & Zhang, X. (2019). Authoritarian personality and subjective well-being in Chinese college students: The moderation effect of the organizational culture context. *Personality and Individual Differences, 138*, 79–83. doi:10.1016/j.paid.2018.09.030

Lobo, L. (2010). *Malaria in the Social Context: A study in western India*. New Delhi: Routledge.

Lock, M., & Scheper-Hughes, N. (1990). A Critical Interpretive Approach in Medical Anthropology: Rituals and Routines of Discipline and Dissent. In T. M. Johnson & C. F. Sargent (Eds.), *Medical Anthropology. Contemporary Theory and Method* (pp. 47–72). New York: Praeger Publishers.

Loftus, L. S., Sokol, G. H., & Laronga, C. (2017). Breast cancer survivorship: Patient characteristics and plans for high-quality care. *Southern Medical Journal, 110*(10), 673–677. doi:10.14423/SMJ.0000000000000701 PMID:28973710

Lolla, A. (2018). Mantras help the general psychological well-being of college students: A pilot study. *Journal of Religion and Health, 57*(1), 110–119. doi:10.100710943-017-0371-7 PMID:28271341

Lone, A. H., Ahmad, T., Anwar, M., Sofi, G., Imam, H., & Habib, S. (2012). Perception of health promotion in Unani herbal medicine. *Journal of Herbal Medicine, 2*(1), 1–5. doi:10.1016/j.hermed.2012.02.003

Loucas, T., Charman, T., Pickles, A., Simonoff, E., Chandler, S., Meldrum, D., & Baird, G. (2008). Autistic symptomatology and language ability in autism spectrum disorder and specific language impairment. *Journal of Child Psychology and Psychiatry, 49*(11), 1184–1192. doi:10.1111/j.1469-7610.2008.01951.x

Lu, S. H., Dear, B. F., Johnston, L., Wootton, B. M., & Titov, N. (2014). An Internet survey of emotional health, treatment seeking, and barriers to accessing mental health treatment among Chinese-speaking international students in Australia. *Counselling Psychology Quarterly, 27*(1), 96–108. doi:10.1080/09515070.2013.824408

Lyubomirsky, S. (2001). Why are some people happier than others? The role of cognitive and motivational processes in well-being. *The American Psychologist, 56*(3), 239–249. doi:10.1037/0003-066X.56.3.239 PMID:11315250

Mahal, D. G., & Matsoukas, I. G. (2017). Y-STR Haplogroup Diversity in the Jat Population Reveals Several Different Ancient Origins. *Frontiers in Genetics*, *8*, 121. doi:10.3389/fgene.2017.00121 PMID:28979290

Manne, S. L., Ostroff, J. S., Norton, T. R., Fox, K., Goldstein, L., & Grana, G. (2006). Cancer-related relationship communication in couples coping with early stage breast cancer. *Psycho-Oncology*, *15*(3), 234–247. doi:10.1002/pon.941 PMID:15926198

Manne, S. L., Siegel, S. D., Heckman, C. J., & Kashy, D. A. (2016). A randomized clinical trial of a supportive versus a skill-based couple-focused group intervention for breast cancer patients. *Journal of Consulting and Clinical Psychology*, *84*(8), 668–681. doi:10.1037/ccp0000110 PMID:27228264

Manne, S., Ostroff, J., Rini, C., Fox, K., Goldstein, L., & Grana, G. (2004). The interpersonal process model of intimacy: The role of self-disclosure, partner disclosure, and partner responsiveness in interactions between breast cancer patients and their partners. *Journal of Family Psychology*, *18*(4), 589–599. doi:10.1037/0893-3200.18.4.589 PMID:15598164

Manns, P. J., & Darrah, J. (2006). Linking research and clinical practice in physical therapy: Strategies for integration. *Physiotherapy*, *92*(2), 88–94. doi:10.1016/j.physio.2005.09.006

Mann, W. C., Ottenbacher, K. J., Fraas, L., Tomita, M., & Granger, C. V. (1999). Effectiveness of assistive technology and environmental interventions in maintaining independence and reducing home care costs for the frail elderly: A randomized controlled trial. *Archives of Family Medicine*, *8*(3), 210–217. doi:10.1001/archfami.8.3.210 PMID:10333815

Marcotte, J., & Lévesque, G. (2018). Anxiety and well-being among students in a psychoeducation program: The mediating role of identity. *Journal of College Student Development*, *59*(1), 90–104. doi:10.1353/csd.2018.0006

Marshall, S. (2016). Predicting college students' positive psychology associated traits with executive functioning dimensions. *College Student Journal*, *50*(2), 179–190. Retrieved from https://search-ebscohost-com.ezp.waldenulibrary.org/login.aspx?direct=true&db=a9h&AN=116190967&site=eds-live&scope=site

Martin-Yellow, I. S. (1992). The burden of schizophrenia on the family. A study from Nigeria. *The British Journal of Psychiatry*, *161*, 779–782.

Maslach, C. (2003). Job burnout: New directions in research and intervention. *Current Directions in Psychological Science*, *12*(5), 189–192. doi:10.1111/1467-8721.01258

Matel-Anderson, D. M., Bekhet, A. K., & Garnier-Villarreal, M. (2019). Mediating effects of positive thinking and social support on suicide resilience. *Western Journal of Nursing Research*, *41*(1), 25–41. doi:10.1177/0193945918757988 PMID:29460692

Math, S. B., & Srinivasaraju, R. (2010). Indian psychiatric epidemiological studies: Learning from the past. *Indian Journal of Psychiatry*, *52*(7), S95–S103. doi:10.4103/0019-5545.69220 PMID:21836725

Matlin, M. W., & Stang, D. J. (1978). *The Pollyanna principle. Selectivity in language, memory, and thought.* Cambridge, MA: Schenkman.

Matsuda, A., Yamaoka, K., Tango, T., Matsuda, T., & Nishimoto, H. (2014). Effectiveness of psychoeducational support on quality of life in early-stage breast cancer patients: A systematic review and meta-analysis of randomized controlled trials. *Quality of Life Research: An International Journal of Quality of Life Aspects of Treatment, Care and Rehabilitation, 23*(1), 21–30. doi:10.100711136-013-0460-3 PMID:23881515

Mayer, J. D., & Salovey, P. (1997). What is emotional intelligence? *Emotional development and emotional intelligence: Educational implications, 3*, 31.

Mayer, J. D., Caruso, D. R., & Salovey, P. (1999). Emotional intelligence meets traditional standards for an intelligence. *Intelligence, 27*(4), 267–298. doi:10.1016/S0160-2896(99)00016-1

Mazzola, A. (2018). Psicoterapia nei contesti: Quale rapporto tra il mandato dei servizi di salute mentale e le domande ad essi rivolte? Resoconto di un intervento in un CSM [Psychotherapy in contexts: What relationship between MentalHealth Services and their users' demands? Report of a clinical intervention in a MentalHealth Center]. *Rivista di Psicologia Clinica, 1*, 66–84. doi:10.14645/RPC.2018.1.716

McCallum, F., & Price, D. (2010). Well teachers, well students. *Journal of Student Wellbeing, 4*(1), 19–34. doi:10.21913/JSW.v4i1.599

McCallum, F., Price, D., Graham, A., & Morrison, A. (2017). *Teacher wellbeing: A review of the literature.* The University of Adelaide.

Mccoy, A., Holloway, J., Healy, O., Rispoli, M., & Neely, L. (2016). *A Systematic Review and Evaluation of Video Modeling, Role-Play and Computer-Based Instruction as Social Skills Interventions for Children and Adolescents with High-Functioning Autism.* doi:10.100740489-015-0065-6

McDermott, R. C., Cheng, H.-L., Wong, J., Booth, N., Jones, Z., & Sevig, T. (2017). Hope for help-seeking: A positive psychology perspective of psychological help-seeking intentions. *The Counseling Psychologist, 45*(2), 237–265. doi:10.1177/0011000017693398

McLafferty, M., Lapsley, C. R., Ennis, E., Armour, C., Murphy, S., Bunting, B. P., ... O'Neill, S. M. (2017). Mental health, behavioural problems, and treatment seeking among students commencing university in Northern Ireland. *PLoS One, 12*(12), e0188785. doi:10.1371/journal.pone.0188785 PMID:29236727

Meadan, H., Snodgrass, M. R., Meyer, L. E., Fisher, K. W., Chung, M. Y., & Halle, J. W. (2016). Internet-Based Parent-Implemented Intervention for Young Children With Autism. *Journal of Early Intervention, 38*(1), 3–23. doi:10.1177/1053815116630327

Mechling, L. C., & Savidge, E. J. (2011). Using a personal digital assistant to increase completion of novel tasks and independent transitioning by students with autism spectrum disorder. *Journal of Autism and Developmental Disorders, 41*(6), 687–704. doi:10.100710803-010-1088-6 PMID:20714798

Meera, S., Rani, M. V., Sreedhar, C., & Robin, D. T. (2019). A review on the therapeutic effects of NetiKriya with special reference to JalaNeti. *Journal of Ayurveda and Integrative Medicine.*

Mendes-Santos, C., Weiderpass, E., Santana, R., & Andersson, G. (2019). A guided internet-delivered individually-tailored ACT-influenced cognitive behavioural intervention to improve psychosocial outcomes in breast cancer survivors (iNNOVBC): Study protocol. *Internet Interventions, 17*(1), 100236. doi:10.1016/j.invent.2019.01.004 PMID:30949435

Meneses-Echávez, J. F., González-Jiménez, E., & Ramírez-Vélez, R. (2015). Effects of supervised exercise on cancer-related fatigue in breast cancer survivors: A systematic review and meta-analysis. *BMC Cancer, 15*(1), 77. doi:10.118612885-015-1069-4 PMID:25885168

Mental health policy, plans and programmes—updated version 2. (2005). *Mental health policy and service guidance package.* World Health Organization.

Mental Health. (2019, June 20). Retrieved from https://www.who.int/mental_health/en/

Meredith, L. N., Frazier, P. A., Paulsen, J. A., Greer, C. S., Howard, K. G., Belgrade, A., & Kim, S. (2014). *Assessing the efficacy of an online stress management intervention for community college students.* doi:10.1037/e555772014-001

Meyer, W., Moore, C., & Viljoen, H. (2002). *Personology: From Individual to Ecosystem.* Johannesburg: Heinemann.

Mijočević, I., & Rijavec, M. (2006). Optimistični i pesimistični eksplanatorni stil i školski uspjeh u višim razredima osnovne škole [Optimistic and pessimistic explanatory styles and school performance in the higher forms of elementary school]. *Odgojne Znanosti, 8*(2), 347–360.

Miljković, D., & Rijavec, M. (2009). Važnost pozitivnih emocija u odgoju i obrazovanju [The Significance of Positive Emotions in Education]. Napredak, 150(3-4), 488-506.

Miller, G. D., & Foster, L. T. (2010). *Critical synthesis of wellness literature.* University of Victoria. Retrieved from http://www.geog.uvic.ca/wellness

Miller, W. R., Forcehimes, A., O'Leary, M. J., & LaNoue, M. D. (2008). Spiritual direction in addiction treatment: Two clinical trials. *Journal of Substance Abuse Treatment, 35*(4), 434–442. doi:10.1016/j.jsat.2008.02.004 PMID:18657945

Miller, W. R., & Thoresen, C. E. (2003). Spirituality, religion, and health: An emerging research field. *The American Psychologist, 58*(1), 24–35. doi:10.1037/0003-066X.58.1.24 PMID:12674816

Mills, P. J., Peterson, C. T., Pung, M. A., Patel, S., Weiss, L., Wilson, K. L., ... Chopra, D. (2018). Change in sense of nondual awareness and spiritual awakening in response to a multidimensional well-being program. *Journal of Alternative and Complementary Medicine (New York, N.Y.)*, *24*(4), 343–351. doi:10.1089/acm.2017.0160 PMID:29216441

Ministero della Salute. (2006). *I servizi di salute mentale* [Mental Health services]. Retrieved May 14, 2019, from http://www.salute.gov.it/portale/temi/p2_6.jsp?id=168&area=salute%20 mentale&menu=rete

Ministry of AYUSH, Government of India. (2015). Available from: http://www. indianmedicine. nic.in/

Ministry of Health and Family Welfare Government of India. (2011). Available from: http:// www.mohfw.nic.in/

Ministry of Health and Family Welfare, Government of India. (1983). *National Health Policy 1983*. New Delhi: MoHFW. Available from: http://www. communityhealth.in/~commun26/wiki/ images/6/64/Nhp_1983.pdf

Ministry of Health and family Welfare, Government of India. (2002). *National Health Policy 2002*. New Delhi: MoHFW. Available from: http://mohfw.nic.in/ WriteReadData/l892s/180488 92912105179110National%20Health%20policy2002.pdf

Ministry of Health and Family Welfare, Government of India. (2014). *New Pathways New Hope*. National Mental Health Policy of India. Retrieved from https://mohfw.gov.in/sites/default/ files/34711242651412939786%20%281%29.pdf

Mirowsky, J., & Ross, C. E. (2002). Selecting outcomes for the sociology of mental health: Issues of measurement and dimensionality. *Journal of Health and Social Behavior*, (43), 152–170. doi:10.2307/3090194 PMID:12096697

Mo, Y. Y. (2010). *Measuring and enhancing the emotional intelligence of built environment students* (Doctoral dissertation).

Moattari, M., Soltani, A., Mousavinasab, M., & Aiattollahi, A. (2005). The effect of problem solving skill training on self-concept of nursing students of the Shiraz faculty of nursing & midwifery. *Iran J Educ Med Sci., 5*(14), 147-55. (in Persian)

Mobile, B. (2010, August 30). *Twenty-Four Hours a Day*. Retrieved from https://apps.apple.com/ us/app/twenty-four-hours-a-day/id389029534

Moghnie, L., & Kazarian, S. S. (2012). Subjective happiness of Lebanese college youth in Lebanon: Factorial structure and invariance of the Arabic Subjective Happiness Scale. *Social Indicators Research, 109*(2), 203–210. doi:10.100711205-011-9895-5

Mohanadasan, T. (2014). *Emotional intelligence and managerial skills: A comparative study on the managers of selected public sector and private sector banks in Kerala*. Academic Press.

Mongrain, M., & Anselmo-Matthews, T. (2012). Do positive psychology exercises work? A replication of Seligman et al. (2005). *Journal of Clinical Psychology*, *382*(4). doi:10.1002/jclp.21839 PMID:24469930

Monier-Williams, M. (2008). *A Sanskrit-English Dictionary (revised)*. Delhi: Motilal Banarsidas Publication.

Montazeri, A. (2008). Health-related quality of life in breast cancer patients: A bibliographic review of the literature from 1974 to 2007. *Journal of Experimental & Clinical Cancer Research*, *27*(1), 32. doi:10.1186/1756-9966-27-32 PMID:18759983

Mood kit app. (n.d.). Retrieved from http://www.thriveport.com/products/moodkit/

Morsy, S. (1990). Political Economy and Medical Anthropology. In T. M. Johnson & C. F. Sargent (Eds.), *Medical Anthropology. Contemporary Theory and Method* (pp. 26–46). New York: Praeger Publishers.

Mortenson, W. B., Demers, L., Fuhrer, M. J., Jutai, J. W., Lenker, J., & DeRuyter, F. (2012). How assistive technology use by individuals with disabilities impacts their caregivers: A systematic review of the research evidence. *American Journal of Physical Medicine & Rehabilitation*, *91*(11), 984–998. doi:10.1097/PHM.0b013e318269eceb PMID:22955027

Mroczek, D. K., & Kolarz, C. M. (1998). The effect of age on positive and negative affect: A developmental perspective on happiness. *Journal of Personality and Social Psychology*, *75*(5), 1333–1349. doi:10.1037/0022-3514.75.5.1333 PMID:9866191

Mudaliar Committee Report Government of India. (1961). Report of the Health Survey and Planning Committee. New Delhi: Ministry of Health.

Munzel, A., Meyer-Waarden, L., & Galan, J.-P. (2018). The social side of sustainability: Well-being as a driver and an outcome of social relationships and interactions on social networking sites. *Technological Forecasting and Social Change*, *130*, 14–27. doi:10.1016/j.techfore.2017.06.031

Murray, C. J. L., & Lopez, A. D. (1996). *The Global Burden of Disease*. Cambridge, MA: Harvard School of Public Health.

Musiat, P., & Tarrier, N. (2014). Collateral outcomes in e-mental health: A systematic review of the evidence for added benefits of computerized cognitive behavior therapy interventions for mental health. *Psychological Medicine*, *44*(15), 3137–3150. doi:10.1017/S0033291714000245 PMID:25065947

Must, A., Phillips, S. M., Curtin, C., Anderson, S. E., Maslin, M., Lividini, K., & Bandini, L. G. (2014). Comparison of sedentary behaviors between children with autism spectrum disorders and typically developing children. *Autism*, *18*(4), 376–384. doi:10.1177/1362361313479039 PMID:24113339

Mustafa, M., Carson-Stevens, A., Gillespie, D., & Edwards, A. G. (2013). Psychological interventions for women with metastatic breast cancer. *Cochrane Database of Systematic Reviews*, *4*(6), CD004253. doi:10.1002/14651858.CD004253.pub4 PMID:23737397

Muszalik, M., Kołucka-Pluta, M., Kędziora-Kornatowska, K., & Robaczewska, J. (2016). Quality of life of women with breast cancer undergoing radiotherapy using the Functional Assessment of Chronic Illness Therapy-Fatigue questionnaire. *Clinical Interventions in Aging*, *11*, 1489–1494. doi:10.2147/CIA.S113530 PMID:27799754

Myers, D. G., & Diener, E. (1995). Who is happy*? Psychological Science*, *6*(1), 10–19. doi:10.1111/j.1467-9280.1995.tb00298.x

Myers, J. E., Sweeney, T. J., & Witmer, J. M. (2000). The Wheel of Wellness Counselling for Wellness: A Holistic Model For Treatment Planning. *Journal of Counseling and Development*, *78*(3), 251–266. doi:10.1002/j.1556-6676.2000.tb01906.x

Nacionalni kurikulum za rani i predškolski odgoj i obrazovanje. (2014). *Ministarstvo znanosti, obrazovanja i sporta* [The National Framework Curriculum of the Pre-school Education. Ministry for science, education and sport: Republic of Croatia]. Retrieved from http://www.azoo.hr/images/strucni2015/Nacionalni-kurikulum-za-rani-i-predskolski-odgoj-i-obrazovanje.pdf

Nagata, C. M., Conoley, C., Arnadottir, V., White, S., & Shishim, M. (2011). *Using positive psychology interventions in a college prevention context*. doi:10.1037/e708082011-001

Nagy, J., & McDonald, J. (2007). New models for learning flexibility: Negotiated choices for both academics and students. In *Proceedings ASCILITE 2007: 24th Annual Conference of the Australasian Society for Computers in Learning in Tertiary Education: ICT: Providing Choices for Learners and Learning* (pp. 737-746). Nanyang Technological University, Centre for Educational Development.

Nakamura, J., & Csikszentmihalyi, M. (2002). The concept of flow. In C. R. Snyder & S. J. Lopez (Eds.), *Handbook of positive psychology* (pp. 89–105). New York: Oxford University Press.

Namkoong, K., McLaughlin, B., Yoo, W., Hull, S. J., Shah, D. V., Kim, S. C., ... Gustafson, D. H. (2013). … Gustafson, D. H. (2013). The effects of expression: How providing emotional support online improves cancer patients' coping strategies. *Journal of the National Cancer Institute. Monographs*, *2013*(47), 169–174. doi:10.1093/jncimonographs/lgt033 PMID:24395987

Natalie, C., Ian, M.D., Steve, H., & Paul, H. (2003). Measuring chronic patient's feelings of being a burden to their caregivers: Development and preliminary validation of a scale. *Official Journal of Medical Care Section, American Public Health Association, 41*(1), 110-118.

National Alliance on Mental Illness. (n.d.). Retrieved from https://www.nami.org/

Nauffal, D., Ammar, D., & Sbeity, R. (2013). The role of perceived social support in predicting subjective well-being in Lebanese college students. *Happiness & Well-Being, 116*. Retrieved from: https://laur.lau.edu.lb:8443/xmlui/handle/10725/4075?show=full

Naz, S. (2015). Relationship of life satisfaction and job satisfaction among pakistani army soldiers. *Journal of Business Research-Turk*, *7*(1), 7–25. doi:10.20491/isader.2015115749

Neki, J. S. (1974). A reappraisal of the guru-chela relationship as a therapeutic paradigm. *International Mental Health Research Newsletter*, *16*(2), 2–7.

Neki, J. S. (1984). Psychotherapy in India traditions and trends. In A. De Souza & M. D. A. De Souse (Eds.), *Psychiatry in India* (pp. 339–342). Bhalani Book Depot.

Neuliep, J. W. (1996). The Influence of Theory X and Y Management Style on the Perception of Ethical Behavior in Organizations. *Journal of Social Behavior and Personality*, (11): 301–311.

New MindShift™ CBT App Gives Canadians Free Anxiety Relief. (n.d.). Retrieved from https://anxietycanada.com/articles/new-mindshift-cbt-app-gives-canadians-free-anxiety-relief/

Ngar, S., Yuan, V., Ho, H., & Ip, S. (2018). Using virtual reality to train emotional and social skills in children with autism spectrum disorder. *London Journal of Primary Care*, *1472*, 1–3. doi:10.1080/17571472.2018.1483000 PMID:30083244

Nguyen, J., Popovic, M., Chow, E., Cella, D., Beaumont, J. L., Chu, D., ... Bottomley, A. (2015). EORTC QLQ-BR23 and FACT-B for the assessment of quality of life in patients with breast cancer: A literature review. *Journal of Comparative Effectiveness Research*, *4*(2), 157–166. doi:10.2217/cer.14.76 PMID:25825844

Nobile, M., Perego, P., Piccinini, L., Mani, E., Rossi, A., Bellina, M., & Molteni, M. (2011). Further evidence of complex motor dysfunction in drug naïve children with autism using automatic motion analysis of gait. *Autism*, *15*(3), 263–283. doi:10.1177/1362361309356929 PMID:21478224

Noreau, L., Fougeyrollas, P., Labbé, A., & Laramée, M. T. (1998). Comparison of 2 measurement tools addressing the concept of handicap: CHART and LIFE-H. *The Journal of Spinal Cord Medicine*, *21*(2), 192.

Noreau, L., Fougeyrollas, P., & Vincent, C. (2002). The LIFE-H: Assessment of the quality of social participation. *Technology and Disability*, *14*(3), 113–118. doi:10.3233/TAD-2002-14306

Northrup, C. M., Lantz, J., Hamlin, T., & Case, N. (2016). *Wearable Stress Sensors for Children with Autism Spectrum Disorder with In Situ Alerts to Caregivers via a Mobile Phone*. Academic Press.

Norton, R., & Warnick, B. (1976). Assertiveness as communication construct. *Human Communication Research*, *3*(1), 62–66. doi:10.1111/j.1468-2958.1976.tb00504.x

Norvilitis, J. M., & Mao, Y. (2013). Attitudes towards credit and finances among college students in China and the United States. *International Journal of Psychology*, *48*(3), 389–398. doi:10.1080/00207594.2011.645486 PMID:22397472

Nwanze, K. (2011) *Closing the gender gap in rural development*. President, International Fund for Agriculture Development. Retrieved from http://www.intracen.org/Closing-the-gender-gap-in-ruraldevelopment/#sthash.F2p63fz1.dpuf

O'Reilly, A., Ryan, D., & Hickey, T. (2010). The psychological well-being and sociocultural adaptation of short-term international students in Ireland. *Journal of College Student Development*, *51*(5), 584–598. doi:10.1353/csd.2010.0011

O'Toole, J. A., Ferguson, C. M., Swaroop, M. N., Horick, N., Skolny, M. N., Brunelle, C. L., ... Taghian, A. G. (2015). The impact of breast cancer-related lymphedema on the ability to perform upper extremity activities of daily living. *Breast Cancer Research and Treatment*, *150*(2), 381–388. doi:10.100710549-015-3325-3 PMID:25749734

Oldridge, N. B. (1996). Outcomes measurement: Health-related quality of life. *Assistive Technology*, *8*(2), 82–93. doi:10.1080/10400435.1996.10132278 PMID:10163932

Olive, M. L., De La Cruz, B., Davis, T. N., Chan, J. M., Lang, R. B., O'Reilly, M. F., & Dickson, S. M. (2007). The effects of enhanced milieu teaching and a voice output communication aid on the requesting of three children with autism. *Journal of Autism and Developmental Disorders*, *37*(8), 1505–1513. doi:10.100710803-006-0243-6 PMID:17066309

Omar, S., & Bidin, A. (2015). The Impact of Multimedia Graphic and Text with Autistic Learners in Reading. *Universal Journal of Educational Research*, *3*(12), 989–996. doi:10.13189/ujer.2015.031206

Opic, S. (2016). Interpersonal relations in school. *International Journal of Cognitive Research in Science, Engineering and Education*, *4*(2), 9-21.

Orellano, E. M., & Jutai, J. W. (2013). Cross-cultural adaptation of the psychosocial impact of assistive device scale (PIADS) for Puerto Rican assistive technology users. *Assistive Technology*, *25*(4), 194–203. doi:10.1080/10400435.2012.761292 PMID:24620702

Ornish, D. (1999). *Love and survival: 8 pathways to intimacy and health*. New York: HarperCollins.

Ostman, M., & Kjelin, L. (2002). Stigma by association: Psychological factors in relatives of people with mental illness. *The British Journal of Psychiatry*, *181*(6), 494–498. doi:10.1192/bjp.181.6.494 PMID:12456519

Ottaviani, C., Thayer, J. F., Verkuil, B., Lonigro, A., Medea, B., Couyoumdjian, A., & Brosschot, J. F. (2016). Physiological concomitants of perseverative cognition: A systematic review and meta-analysis. *Psychological Bulletin*, *142*(3), 231–259. doi:10.1037/bul0000036 PMID:26689087

Overcome stress and negative thoughts. Build resilience. (n.d.). Retrieved from https://www.happify.com/

Pajouhandeh, E. (2013). Personal Development and Self-Actualization of Students in the New Environment. *International Journal (Toronto, Ont.)*, *2*(1), 2307–227X.

Palmore, E., & Luikart, C. (1972). Health and social factors related to life satisfaction. *Journal of Health and Social Behavior*, *13*(1), 68–80. doi:10.2307/2136974 PMID:5025756

Panda, M. (2015). Emotional intelligence as a correlate of self-actualization among teachers at secondary teachers training college. *International Journal of Multidisciplinary Research and Development.*, *2*(12), 158–168.

Pandia Rajan, J., & Edward Rajan, S. (2018). An Internet of Things based physiological signal monitoring and receiving system for virtual enhanced health care network. *Technology and Health Care*, *26*(2), 379–385. doi:10.3233/THC-171173 PMID:29526864

Panyan, M. V. (1984). Computer technology for autistic students. *Journal of Autism and Developmental Disorders*, *14*(4), 375–382. doi:10.1007/BF02409828 PMID:6549182

Park, C. L., Masters, K. S., Salsman, J. M., Wachholtz, A., Clements, A. D., Salmoirago-Blotcher, E., ... Wischenka, D. M. (2017). Advancing our understanding of religion and spirituality in the context of behavioral medicine. *Journal of Behavioral Medicine*, *40*(1), 39–51. doi:10.100710865-016-9755-5 PMID:27342616

Parker, J. D., Summerfeldt, L. J., Hogan, M. J., & Majeski, S. A. (2004). Emotional intelligence and academic success: Examining the transition from high school to university. *Personality and Individual Differences*, *36*(1), 163–172. doi:10.1016/S0191-8869(03)00076-X

Parkerson, G. R. Jr, Connis, R. T., Broadhead, W. E., Patrick, D. L., Taylor, T. R., & Tse, C. K. J. (1993). Disease-specific versus generic measurement of health-related quality of life in insulin-dependent diabetic patients. *Medical Care*, *31*(7), 629–639. doi:10.1097/00005650-199307000-00005 PMID:8326776

Passmore, H. A., & Holder, M. D. (2017). Noticing nature: Individual and social benefits of a two-week intervention. *The Journal of Positive Psychology*, *12*(6), 537–546. doi:10.1080/17439760.2016.1221126

Paterson, C. L., Lengacher, C. A., Donovan, K. A., Kip, K. E., & Tofthagen, C. S. (2015). Body image in younger breast cancer survivors. *Cancer Nursing*, *31*(2), 1. doi:10.1097/NCC.0000000000000251 PMID:25881807

Patrick, D. L., & Deyo, R. A. (1989). Generic and disease-specific measures in assessing health status and quality of life. *Medical Care*, *27*(Supplement), S217–S232. doi:10.1097/00005650-198903001-00018 PMID:2646490

Paulo, T. R. S., Rossi, F. E., Viezel, J., Tosello, G. T., Seidinger, S. C., Simões, R. R., ... Freitas, I. F. (2019). The impact of an exercise program on quality of life in older breast cancer survivors undergoing aromatase inhibitor therapy: A randomized controlled trial. *Health and Quality of Life Outcomes*, *17*(1), 17. doi:10.118612955-019-1090-4 PMID:30658629

Pavot, W., & Diener, E. (1993). Review of satisfaction with life scale. *Psychological Assessment*, *5*(2), 164–172. doi:10.1037/1040-3590.5.2.164

Peko, A., Mlinarević, V., & Gajger, V. (2009). Učinkovitost vođenja u osnovnim školama. *Odgojne Znanosti*, *11*(2), 67–84.

Pekrun, R., Goetz, T., Frenzel, A. C., Barchfeld, P., & Perry, R. P. (2011). Measuring emotions in students' learning and performance: The Achievement Emotions Questionnaire (AEQ). *Contemporary Educational Psychology*, *36*(1), 36–48. doi:10.1016/j.cedpsych.2010.10.002

Pekrun, R., Lichtenfeld, S., Marsh, H. W., Murayama, K., & Goetz, T. (2017). Achievement emotions and academic performance: Longitudinal models of reciprocal effects. *Child Development*, *88*(5), 1653–1670. doi:10.1111/cdev.12704 PMID:28176309

Penezić, Z. (2006). Zadovoljstvo životom u adolescentnoj i odrasloj dobi. *Društvena istraživanja, 15*(4-5), 643-669. Retrieved from hrcak.srce.hr/10864

Peng, L., Zhang, J., Li, M., Li, P., Zhang, Y., Zuo, X., ... Xu, Y. (2012). Negative life events and mental health of Chinese medical students: The effect of resilience, personality, and social support. *Psychiatry Research, 196*(1), 138–141. doi:10.1016/j.psychres.2011.12.006 PMID:22405636

Perlick, D., Clarkin, J.F., Sirey, J., Raue, P., Greenfield, S., Struening, E., & Rosenheck, R. (1999). Burden experienced by caregiver of persons with bipolar affective disorders. *The British Journal of Psychiatry Journal, 175*, 56-62.

Peter, J., Kühne, R., Barco, A., Jong, C. De, & Straten, C. L. Van. (2016). Asking Today the Crucial Questions of Tomorrow: Social Robots and the Internet of Toys. *Studies in Childhood and Youth*, 25–46. doi:10.1007/978-3-030-10898-4

Peterson, T. (2015, October 13). What is Emotional Health? And How to improve it. *Healthy Place.* Retrieved on 2019, July 2 from https://www.healthyplace.com/other-info/mental-illness-overview/what-is-emotional-health-and-how-to-improve-it

Peterson, C., & de Avila, M. E. (1995). Optimistic explanatory style and the perception of health problems. *Journal of Clinical Psychology, 51*(1), 128–132. doi:10.1002/1097-4679(199501)51:1<128::AID-JCLP2270510120>3.0.CO;2-1 PMID:7782467

Peterson, L. L., & Ligibel, J. A. (2018). Physical activity and breast cancer: An opportunity to improve outcomes. *Current Oncology Reports, 20*(7), 50. doi:10.100711912-018-0702-1 PMID:29713835

Petric, F., Hrvatini, K., Babic, A., Malovan, L., Miklic, D., Kovacic, Z., … Simlesa, S. (2014). Four tasks of a robot-assisted autism spectrum disorder diagnostic protocol: First clinical tests. *Proceedings of the 4th IEEE Global Humanitarian Technology Conference, GHTC 2014*, 510–517. 10.1109/GHTC.2014.6970331

Pettay, R. F. (2008). *Health behaviors and life satisfaction in college students* (Doctoral dissertation). Kansas State University.

Phillips, B., & Zhao, H. (1993). Predictors of assistive technology abandonment. *Assistive Technology, 5*(1), 36–45. doi:10.1080/10400435.1993.10132205 PMID:10171664

Phillips, M. R. (2009). Is distress a symptom of mental disorders, a marker of impairment, both or neither? *World Psychiatry; Official Journal of the World Psychiatric Association (WPA)*, (8), 91–92. PMID:19516930

Pinto-Carral, A., Molina, A. J., de Pedro, Á., & Ayán, C. (2018). Pilates for women with breast cancer: A systematic review and meta-analysis. *Complementary Therapies in Medicine, 41*(7), 130–140. doi:10.1016/j.ctim.2018.09.011 PMID:30477829

Pioggia, G., Sica, M. L., Ferro, M., Igliozzi, R., Muratori, F., Ahluwalia, A., & De Rossi, D. (2007). Human-robot interaction in autism: FACE, an android-based social therapy. *Proceedings - IEEE International Workshop on Robot and Human Interactive Communication*, 605–612. 10.1109/ROMAN.2007.4415156

Pirinççi, E., Rahman, S., Durmus, A. B., & Erdem, R. (2008). Factors affecting health-promoting behaviours in academic staff. *Public Health*, *122*(11), 1261–1263. doi:10.1016/j.puhe.2008.04.006 PMID:18849056

Pits, S., & Hansen, V. (2015). The relationship between lifestyle, occupational health and work related factors with presenteeism among general practitioners. *Archives of Environmental & Occupational Health*. Retrieved from www.ncbi.nlm.nih.gov/pubmed/25892305

Plienis, A. J., & Romanczyk, R. G. (1985). Analyses of performance, behavior, and predictors for severely disturbed children: A comparison of adult vs. computer instruction. *Analysis and Intervention In Developmental Disablities*, *5*(4), 345–356. doi:10.1016/0270-4684(85)90004-7

Plomin, R., Scheier, M. F., Bergeman, C. S., Pedersen, N. L., Nesselroade, J. R., & McClearn, G. E. (1992). Optimism, pessimism and mental health: A twin/adoption analysis. *Personality and Individual Differences*, *13*(8), 921–930. doi:10.1016/0191-8869(92)90009-E

Pollard, E. L., & Lee, P. D. (2003). Child Well-being: A Systematic Review of the Literature. *Social Indicators Research*, *61*(1), 59–78. doi:10.1023/A:1021284215801

Por, J., Barriball, L., Fitzpatrick, J., & Roberts, J. (2011). Emotional intelligence: Its relationship to stress, coping, well-being and professional performance in nursing students. *Nurse Education Today*, *31*(8), 855–860. doi:10.1016/j.nedt.2010.12.023 PMID:21292360

Pradhan, M. C. (1965, Dec. 11). The Jats of Northern India: Their Traditional Political System-II. *The Economic Weekly*, 1821–1824.

Prasad, J., Abraham, S., Akila, B., Joseph, A., & Jacaob, K. S. (2003). Symptoms related to the reproductive tract and mental health among women in rural southern India. *The National Medical Journal of India*, *16*(6), 303–308. PMID:14765620

Procter, P. (Ed.). (2002). *Cambridge International Dictionary of English*. Cambridge, UK: Cambridge University Press.

Prosen, S., Smrtnik Vitulić, H., & Poljšak Škraban, O. (2011). Teachers' Emotional Expression in Interaction with Students of Different Ages. *Center for Educational Policy Studies Journal*, *1*(3), 141–157.

Ptaznik, H., & Nelson, G. (1984). Stress and Social Support: The burden experienced by the family of a mentally ill person. *American Journal of Community Psychology*, *12*, 589–607. PMID:6496414

Qanungo, K. (1982). *History of the Jats: Contribution to the history of northern India*. New Delhi: Surajmal Memorial Education Society.

Raboteg-Šarić, Z., Merkaš, M., & Majić, M. (2011). Nada *i* optimizam adolescenata u odnosu na roditeljski odgojni stil. *Napredak, 152*(3 - 4), 373 – 388. Retrieved from hrcak.srce.hr/file/123149

Radhakrishnan, S. (1923). *Indian Philosophy* (Vol. 1). New Delhi: Oxford University Press.

Raguram, R., Weiss, M. G., Channabasavanna, S. M., & Devins, G. M. (1996). Stigma, depression, and somatization in South India. *The American Journal of Psychiatry, 153*(8), 1043–1049. doi:10.1176/ajp.153.8.1043 PMID:8678173

Raj, E. A., Shiri, S., & Jangam, K. V. (2016). Subjective burden, psychological distress, and perceived social support among caregivers of persons with schizophrenia. *Indian Journal of Social Psychiatry, 32*(1), 42. doi:10.4103/0971-9962.176767

Raju, P. T. (1992). *The philosophical traditions of India*. New Delhi: Motilal Banarasidass Pub. Ltd.

Raj-Yoga Meditation. (n.d.). *The Science of Peace and of Social, Economic and over-all Development*. Available from https://www.brahma-kumaris.com/rajyoga-meditation

Ramiro, S. L., Hassan, F., & Peedicayil, A. (2004). Risk markers of severe psychological violence against women: A world safe multi- country study. *Injury Control and Safety Promotion, 11*(2), 131–137. doi:10.1080/15660970412331292360 PMID:15370350

Randell, T., Hall, M., Bizo, L., & Remington, B. (2007). DTkid: Interactive simulation software for training tutors of children with autism. *Journal of Autism and Developmental Disorders, 37*(4), 637–647. doi:10.100710803-006-0193-z PMID:17019627

Ranney, M., Kleinpeter, C. B., & Potts, M. (2018). Personal well-being, depression, and alcohol use among community college students receiving services from a student health center. *The International Journal of Health, Wellness & Society, 8*(2), 9–16. doi:10.18848/2156-8960/CGP/v08i02/9-16

Rao, K. (2017). Empirical studies of Meditation. In *Foundations of Yoga Psychology* (pp. 137–174). Singapore: Springer. doi:10.1007/978-981-10-5409-9_6

Ratajczak, H. V. (2011). Theoretical aspects of autism: Causes—A review. *Journal of Immunotoxicology, 8*(1), 68–79. doi:10.3109/1547691X.2010.545086 PMID:21299355

Ratelle, C. F., Simard, K., & Guay, F. (2013). University students' subjective well-being: The role of autonomy support from parents, friend, and the romantic partner. *Journal of Happiness Studies, 14*(3), 803–910. doi:10.100710902-012-9360-4

Rauktis, M., Koeske, G. F., & Tereshko, O. (1995). Negative social interactions, distress & depression among those caring for a seriously and persistently mentally ill relative. *American Journal of Community Psychology, 23*(2), 279–299. doi:10.1007/BF02506939 PMID:7572833

Ravi Shankar, S. S. (2008). *God Loves Fun*. Bangalore: Sri Sri Publications.

Razza, R., Dessa, B., & Raymond, K. (2015). Enhancing preschoolers' Self-regulation via Mindful yoga. *Journal of Child and Family Studies, 24*(2), 372–385. doi:10.100710826-013-9847-6

Reeves, M. J., & Rafferty, A. P. (2005). Healthy lifestyle characteristics among adults in the united states, 2000. *Archives of Internal Medicine*, *165*(8), 854. doi:10.1001/archinte.165.8.854 PMID:15851634

Regan, T., Levesque, J. V., Lambert, S. D., & Kelly, B. (2015). A qualitative investigation of health care professionals', patients' and partners' views on psychosocial issues and related interventions for couples coping with cancer. *PLoS One*, *10*(7), e0133837. doi:10.1371/journal.pone.0133837 PMID:26222890

Reinares, M., Vieta, E., Colom, F., Martinez-Aran, A., Torrent, C., Comes, M., ... Sanchezmoreno, J. (2006). What really matters to bipolar patients' caregivers: Sources of family burden. *Journal of Affective Disorders*, *94*(1-3), 157–163. doi:10.1016/j.jad.2006.04.022 PMID:16737741

Renshaw, T. L. (2018). Psychometrics of the revised college student subjective well-being questionnaire. *Canadian Journal of School Psychology*, *33*(2), 136–149. doi:10.1177/0829573516678704

Renshaw, T. L., & Rock, D. K. (2018). Effects of a brief grateful thinking intervention on college students' mental health. *Mental Health and Prevention*, *9*, 19–24. doi:10.1016/j.mhp.2017.11.003

Respondek, L., Seufert, T., Stupnisky, R., & Nett, U. E. (2017). Perceived academic control and academic emotions predict undergraduate university student success: Examining effects on dropout intention and achievement. *Frontiers in Psychology*, *8*, 243. doi:10.3389/fpsyg.2017.00243 PMID:28326043

Rettew, D., & Reivich, K. (1995). Sports and explanatory style. In G. M. Buchanan & M. E. P. Seligman (Eds.), *Explanatory style* (pp. 173–185). Hillsdale, NJ: Lawrence Erlbaum Associates, Inc.

Reymann, L. S., Fialkowski, G. M., & Stewart-Sicking, J. A. (2015). Exploratory study of spirituality and psychosocial growth in college students. *Journal of College Counseling*, *18*(2), 103–115. doi:10.1002/jocc.12008

Rice, L. M., Wall, C. A., Fogel, A., & Shic, F. (2015). Computer-Assisted Face Processing Instruction Improves Emotion Recognition, Mentalizing, and Social Skills in Students with ASD. *Journal of Autism and Developmental Disorders*, *45*(7), 2176–2186. doi:10.100710803-015-2380-2 PMID:25694364

Riemer-Reiss, M. L., & Wacker, R. R. (2000). Factors associated with assistive technology discontinuance among individuals with disabilities. *Journal of Rehabilitation*, *66*(3).

Rietman, J. S., Dijkstra, P. U., Debreczeni, R., Geertzen, J. H., Robinson, D. P., & de Vries, J. (2004). Impairments, disabilities and health related quality of life after treatment for breast cancer: A follow-up study 2.7 years after surgery. *Disability and Rehabilitation*, *26*(2), 78–84. doi:10.1080/09638280310001629642 PMID:14668143

Rijavec, M., & Miljković, D. (2008). Pozitivna psihologija na poslu [Positive psychology at work]. Zagreb: IEP – D2.

Rijavec, M., Miljković, D., & Brdar, I. (2008). Pozitivna psihologija [Positive psychology]. Zagreb: IEP-D2.

Rivera, D., Garc, A., Mart, L., Alarcos, B., & Ana, G. (2019). Secure Communications and Protected Data for a Internet of Things Smart Toy Platform. *Journal of IEEE Internet of Things*, *4662*, 1–11. doi:10.1109/JIOT.2019.2891103

Rizzolo, D., Zipp, G. P., Stiskal, D., & Simpkins, S. (2009). Stress management strategies for students: The immediate effects of yoga, humor, and reading on stress. *Journal of College Teaching and Learning*, *6*(8), 79–88.

Robino, A., & Foster, T. (2018). Psychosocial predictors of wellness in college students. *Adultspan Journal*, *17*(1), 3–13. doi:10.1002/adsp.12049

Robins, B., Dautenhahn, K., & Dickerson, P. (2009). From isolation to communication: A case study evaluation of robot assisted play for children with autism with a minimally expressive humanoid robot. *Proceedings of the 2nd International Conferences on Advances in Computer-Human Interactions, ACHI 2009*, 205–211. 10.1109/ACHI.2009.32

Robins, C. J., & Hayes, A. M. (1995). An appraisal of cognitive therapy. In M. J. Mahoney (Ed.), *Cognitive and constructive psychotherapies* (pp. 41–65). New York: Springer.

Rockey, M., & Congleton, R. (2016). *Exploring the role of first-year experiences in enhancing equity & outcomes. Insights on Equity and Outcomes, 14*. Office of Community College Research and Leadership.

Rogers, J. (1997). Homoeopathy and the treatment of alcohol-related problems. *Complementary Therapies in Nursing & Midwifery*, *3*(1), 21–28. doi:10.1016/S1353-6117(97)80030-3 PMID:9432423

Rogers, K. A., & MacDonald, M. (2015). Therapeutic Yoga: Symptom Management for Multiple Sclerosis. *Journal of Alternative and Complementary Medicine (New York, N.Y.)*, *21*(11), 655–659. doi:10.1089/acm.2015.0015 PMID:26270955

Roh, S. Y. (2018). The influence of physical self-perception of female college students participating in Pilates classes on perceived health state and psychological well-being. *Journal of Exercise Rehabilitation*, *14*(2), 192–198. doi:10.12965/jer.1836088.044 PMID:29740551

Roh, S., Kim, Y., Lee, K. H., Lee, Y. S., Burnette, C. E., & Lawler, M. J. (2015). Religion, Social Support, and Life Satisfaction Among American Indian Older Adults. *Journal of Religion & Spirituality in Social Work*, *34*(4), 414–434. doi:10.1080/15426432.2015.1097094

Roosevelt, E. (2017). Emotional Intelligence Skills – Self-Regard. *Apex Leadership Mastery*. Retrieved from https://www.apexmastery.com/emotional-intelligence-skills-self-regard-1/

Rosenthal, D. A., Russell, J., & Thomson, G. (2008). The health and well-being of international students at an Australian university. *Higher Education*, *55*(1), 51–67. doi:10.100710734-006-9037-1

Rottmann, N., Dalton, S. O., Christensen, J., Frederiksen, K., & Johansen, C. (2010). Self-efficacy, adjustment style and well-being in breast cancer patients: A longitudinal study. *Quality of Life Research: An International Journal of Quality of Life Aspects of Treatment, Care and Rehabilitation, 19*(6), 827–836. doi:10.100711136-010-9653-1 PMID:20401551

Rowniyar, P. (2016). Emotional intelligence as a key to reduce academic stress among adolescence student. *The Signage, 4*(1), 2455–0051.

Roy, G. (2018). *To construct and test multi-component trait model of personality in Indian psychology* (Unpublished thesis). The Maharaja Sayajirao University of Baroda, Vadodara.

Roy, K., Shinde, S., Sarkar, B. K., Malik, K., Parikh, R., & Patel, V. (2019). India's response to adolescent mental health: A policy review and stakeholder analysis. *Social Psychiatry and Psychiatric Epidemiology*, 1–10. PMID:30607452

Roy, N., Tanner, K., Merrill, R. M., Wright, C., Miller, K. L., & Kendall, K. A. (2016). Descriptive epidemiology of voice disorders in rheumatoid arthritis: Prevalence, risk factors, and quality of life burden. *Journal of Voice, 30*(1), 74–87. doi:10.1016/j.jvoice.2015.02.011 PMID:25888079

Rutgers, A. H., Van IJzendoorn, M. H., Bakermans-Kranenburg, M. J., Swinkels, S. H. N., Van Daalen, E., Dietz, C., ... Van Engeland, H. (2007). Autism, attachment and parenting: A comparison of children with autism spectrum disorder, mental retardation, language disorder, and non-clinical children. *Journal of Abnormal Child Psychology, 35*(5), 859–870. doi:10.100710802-007-9139-y PMID:17505877

Rutherford, M. D., Pennington, B. F., & Rogers, S. J. (2006). The perception of animacy in young children with autism. *Journal of Autism and Developmental Disorders, 36*(8), 983–992. doi:10.100710803-006-0136-8 PMID:16897392

Rye, S. A. (2008). Dimensions of flexibility-students, communication technology and distributed education. Seminar.net, 4(1), 1-18.

Ryff, C. D., & Singer, B. (1998). The Contours of Positive Human Health. *Psychological Inquiry, 9*(1), 1–28. doi:10.120715327965pli0901_1

Sabbah, I., Sabbah, H., Khamis, R., Sabbah, S., & Droubi, N. (2013). Health related quality of life of university students in Lebanon: Lifestyles behaviors and socio-demographic predictors. *Health, 5*(7), 1–12. doi:10.4236/health.2013.57A4001

Saki, A., Ebrahim, H., & Tehranian, N. (2011, January 1). Evaluating the risk factors of breast cancer using the analysis of tree models. *OFOGH-E-DANESH, 17*(2), 61-68. Retrieved from https://www.sid.ir/en/journal/ViewPaper.aspx?id=196820

Sakuma, A., Takahashi, Y., Veda, I., Sato, H., Ketsura, M., Abe, M., ... Matsumoto, K. (2015). Post–Traumatic Stress Disorder and Depression prevalence and associated risk factors among local disaster relief and reconstruction worker fourteen months after the Great East Japan Earthquake: A cross sectional study. *BMC Psychiatry, 15*(1), 58. doi:10.118612888-015-0440-y PMID:25879546

Salehi, M., Zadeh, M. A., Ghaderi, A., & Tabasi, A. Z. (2016). Study of the Effect of Education and Academic Environment on Emotional Intelligence on Accounting Students in Iran. *International Education Studies*, *9*(1), 182–188. doi:10.5539/ies.v9n1p182

Salovey, P., & Mayer, J.D. (1990). Emotional Intelligence. *Imagination, Cognition and Personality*, *9*, 185-211.

Salovey, P., & Mayer, J. D. (1990). Emotional intelligence. *Imagination, Cognition and Personality*, *9*(3), 185–211. doi:10.2190/DUGG-P24E-52WK-6CDG

Sandroff, B., Hillman, C., Benadict, R., & Molt, R. (2015). acute effects of walking, cycling and yoga exercise on cognition in person with relapsing-remitting multiple sclerosis without impaired cognitive processing speed. *Neuropsychology*, *37*(2), 209–219. PMID:25658772

Sani-bozkurt, S., Vuran, S., & Akbulut, Y. (2017). *Design and Use of Interactive Social Stories for Children with Autism Spectrum Disorder*. Academic Press.

Sansosti, F. J., & Powell-Smith, K. (2008). Using Computer-Presented Social Stories and Video Models to Increase the Social Communication Skills of Children With High-Functioning Autism Spectrum Disorders. *Journal of Positive Behavior Interventions*, *10*(3), 162–178. doi:10.1177/1098300708316259

Sanuade, O. A., & Boatemaa, S. (2015). Caregiver profiles and determinants of caregiving burden in Ghana. *Public Health*, *129*(7), 941–947. doi:10.1016/j.puhe.2015.05.016 PMID:26115592

Sarita, S. (2015). Academic stress among students: Role and responsibilities of parents. *International Journal of Applied Research*, *1*(10), 385–388.

Sarkar, S., & Varshney, M. (2017). Yoga and substance use disorders: A narrative review. *Asian Journal of Psychiatry*, *25*, 191–196. doi:10.1016/j.ajp.2016.10.021 PMID:28262148

Sasanpour, M., Khodabakhshi, M., & Kh, N. (2012). The relationship between emotional intelligence, happiness and mental health in students of medical sciences of Isfahan University. *International Journal of Collaborative Research on Internal Medicine & Public Health*, *4*(9), 1614–1620.

Saxena, K. B. (2009). The naxalite movement and the crisis of governance: Reform measures for regaining people's trust. *Social Change*, *39*(4), 475–503.

Sayler, M. F., Boazman, J., Natesan, P., & Periathiruvadi, S. (2015). Subjective well-being of gifted American college students: An examination of psychometric properties of the PWI-A. *Gifted Child Quarterly*, *59*(4), 236–248. doi:10.1177/0016986215597748

Scheier, M. F., Carver, C. S., & Bridges, M. W. (1994). Distinguishing optimism from neuroticism (and trait anxiety, self-mastery, and self-esteem): A re-evaluation of the Life Orientation Test. *Journal of Personality and Social Psychology*, *67*(6), 1063–1078. doi:10.1037/0022-3514.67.6.1063 PMID:7815302

Scheier, M. F., Carver, C. S., & Bridges, M. W. (2001). Optimism, pessimism, and psychological well-being. In E. C. Chang (Ed.), *Optimism and Pessimism: Implications for theory, research, and practice* (pp. 189–216). Washington, DC: American Psychological Association. doi:10.1037/10385-009

Scherer, M. J. (1996). Outcomes of assistive technology use on quality of life. *Disability and Rehabilitation, 18*(9), 439–448. doi:10.3109/09638289609165907 PMID:8877302

Schmuck, R. A., & Schmuck, P. A. (1975). *Group processes in the classroom.* Academic Press.

Schulman, P. (1995). Explanatory style and achievement in school and work. In G. McC. Buchanan & M. E. P. Seligman (Eds.), *Explanatory style* (pp. 159–171). Hillsdale, NJ: Lawrence Erlbaum Associates.

Schultz-Ross, R. A., & Gutheil, T. G. (1997). Difficulties in integrating spirituality into psychotherapy. *The Journal of Psychotherapy Practice and Research, 6*(2), 130–138. PMID:9071663

Schulz, R., & Williamson, G. (1991). A Two-year longitudinal study of depression among Alzheimer's caregivers. *Psychology and Aging, 6*(4), 569–578. doi:10.1037/0882-7974.6.4.569 PMID:1777145

Schuster, C. S., & Ashburn, S. S. (1992). *The process of human development: A holistic lifespan approach* (3rd ed.). New York: Lippincott.

Schutte, N. S., Malouff, J. M., Thorsteinsson, E., Bhullar, N., & Rooke, S. (2007). A meta investigation of the relationship between emotional intelligence and health. *Personality and Individual Differences, 42*(6), 921–933. doi:10.1016/j.paid.2006.09.003

Schwartz, M., Oppold, P., & Hancock, P. A. (2019). Wearables and Workload. In Critical Issues Impacting Science, Technology, Society (STS), and Our Future (pp. 145-170). IGI Global.

Schwartz, M., & Oppold, P. (in press). Cross-cultural Adaptation of the Psychosocial Impact of Assistive Devices Scale (PIADS) for South African Exoskeleton Users. *Human Factors.* doi:10.4018/978-1-5225-7949-6.ch007

Schweitzer, A. L., Ross, J. T., Klein, C. J., Lei, K. Y., & Mackey, E. R. (2016). An electronic wellness program to improve diet and exercise in college students: A pilot study. *JMIR Research Protocols, 5*(1), e29. doi:10.2196/resprot.4855 PMID:26929118

Scott, D. L., & Garrood, T. (2000). Quality of life measures: Use and abuse. *Best Practice & Research. Clinical Rheumatology, 14*(4), 663–687. doi:10.1053/berh.2000.0106 PMID:11092795

Seale, J., & Turner-Smith, A. (2003). 8: Measuring the impact of assistive technologies on quality of life: can rehabilitation professionals rise to the challenge? *Alison J Carr,* 79.

Seligman, M. (2011). *Flourish: A visionary new understanding of happiness and well-being.* New York, NY: Simon & Schuster.

Seligman, M. E. P. (1998). *Learned optimism.* New York: Pocket Books.

Seligman, M. E. P. (2002). *Authentic happiness: Using the new positive psychology to realize your potential for lasting fulfillment*. New York, NY: Free Press.

Seligman, M. E. P., & Csikszentmihalyi, M. (2000). Positive psychology: An Introduction. *The American Psychologist, 55*(1), 5–14. doi:10.1037/0003-066X.55.1.5 PMID:11392865

Seligman, M. E. P., Ernst, R. M., Gillham, J., Reivich, K., & Linkins, M. (2009). Positive education: Positive psychology and classroom interventions. *Oxford Review of Education, 35*(3), 293–311. doi:10.1080/03054980902934563

Seligman, M. E. P., Reivich, K., Jaycox, L., & Gillham, J. (1995). *The Optimistic Child*. Boston, MA: Houghton Mifflin.

Seligman, M. E. P., Steen, T. A., Park, N., & Peterson, C. (2005). Positive psychology progress: Empirical validation of interventions. *The American Psychologist, 60*(5), 410–421. doi:10.1037/0003-066X.60.5.410 PMID:16045394

Seltzer, M. M., Krauss, M. W., Shattuck, P. T., Orsmond, G., Swe, A., & Lord, C. (2003). The symptoms of autism spectrum disorders. *Journal of Autism and Developmental Disorders, 33*(6), 565–581. doi:10.1023/B:JADD.0000005995.02453.0b PMID:14714927

Selvaraj, P. R., & Bhat, C. S. (2018). Predicting the mental health of college students with psychological capital. *Journal of Mental Health (Abingdon, England), 27*(3), 279–287. doi:10.1080/09638237.2018.1469738 PMID:29733236

Senato della Repubblica. (1948). *La Costituzione della Repubblica Italiana* [The Constitution of the Italian Republic]. Retrieved May 14, 2019, from http://www.senato.it/application/xmanager/projects/leg18/file/repository/relazioni/libreria/novita/XVII/COST_INGLESE.pdf

Şener, H. Ö., Malkoç, M., Ergin, G., Karadibak, D., & Yavuzşen, T. (2017). Effects of clinical Pilates exercises on patients Developing lymphedema after breast cancer treatment: A randomized clinical trial. *The Journal of Breast Health, 13*(1), 16–22. doi:10.5152/tjbh.2016.3136 PMID:28331763

Seven Dimensions of Wellness. (n.d.). Retrieved from https://wellness.ucr.edu/seven_dimensions.html

Shah, J. A., Wadoo, O., & Latoo, J. (2010). Psychological Distress in Carers with Mental Disorders. *British Journal of Medical Practitioners, 3*(3), 327.

Shapiro, D. (2017). *Meditation: Classic and Contemporary perspectives*. New York: Routledge. doi:10.4324/9780203785843

Sharma, N., Chakrabarti, S., & Grover, S. (2016). Gender differences in care giving among family-caregivers of people with mental illness. *World Journal of Psychiatry, 6*(1), 7–17. doi:10.5498/wjp.v6.i1.7 PMID:27014594

Sharma, R., Kabra, A., Rao, M. M., & Prajapati, P. K. (2018). Herbal and holistic solutions for neurodegenerative and depressive disorders: Leads from Ayurveda. *Current Pharmaceutical Design, 24*(22), 2597–2608. doi:10.2174/1381612824666180821165741 PMID:30147009

Shenoi, S. D., & Prabhu, S. S. (2018). Psychodermatology: An Indian perspective. *Clinics in Dermatology*, *36*(6), 737–742. doi:10.1016/j.clindermatol.2018.08.013 PMID:30446197

Shewchuk, R. M., Johnson, M. O., & Elliott, T. R. (2000). Self-appraised social problem solving abilities, emotional reactions and actual problem solving performance. *Behaviour Research and Therapy*, *38*(7), 727–740. doi:10.1016/S0005-7967(99)00122-9 PMID:10875194

Shin, D. C., & Johnson, D. M. (1978). Avowed happiness as an overall assessment of the quality of life. *Social Indicators Research*, *5*(1-4), 475–492. doi:10.1007/BF00352944

Shipley-Benamou, R., Lutzker, J. R., & Taubman, M. (2002). Teaching Daily Living Skills to Children with Autism Through Instructional Video Modeling. *Journal of Positive Behavior Interventions*, *4*(3), 166–177. doi:10.1177/10983007020040030501

Shushok, J. F. Jr, & Hulme, E. (2006). What's right with you: Helping students find and use their personal strengths. *About Campus: Enriching the Student Learning Experience*, *11*(4), 2–8. doi:10.1002/abc.173

Sigafoos, J., & Drasgow, E. (2001). Conditional Use of Aided and Unaided AAC: A Review and Clinical Case Demonstration. *Focus on Autism and Other Developmental Disabilities*, *16*(3), 152–161. doi:10.1177/108835760101600303

Šimić Šašić, S., Klarin, M., & Lapić, L. (2011). Percepcija odgovornosti, društvenog statusa i zadovoljstvo poslom kod odgojiteljica. *Magistra Iadertina, 6,* 17-32. Retrieved from http://hrcak.srce.hr/87329

Simpionato De Paula, É., Castanheira Nascimento, L., Melani, S., & Rocha, M. (n.d.). *The influence of social support on strengthening families of children with chronic renal failure.* Retrieved from www.eerp.usp.br/rlae

Sinclair, J. M. (Ed.). (1998). *Collins Concise Dictionary.* Glasgow, UK: Collins.

Singer, M. (1990). Postmodernism and Medical Anthropology: Words of Caution. *Medical Anthropology*, *12*(3), 289–304. doi:10.1080/01459740.1990.9966027 PMID:2233174

Singh, A., & Srinivasan, N. (2019). Concentrative (Sahaj Samadhi) meditation expands subjective time. *PsyCh Journal*, *8*(1), 28–35. doi:10.1002/pchj.265 PMID:30788909

Sinha, D. (1990). Concept of Psychological Well-being: Western and Indian Perspective. *Nimhans Journal*, *8*, 1–11.

Sintayehu, M., Mulat, H., Yohannis, Z., Adera, T., & Fekade, M. (2015). Prevalence of mental distress and associated factors among caregivers of patients with severe mental illness in the outpatient unit of Amanuel Hospital, Addis Ababa, Ethiopia, 2013: Cross-sectional study. *Journal of Molecular Psychiatry*, *3*(1), 9. doi:10.118640303-015-0014-4 PMID:26457184

Sivis-Cetinkaya, R. (2013). Turkish college students' subjective wellbeing in regard to psychological strengths and demographic variables: Implications for college counseling. *International Journal for the Advancement of Counseling*, *35*(4), 317–330. doi:10.100710447-013-9185-9

Škrinjar, J. (1994). *Profesionalna opterećenost i sindrom burnout djelatnika u ustanovama za rehabilitaciju osoba s težom mentalnom retardacijom* (Disertation). Zagreb: Fakultet za defektologiju, Sveučilište u Zagrebu.

Slevin, M. L., Plant, H., Lynch, D. A., Drinkwater, J., & Gregory, W. M. (1988). Who should measure quality of life, the doctor or the patient? *British Journal of Cancer, 57*(1), 109–112. doi:10.1038/bjc.1988.20 PMID:3348942

Smith, H. (1994). *The world's religions: A guide to our windows traditions.* San Francisco: Harper Collines.

Snyder, C. R., Rand, K. L., & Sigmon, D. R. (2005). Hope Theory: A Member of the Positive Psychology Family. In Handbook of Positive Psychology. Oxford University Press.

Sohl, S. J., Levine, B., & Avis, N. E. (2015). Evaluation of the quality of life in adult cancer survivors (QLACS) scale for early post-treatment breast cancer survivors. *Quality of Life Research: An International Journal of Quality of Life Aspects of Treatment, Care and Rehabilitation, 24*(1), 205–212. doi:10.100711136-014-0749-x PMID:24996392

SolutionsV. W. (n.d.). *PTSD Coach.* Retrieved from https://mobile.va.gov/app/ptsd-coach

Southall, K., Tuazon, J. R., Djokhdem, A. H., van den Heuvel, E. A., Wittich, W., & Jutai, J. W. (2017). Assessing the stigma content of urinary incontinence intervention outcome measures. *Journal of Rehabilitation and Assistive Technologies Engineering, 4.*

Spatuzzi, R., Vespa, A., Lorenzi, P., Miccinesi, G., Ricciuti, M., Cifarelli, W., ... Aieta, M. (2016). Evaluation of social support, quality of life, and body image in women with breast cancer. *Breast Care (Basel, Switzerland), 11*(1), 28–32. doi:10.1159/000443493 PMID:27051393

Sreeja, I., Sandhya, G., Rakesh, L., & Singh, M. (2009). Comparison of burden between family caregivers of patients having schizophrenia and epilepsy. *International Journal of Epidemiology, 6*, 2.

Srivastava Committee Report Government of India. (1975). Health series and medical education: a programme for immediate action: a report of the group on medical education and support manpower. New Delhi: Ministry of Health and Family Planning.

Steer, E. (2019). A cross comparison between Ayurvedic etiology of Major Depressive Disorder and bidirectional effect of gut dysregulation. *Journal of Ayurveda and Integrative Medicine, 10*(1), 59–66. doi:10.1016/j.jaim.2017.08.002 PMID:30655102

Stein, S. J., & Book, H. E. (2011). *The EQ edge: Emotional intelligence and you success.* John Wiley.

Stephen, J., Rojubally, A., Macgregor, K., McLeod, D., Speca, M., Taylor-Brown, J., ... Mackenzie, G. (2013). Evaluation of CancerChatCanada: A program of online support for Canadians affected by cancer. *Current Oncology (Toronto, Ont.), 20*(1), 39–47. doi:10.3747/co.20.1210 PMID:23443892

Stephens, I. (2019). Case report: The use of medical yoga for adolescent mental health. *Complementary Therapies in Medicine*, *43*, 60–65. doi:10.1016/j.ctim.2019.01.006 PMID:30935556

Sternfeld, B., Weltzien, E., Quesenberry, C. P. Jr, Castillo, A. L., Kwan, M., Slattery, M. L., & Caan, B. J. (2009). Physical activity and risk of recurrence and mortality in breast cancer survivors: Findings from the LACE study. *Cancer Epidemiology, Biomarkers & Prevention*, *18*(1), 87–95. doi:10.1158/1055-9965.EPI-08-0595 PMID:19124485

Strachey, J., & Freud, A. (Eds.). (1953-1964). The Standard Edition of the Complete Psychological Works of Sigmund Freud (pp. 1-24). London: Academic Press.

Straus, S. E., Glasziou, P., Richardson, W. S., & Haynes, R. B. (2018). *Evidence-Based Medicine E-Book: How to Practice and Teach EBM*. Elsevier Health Sciences.

Strine, T. W., Chapman, D. P., Balluz, L. S., Moriarty, D. G., & Mokdad, A. H. (2008). The associations between life satisfaction and health related quality of life, chronic illness, and health behaviors among U.S. community-dwelling adults. *Journal of Community Health*, *33*(1), 40–50. doi:10.100710900-007-9066-4 PMID:18080207

Subjective. (n.d.). In *Merriam-Webster's dictionary*. Retrieved from https://www.merriam-webster.com/dictionary/subjective

Subramanyam, K. (2016). Impact of emotional intelligence, nature of course and gender on academic stress among college students. *The International Journal of Indian Psychology, Volume 3, Issue 4, No. 60*, 120.

Sudarshan, M., Petrucci, A., Dumitra, S., Duplisea, J., Wexler, S., & Meterissian, S. (2013). Yoga therapy for breast cancer patients: A prospective cohort study. *Complementary Therapies in Clinical Practice*, *19*(4), 227–229. doi:10.1016/j.ctcp.2013.06.004 PMID:24199978

Suicide data. (2018, November 5). Retrieved from https://www.who.int/mental_health/prevention/suicide/suicideprevent/en/

Suicide Prevention App for Android and iPhone - MY3. (n.d.). Retrieved from https://my3app.org/

Sujoy, B. K. (2018). We are Spiritual Butterflies Having a Caterpillar Experience. *The World Renewal*, *49*(3), 13–15.

Sula, A., Spaho, E., Matsuo, K., Barolli, L., Miho, R., & Xhafa, F. (2013). An IoT-based System for Supporting Children with Autism Spectrum Disorder. In *8th International Conference on Automatic Face and Gesture Recognition International Conference on Broadband, Wireless Computing, Communication and Applications* (pp. 282–289). 10.1109/BWCCA.2013.51

Sulmasy, D. P. (2002). A Biopsychosocial-Spiritual Model for the Care of Patients at the End of Life. *The Gerontologist*, *42*(3suppl_3), 24–33. doi:10.1093/geront/42.suppl_3.24 PMID:12415130

Sundaram, S. K., & Kumar, S. (2018). Tracing the development of psychosocial rehabilitation from its origin to the current with emphasis on the Indian context. *Indian Journal of Psychiatry, 60*(6), S253–S256. PMID:29527057

Sunil, K., & Rooprai, K. Y. (2009). Role of emotional intelligence in managing stress and anxiety at workplace. *Proceedings of ASBBS, 16*(1), 163–172.

Sun, P., Jiang, H., Chu, M., & Qian, F. (2014). Gratitude and school well-being among Chinese university students: Interpersonal relationships and social support as mediators. *Social Behavior and Personality, 42*(10), 1689–1698. doi:10.2224bp.2014.42.10.1689

Swami Nikhilananda. (1996). *Vivekanana: Yogas and other works.* Chennai Mission Publication.

Swinburne, R. (1986). *The evolution of the soul.* Oxford, UK: Oxford University Press.

Sylva, K. (2000). School influences on children's development. *Psychology of Education: Schools. Teachers and Parents, 1*, 51.

Tabrizi, F. M., & Radfar, M. (2015). Fatigue, sleep quality, and disability in relation to quality of life in multiple sclerosis. *International Journal of MS Care, 17*(6), 268–274. doi:10.7224/1537-2073.2014-046 PMID:26664332

Tackett, S., Wright, S., Lubin, R., Li, J., & Pan, H. (2017). International study of medical school learning environments and their relationship with student well-being and empathy. *Medical Education, 51*(3), 280–289. doi:10.1111/medu.13120 PMID:27896846

Talkspace. (n.d.). *Online Therapy: Counseling Online: Marriage Counseling*. Retrieved from https://www.talkspace.com/

Tambağ, H., & Öz, F. (2013). Evaluation of the psychoeducation given to the elderly at nursing homes for a healthy lifestyle and developing life satisfaction. *Community Mental Health Journal, 49*(6), 742–747. doi:10.100710597-013-9602-x PMID:23400690

Tan, M. L., Idris, D. B., Teo, L. W., Loh, S. Y., Seow, G. C., Chia, Y. Y., & Tin, A. S. (2014). Validation of EORTC QLQ-C30 and QLQ-BR23 questionnaires in the measurement of quality of life of breast cancer patients in Singapore. *Asia-Pacific Journal of Oncology Nursing, 1*(1), 22-32. doi:10.4103/2347-5625.135817

Tanaka, J. W., Wolf, J. M., Klaiman, C., Koenig, K., Cockburn, J., Herlihy, L., ... Schultz, R. T. (2012). The perception and identification of facial emotions in individuals with autism spectrum disorders using the Let's Face It! Emotion Skills Battery. *Journal of Child Psychology and Psychiatry, and Allied Disciplines, 53*(12), 1259–1267. doi:10.1111/j.1469-7610.2012.02571.x PMID:22780332

Tanesini, A. (2016). 'Calm Down, Dear': Intellectual Arrogance, Silencing and Ignorance. *Aristotellian Society Supplementary, 90*(1), 71–92. doi:10.1093/arisup/akw011

Tangmunkongvorakul, A., Musumari, P. M., Thongpibul, K., Srithanaviboonchai, K., Techasrivichien, T., Suguimoto, S. P., ... Kihara, M. (2019). Association of excessive smartphone use with psychological well-being among university students in Chiang Mai, Thailand. *PLoS One*, *14*(1), e0210294. doi:10.1371/journal.pone.0210294 PMID:30615675

Tao, Z., Shi, A., Lu, C., Song, T., Zhang, Z., & Zhao, J. (2015). Breast cancer: Epidemiology and etiology. *Cell Biochemistry and Biophysics*, *72*(2), 333–338. doi:10.100712013-014-0459-6 PMID:25543329

Tatalović Vorkapić, S. (2015). How much personality is important in educational context? In *International Conference EDUvision 2015: "Modern Approaches to Teaching Coming Generation"* (pp. 75-83). EDUvision, Stanislav Jurjevčič. Retrieved from http://eduvision.si/Content/Docs/Zbornik%20prispevkov%20EDUvision%202015.pdf

Tatalović Vorkapić, S., & Gović, A. (2016). Relationship between flow and personality traits among preschool teachers. *Metodički obzori, 11*(1), 24-40. Retrieved from https://hrcak.srce.hr/168804

Tatalović Vorkapić, S., & Jelić Puhalo, J. (2016). Povezanost osobina ličnosti, nade, optimizma i zadovoljstva životom odgojitelja predškolske djece [The connection of personality traits of pre-school teachers with their hopes, optimism and life satisfaction]. Napredak, 157(1-2), 205-220.

Tatalović Vorkapić, S. (2012). The significance of preschool teacher's personality in early childhood education: Analysis of Eysenck's and Big Five Dimensions of personality. *International Journal of Psychology and Behavioral Sciences*, *2*(2), 28–37. doi:10.5923/j.ijpbs.20120202.05

Tatalović Vorkapić, S. (2017). Personality and Education: Contemporary issues in Psychological science about Personality in Teacher Education. In C. Martin & D. Polly (Eds.), *Handbook of Research on Teacher Education and Professional Development Professional Development* (pp. 163–186). IGI Global.

Tatalović Vorkapić, S., Čepić, R., & Šekulja, I. (2016). Are there any differences in personality traits and life satisfaction between preschool and primary school teachers? *Journal of Research in Childhood Education*, *30*(3), 361–373. doi:10.1080/02568543.2016.1179236

Tatalović Vorkapić, S., & Lončarić, D. (2013). Posreduje li profesionalno sagorijevanje učinke osobina ličnosti na zadovoljstvo životom odgajatelja predškolske djece? [Does Professional Burnout Mediate the Effects of Personality Traits on Life Satisfaction among Preschool Teachers?]. *Psihologijske Teme*, *22*(3), 431–455.

Tatalović Vorkapić, S., & Peloza, I. (2017). Exploring the personality traits and well-being among pre-school and primary school teachers in Croatia. *Current Issues in Personality Psychology*, *5*(1), 21–31. doi:10.5114/cipp.2017.65830

Technology enabled best practice for eating disorder treatment. (n.d.). Retrieved from https://www.recoveryrecord.com/

Tehrani, N., Humpage, S., Willmott, B., & Haslam, I. (2011). *What's happening with well-being at work?* London, UK: Chartered Institute of Personnel and Development.

Teven, C. M., Schmid, D. B., Sisco, M., Ward, J., & Howard, M. A. (2017). Systemic therapy for early-stage breast cancer: What the plastic surgeon should know. *Eplasty*, *17*, e7. PMID:28293332

Tewey, B. P., Barnicle, K., & Perr, A. (1994). The wrong stuff. *Mainstream*, *19*(2), 19–23.

The Dahlgren-Whitehead Rainbow. (n.d.). Retrieved from http://www.esrc.ac.uk/about-us/50-years-of-esrc/50-achievements/the-dahlgren-whitehead-rainbow

The New Oxford Dictionary of English. (1998). London: Oxford University Press.

Thirthalli, J., Zhou, L., Kumar, K., Gao, J., Vaid, H., Liu, H., ... Nichter, M. (2016). Traditional, complementary, and alternative medicine approaches to mental health care and psychological wellbeing in India and China. *The Lancet. Psychiatry*, *3*(7), 660–672. doi:10.1016/S2215-0366(16)30025-6 PMID:27209157

Thomas, G. A., Cartmel, B., Harrigan, M., Fiellin, M., Capozza, S., Zhou, Y., ... Irwin, M. L. (2016). The effect of exercise on body composition and bone mineral density in breast Cancer survivors taking aromatase inhibitors. *The Observatory Journal*, *1*, 1–6. PMID:28026901

Thoresen, C. E. (1998). Spiritual health and science, the coming revival? In S Roth Roemer, S Korpivas Robinson, & C. C. (Eds.), The emerging role of counseling psychology in health care. New York: Norton.

Tiemann, G. (1970). The Four-got-Rule among the Jat of Haryana in Northern India. *Anthropos*, *65*(1/2), 166–177.

Tinto, V. (1975). Dropout from higher education: A theoretical synthesis of recent research. *Review of Educational Research*, *45*(1), 89–125. doi:10.3102/00346543045001089

Tinto, V. (1987). *Leaving college: Rethinking the causes and cures of student attrition* (2nd ed.). Chicago, IL: University of Chicago Press.

Topham, P., & Moller, N. (2011). New students' psychological well-being and its relation to first year academic performance in a UK university. *Counselling & Psychotherapy Research*, *11*(3), 196–203. doi:10.1080/14733145.2010.519043

Tran, C. T., Kuhn, E., Walser, R. D., & Drescher, K. D. (2012). The Relationship between religiosity, PTSD, and depressive symptoms in veterans in PTSD residential treatment. *Journal of Psychology and Theology*, *40*(4), 313–322. doi:10.1177/009164711204000406

Traore, B. M., El Fakir, S., Charaka, H., Benaicha, N., Najdi, A., Zidouh, A., . . . Nejjari, C. (2018). Evolution of quality of life in patients with breast cancer during the first year of follow-up in Morocco. *BMC Cancer*, *18*(1), 109. doi:10.118612885-018-4008-3

Trinidad, D. R., & Johnson, C. A. (2002). The association between emotional intelligence and early adolescent tobacco and alcohol use. *Personality and Individual Differences*, *32*(1), 95–105. doi:10.1016/S0191-8869(01)00008-3

Tümkaya, S. (2011). Humor styles and socio-demographic variables as predictors of subjective well-being of turkish university students. *Egitim ve Bilim, 36*(160), 158-170. Retrieved from http://search.ebscohost.com/login.aspx?direct=true&db=edselc&AN=edselc.2-52.0-84885637295&site=eds-live&scope=site

Turner, N., Barling, J., Epitropaki, O., Butcher, V., & Milner, C. (2002). Transformational Leadership and Moral Reasoning. *The Journal of Applied Psychology, 87*(2), 304–311. doi:10.1037/0021-9010.87.2.304 PMID:12002958

UCSF. (2016, July 13). *UCSF PRIME*. Retrieved from https://apps.apple.com/us/app/ucsf-prime/id1031402495

University of the West of England. (2013, July 4). *Self-help for Anxiety Management*. Retrieved from https://apps.apple.com/us/app/self-help-for-anxiety-management/id666767947

Utting, D. (2007). *Parenting and the different ways it can affect children's lives: research evidence*. Joseph Rowntree Foundation.

Vaksh, S., Pandey, M., & Kumar, R. (2016). Study the Effect of Pranayam on Academic Performance of School Students of IX and XI Standards. *Scholars Journal of Applied Medical Sciences, 4*(5D), 1703–1705.

Van Der Aa, C., Pollmann, M. M. H., Plaat, A., & Van Der Gaag, R. J. (2016). Computer-mediated communication in adults with high-functioning autism spectrum disorders and controls. *Research in Autism Spectrum Disorders, 23*, 15–27. doi:10.1016/j.rasd.2015.11.007

van der Willik, K. D., Koppelmans, V., Hauptmann, M., Compter, A., Ikram, M. A., & Schagen, S. B. (2018). Inflammation markers and cognitive performance in breast cancer survivors 20 years after completion of chemotherapy: A cohort study. *Breast Cancer Research: BCR, 20*(1), 135. doi:10.118613058-018-1062-3 PMID:30442190

van Londen, G. J., Perera, S., Vujevich, K., Rastogi, P., Lembersky, B., Brufsky, A., ... Greenspan, S. L. (2011). The impact of an aromatase inhibitor on body composition and gonadal hormone levels in women with breast cancer. *Breast Cancer Research and Treatment, 125*(2), 441–446. doi:10.100710549-010-1223-2 PMID:21046232

van Nes, J. G. H., Fontein, D. B. Y., Hille, E. T. M., Voskuil, D. W., van Leeuwen, F. E., de Haes, J. C. J. M., ... van de Velde, C. J. H. (2012). Quality of life in relation to tamoxifen or exemestane treatment in postmenopausal breast cancer patients: A Tamoxifen Exemestane Adjuvant Multinational (TEAM) trial side study. *Breast Cancer Research and Treatment, 134*(1), 267–276. doi:10.100710549-012-2028-2 PMID:22453754

Van Slingerland, K. J., Durand-Bush, N., & Rathwell, S. (2018). Levels and prevalence of mental health functioning in Canadian university student-athletes. *Canadian Journal of Higher Education, 48*(2), 149–168. doi:10.7202/1057108ar van Vulpen, J. K., Peeters, P. H. M., Velthuis, M. J., van der Wall, E., & May, A. M. (2016). Effects of physical exercise during adjuvant breast cancer treatment on physical and psychosocial dimensions of cancer-related fatigue: A meta-analysis. *Maturitas*, *85*(4), 104–111. doi:10.1016/j.maturitas.2015.12.007 PMID:26857888

VandenBos, G. R. (Ed.). (2015). *APA Dictionary of Psychology* (2nd ed.). Washington, DC: American Psychological Association; doi:10.1037/14646-000

Vanderveer, P. (2009). Spirituality in Modern Society. *Social Research*, *76*(4), 1097–1120.

VanderWeele, T. J., Balboni, T. A., & Koh, H. K. (2017, August 8). Health and spirituality. *JAMA - Journal of the American Medical Association*. doi:10.1001/jama.2017.8136

Van, H. V., & Neves, D. (2004). Activity Theory as a Framework for Psychological Research and Practice Developing Societies. In *Self, Community and Psychology* (pp. 9–20). Lansdowne: UCT Press.

Vari, R. (2014). Centro di Salute Mentale: La relazione 'individuo/ambiente di convivenza/Servizio' nell'intervento clinico per le malattie mentali [Mental Health Center. The relationship 'individual/ social coexistence milieu/Service' in the clinical intervention for mental illness]. *Rivista di psicologia clinica, 1,* 154-185. Retrieved from http://www.rivistadipsicologiaclinica.it

Varma, P., Cheaskul, U., & Poonpol, P. (2018). The influence of parenting styles on academic adjustment and psychological well-being among Thai university students mediated by Internet addiction and self-regulation: A path model. *Journal for Leadership and Instruction*, *17*(2), 13–24. Retrieved from https://ezp.waldenulibrary.org/login?url=https://search.ebscohost.com/login.aspx?direct=true&db=eric&AN=EJ1199679&site=eds-live&scope=site

Vasold, K. L., Deere, S. J., & Pivarnik, J. M. (2018). Self-reported wellness benefits of recreational sports use in college freshmen: 1328 Board# 136 May 31 9. *Medicine and Science in Sports and Exercise*, *50*(5S), 316. doi:10.1249/01.mss.0000536122.63367.fc

Vaughan, F. (1991). Spiritual issues in psychotherapy. *Journal of Transpersonal Psychology*, *23*(2), 105–119.

Vela, J. C., Smith, W. D., Whittenberg, J. F., Guardiola, R., & Savage, M. (2018). Positive psychology factors as predictors of Latina/o college students' psychological grit. *Journal of Multicultural Counseling and Development*, *46*(1), 2–19. doi:10.1002/jmcd.12089

Verma, S. K., & Verma, A. (1989). *Manual for PGI General Wellbeing Measure*. Lucknow: Ankur Psychological Agency.

Verza, R., Carvalho, M. L., Battaglia, M. A., & Uccelli, M. M. (2006). An interdisciplinary approach to evaluating the need for assistive technology reduces equipment abandonment. *Multiple Sclerosis Journal*, *12*(1), 88–93. doi:10.1191/1352458506ms1233oa PMID:16459724

Vijaylakshmi, P., Reddy, D., Math, S. B., & Thimmaiah, R. (2013). Attitudes of undergraduates towards mental illness: A comparison between the nursing and business managements students in India. *South African Journal of Psychology. Suid-Afrikaanse Tydskrif vir Sielkunde*, *19*(3), 66–73.

Viral, B. K. (2019). Being Happy Always. *The World Renewal*, *49*(9), 27–29.

Vizcarra, B., Hassan, F., Wanda, M., Hunter, Munroz, R.S., Ramiro, L., & Paula De, S.C. (2004). Partner violence as a risk factor for mental health among women from communities in the Philippines, Egypt, Chile & India. *Injury Control & Safety Promotion. Journal*, *11*(2), 125-129.

Wacker, M. E., Jörres, R. A., Karch, A., Wilke, S., Heinrich, J., Karrasch, S., ... Vogelmeier, C. (2016). Assessing health-related quality of life in COPD: Comparing generic and disease-specific instruments with focus on comorbidities. *BMC Pulmonary Medicine*, *16*(1), 70. doi:10.118612890-016-0238-9 PMID:27160582

Waldron-Perrine, B., Rapport, L. J., Hanks, R. A., Lumley, M., Meachen, S. J., & Hubbarth, P. (2011). Religion and Spirituality in Rehabilitation Outcomes Among Individuals With Traumatic Brain Injury. *Rehabilitation Psychology*, *56*(2), 107–116. doi:10.1037/a0023552 PMID:21574729

Walker, S., Noble, K., Sechrist, R., & Pender, N. J. (1987). The Health-Promoting Lifestyle Profile: Development and Psychometric Characteristics. *Nursing Research*, *36*(2), 76–81. doi:10.1097/00006199-198703000-00002 PMID:3644262

Walsh, K., & O'shea, E. (2008). Responding to rural social care needs: Older people empowering themselves, others and their community. *Health & Place*, *14*(4), 795–805. doi:10.1016/j.healthplace.2007.12.006 PMID:18289914

Walsh, P. (2005). Well-being. In T. Honderich (Ed.), *The Oxford Companion to Philosophy* (pp. 955–956). Oxford: Oxford University Press.

Wang, J.-L., Jackson, L. A., Gaskin, J., & Wang, H.-Z. (2014). The effects of social networking site (SNS) use on college students' friendship and well-being. *Computers in Human Behavior*, *37*, 229–236. doi:10.1016/j.chb.2014.04.051

Wang, Y., & Kuchenbecker, K. J. (2012, March). HALO: Haptic alerts for low-hanging obstacles in white cane navigation. In *2012 IEEE Haptics Symposium (HAPTICS)* (pp. 527-532). IEEE. 10.1109/HAPTIC.2012.6183842

Waris, A., & Viraktamath, B. C. (2013). Gender gap and Women's empowerment in India- Issues & Strategies. *International Journal of Scientific and Research Publications*, *3*(9). Retrieved from http://www.ijsrp.org/research-paper-0913/ijsrp-p21116.pdf

Warr, P. (1999). Well-being and the workplace. In D. Kahneman, E. Diener, & N. Schwarz (Eds.), *Well-being: The foundations of hedonic psychology* (pp. 392–412). New York, NY: Russell Sage Foundation.

Wass, A. (2000). *Promoting Health-The Primary Health Care Approach*. Marruckville: Harcourt Australia.

Watson, D. (2009). Differentiating the mood and anxiety disorders: A quadripartite model. *Annual Review of Clinical Psychology*, *5*(5), 221–247. doi:10.1146/annurev.clinpsy.032408.153510 PMID:19327030

Watson, D., Clark, L. A., & Tellegen, A. (1988). Development and validation of brief measures of positive and negative affect: The PANAS Scales. *Journal of Personality and Social Psychology*, *47*(6), 1063–1070. doi:10.1037/0022-3514.54.6.1063 PMID:3397865

Weenk, M., Van Goor, H., Frietman, B., & Engelen, L. J. (2017). Continuous Monitoring of Vital Signs Using Wearable Devices on the General Ward. *Pilot Study Corresponding Author*, *5*(7), 1–14. doi:10.2196/mhealth.7208 PMID:28679490

Wehmeier, S. (Ed.). (2002). *Oxford Advanced Learner's Dictionary*. Oxford, UK: Oxford University Press.

Weinberg, M. K., Seton, C., & Cameron, N. (2018). The measurement of subjective well-being: Item-order effects in the Personal Well-being Index—Adult. *Journal of Happiness Studies*, *19*(1), 315–332. doi:10.100710902-016-9822-1

Well-being. (n.d.). In *Cambridge dictionary*. Retrieved from https://dictionary.cambridge.org/dictionary/english/well-being

Well-being. (n.d.). In *Merriam-Webster's dictionary*. Retrieved from https://www.merriam-webster.com/dictionary/well-being

Welle, P. D., & Graf, H. M. (2011). Effective lifestyle habits and coping strategies for stress tolerance among college students. *American Journal of Health Education*, *42*(2), 96–105. doi:10.1080/19325037.2011.10599177

Wenger, M. A., & Bagchi, B. K. (1961). Studies of autonomic functions in practitioners of yoga in India. *Behavioral Science*, *6*(4), 312–323. doi:10.1002/bs.3830060407 PMID:14006122

Wert, B. Y., & Neisworth, J. T. (2003). Effects of Video Self-Modeling on Spontaneous Requesting in Children with Autism. *Journal of Positive Behavior Interventions*, *5*(1), 30–34. doi:10.1177/10983007030050010501

Westgate, C. E. (1996). Spiritual wellness and depression. *Journal of Counseling and Development*, *75*(1), 26–35. doi:10.1002/j.1556-6676.1996.tb02311.x

Westphal-Hellbusch, S., & Westphal, H. (1964). *The Jat of Pakistan*. Berlin: Duncker & Humbolt.

Whalen, C., Moss, D., Ilan, A. B., Vaupel, M., Fielding, P., Macdonald, K., ... Symon, J. (2010). Efficacy of TeachTown: Basics computer-assisted intervention for the Intensive Comprehensive Autism Program in Los Angeles Unified School District. *Autism*, *14*(3), 179–197. doi:10.1177/1362361310363282 PMID:20484002

What is Emotional Health? And How to Improve it? (n.d.). Retrieved from https://www.healthyplace.com/other-info/mental-illness-overview/what-is-emotional-health-and-how-to-improve-it

What's Up? - Mental Health App – Apps on Google Play. (n.d.). Retrieved from https://play.google.com/store/apps/details?id=com.jacksontempra.apps.whatsup&hl=en_GB

Whelan, T. J., Levine, M., Julian, J., Kirkbride, P., & Skingley, P. (2000). The effects of radiation therapy on quality of life of women with breast carcinoma: Results of a randomized trial. Ontario Clinical Oncology Group. *Cancer*, *88*(10), 2260–2266. doi:10.1002/(SICI)1097-0142(20000515)88:10<2260::AID-CNCR9>3.0.CO;2-M PMID:10820347

Whiteford, H. A., Degenhardt, L., Rehm, J., Baxter, A. J., Ferrari, A. J., Erskine, H. E., ... Vos, T. (2013). Global burden of disease attributable to mental and substance use disorders: Findings from the Global Burden of Disease Study 2010. *Lancet*, *382*(9904), 1575–1586. doi:10.1016/S0140-6736(13)61611-6 PMID:23993280

WHO. (2018). Breast cancer. *WHO*. Retrieved from https://www.who.int/cancer/prevention/diagnosis-screening/breast-cancer/en/

Wig, N. N. (1990). Indian concepts of mental health and their impact on the care of the mentally ill. *International Journal of Mental Health*, *18*(3), 71–80. doi:10.1080/00207411.1989.11449136

Wiley, J. A., & Camacho, T. C. (1980). Lifestyle and future health: Evidence from the alameda county study. *Preventive Medicine*, *9*(1), 1–21. doi:10.1016/0091-7435(80)90056-0 PMID:7360725

Wilson, J. T. (2016). Brightening the mind: The impact of practicing gratitude on focus and resilience in learning. *The Journal of Scholarship of Teaching and Learning*, *16*(4), 1–13. doi:10.14434/josotl.v16i4.19998

Wing, L. (1993). The definition and prevalence of autism: A review. *European Child & Adolescent Psychiatry*, *2*(2), 61–74. doi:10.1007/BF02098832 PMID:21590530

Wing, L., & Gould, J. (1979). Severe impairments of social interaction and associated abnormalities in children: Epidemiology and classification. *Journal of Autism and Developmental Disorders*, *9*(1), 11–29. doi:10.1007/BF01531288 PMID:155684

Winzelberg, A. J., Classen, C., Alpers, G. W., Roberts, H., Koopman, C., Adams, R. E., ... Taylor, C. B. (2003). Evaluation of an internet support group for women with primary breast cancer. *Cancer*, *97*(5), 1164–1173. doi:10.1002/cncr.11174 PMID:12599221

Wissing, M. P. (2000). Wellness: Construct clarification and a framework for future research and practice. *First South African National Wellness Conference*.

World Health Organization. (1978). *Alma-Ata Declaration*. Geneva: WHO.

World Health Organization. (1986). *Young People's Health – A Challenge for Society. Technical Report Series 731*. Geneva: WHO.

World Health Organization. (2000). *General Guidelines for Methodologies on Research and Evaluation of Traditional Medicine*. Geneva: World Health Organization.

World Health Organization. (2004). *Promoting mental health: Concepts, emerging evidence, practice: Summary report*. Author.

World Health Organization. (2018). *Mental health: strengthening our response.* Retrieved May 14, 2019, from https://www.who.int/news-room/fact-sheets/detail/mental-health-strengthening-our-response

World Health Organization. (n.d.). *Definition of Health.* Retrieved from http://www.who.int

Xiao, C., Miller, A. H., Felger, J., Mister, D., Liu, T., & Torres, M. A. (2016). A prospective study of quality of life in breast cancer patients undergoing radiation therapy. *Adv Radiat Oncol.*, *1*(1), 10–16. doi:10.1016/j.adro.2016.01.003 PMID:27453954

Xiao, F., Song, X., Chen, Q., Dai, Y., Xu, R., Qiu, C., & Guo, Q. (2017). Effectiveness of psychological interventions on depression in patients after breast cancer surgery: A meta-analysis of randomized controlled trials. *Clinical Breast Cancer*, *17*(3), 171–179. doi:10.1016/j.clbc.2016.11.003 PMID:28040415

Yamashiro, J. (2015). Brain basis of Samadhi: The Neuroscience of Meditative Absorption. *The New School Psychology Bulletin*, *13*(1), 1–10.

Yan, B., Yang, L. M., Hao, L. P., Yang, C., Quan, L., Wang, L. H., . . . Yuan, J. M. (2016). Determinants of quality of life for breast cancer patients in Shanghai, China. *PLoS One*, *11*(4), e0153714. doi:10.1371/journal.pone.0153714

Yang, J., & Mossholder, K. W. (2004). Decoupling task and relationship conflict: The role of intragroup emotional processing. *Journal of Organizational Behavior*, *25*(5), 589–605. doi:10.1002/job.258

Yasobant, S. (2016). Physical health promotion through modern technologies: challenges to concerns. In Handbook of Research on Advancing Health Education through Technology. Medical Information Science.

Yazdi, S. A. A., Farahi, S. M. M., Farahi, S. M. M. M., & Hosseini, J. (2018). Emotional Intelligence and its role in Cognitive Flexibility of Children with and without Attention Deficit Hyperactivity Disorder. *Anales de Psicología/Annals of Psychology, 34*(2), 299-304.

Yoga Sutra. (n.d.). New Delhi: Vijay Goyal Publisher.

Yucel, B., Akkaş, E. A., Okur, Y., Eren, A. A., Eren, M. F., Karapinar, H., . . . Kiliçkap, S. (2014). The impact of radiotherapy on quality of life for cancer patients: a longitudinal study. *Support Care Cancer, 22*(9), 2479-2487. doi:10.100700520-014-2235-y

Yusuf, A. J., & Nuhu, F. T. (2011). Factors associated with emotional distress among caregivers of patients with schizophrenia in Katsina, Nigeria. *Social Psychiatry and Psychiatric Epidemiology*, *46*(1), 11–16. doi:10.100700127-009-0166-6 PMID:19907909

Yusuf, S., Hawken, S., Ounpuu, S., Dans, T., Avezum, A., Lanas, F., ... Lisheng, L. (2004). Effect of potentially modifiable risk factors associated with myocardial infarction in 52 countries (The INTERHEART study): Case-control study. *Lancet*, *364*(9438), 937–952. doi:10.1016/S0140-6736(04)17018-9 PMID:15364185

Zaraki, A., Wood, L., Robins, B., & Dautenhahn, K. (2018). Development of a Semi-Autonomous Robotic System to Assist Children with Autism in Developing Visual Perspective Taking Skills. *2018 27th IEEE International Symposium on Robot and Human Interactive Communication (RO-MAN)*, 969–976.

Zastro, C., & Kirst-Ashman, K. (1990). *Understanding human behavior and the social environment*. Chicago: Nelson-Hall.

Zendjidjian, X., Richieri, R., Adida, M., Limousin, S., Gaubert, N., Parola, N., ... Boyer, L. (2012). Quality of life among caregivers of individuals with affective disorders. *Journal of Affective Disorders*, *136*(3), 660–665. doi:10.1016/j.jad.2011.10.011 PMID:22100129

Zhang, H., Zhao, Q., Cao, P., & Ren, G. (2017). Resilience and quality of life: Exploring the mediator role of social support in patients with breast cancer. *Medical Science Monitor: International Medical Journal of Experimental and Clinical Research*, *23*, 5969-5979. doi:10.12659/msm.907730

Zhan, Z., & Mei, H. (2013). Academic self-concept and social presence in face-to-face and online learning: Perceptions and effects on students' learning achievement and satisfaction across environments. *Computers & Education*, *69*, 131–138. doi:10.1016/j.compedu.2013.07.002

Zheng, G., Li, M., Lan, X., Yan, X., Lin, Q., Chen, L., ... Fang, Q. (2013). The effect of Baduanjin exercise for physical and psychological wellbeing of college students: Study protocol for a randomized controlled trial. *Trials*, *14*(1), 422. doi:10.1186/1745-6215-14-422 PMID:24308310

Zheng, X., Xie, F., & Ding, L. (2018). Mediating role of self-concordance on the relationship between Internet altruistic behaviour and subjective well-being. *Journal of Pacific Rim Psychology*, *12*, e1. doi:10.1017/prp.2017.14

About the Contributors

Srinivasan Padmanaban is working as Associate Professor in the School of Education, Central University of Tamil Nadu, Tamil Nadu, India. Editor possess 19 years of experience in teacher education at various levels. 10 research scholars have been awarded a doctorate in Education under his guidance. 38 research scholars have been awarded M.Phil. in Education. Has completed 01 Major and 02 Minor research projects. Has published 11 books and 56 research articles in peer-reviewed journals. Has organized 02 national level seminars. Has been a resource person for 80 occasions.

Chittaranjan Subudhi is working as an Assistant Professor, in the Department of Social Work, School of Social Sciences and Humanities, Central University of Tamil Nadu (by an Act of Parliament) Thiruvarur, India. He has Bachelor Degree in Commerce and Master Degree in Social Work from the Utkal University of Odisha, India. He is also pursuing Ph.D. in Mental Health from Department of Humanities and Social Sciences, National Institute of Technology Rourkela, India. He has conducted research in various areas like Health and Mental Health, Medical Anthropology, Family and Child Welfare, Disability studies, and Tribal Health issues. He teaches Psychiatric Social Work, Working with Individuals and Communities, Qualitative Research, ICTs in Social Development and Health System Management. He has written many articles including conference papers and published in national and international reputed peer-reviewed journals. He has extensive professional experiences in university teaching; research consultancy; extensive fieldwork supervision, mentoring postgraduate students; conducted various soft skill training and professional development programmes; organised various national, international conference. He is also associated with various National and International organizations and associations.

* * *

Melisa Anderson is a recipient of the 2017 UK Global Chevening Scholarship and recently completed her Master of Science in Biomedical Sciences at the University of Glasgow, Scotland, UK. She also holds a Master of Art in Teaching from the University of the West Indies Mona and a Bachelor of Science (Honours) from the University of Technology, Jamaica. Melisa is a Lecturer of Clinical Chemistry at the University of Technology, Jamaica.

Lennox Anderson-Jackson holds the Caribbean Diploma in Diagnostic Radiological Science from the University of the West Indies Mona, Kingston, Jamaica; A Bachelor of Science degree with honors in Diagnostic Medical Sonography from Weber State University in Ogden, Utah, USA; A Master of Science degree in Counselling and Consulting Psychology from the International University of the Caribbean, Kingston, Jamaica. Presently Mr. Anderson-Jackson is pursuing the MPhil / PhD in Chemical Pathology at the University of the West Indies, Mona, Kingston, Jamaica. He has over 28 years of experience in the field of radiological science and has worked in 4 countries including Jamaica, United States of America, Cayman Islands and Anguilla. He worked in several Government hospitals and Private hospitals and clinics in Jamaica including: Kingston Public Hospital (1991), Bustamante Hospital for Children, Cornwall Regional Hospital, Montego Bay Hospital, Radiology West (2003-2013), Royale Imaging Centre (2009-2013) and Reddy's Medical Centre. He also worked as a Clinical Ultrasound Instructor at the School of Medical Radiation Technology, University of the West Indies, Mona, Jamaica in collaboration with Michner Institute in Canada (2004-2008). Mr. Anderson-Jackson is presently the CEO and chief Medical Ultrasound Practitioner and Radiographer at the LYL Ultrasound Centre in Lucea, Hanover, Jamaica. He is a member of Who's Who amongst Students of American Universities and Colleges (Edition 1999). He was also a nominee for Crystal Crest Scholar of the year for Weber State University (1997). A Member of the Profession Supplementary to Medicine, Jamaica. He has been involved in some published articles as author and co-author. Mr. Anderson-Jackson was honoured in 2011 with the Distinguished Alumni Award by the Rusea's Old Student Association (ROSA) for achievements in the field of Science and Research.

Manju Bala is Professor and Director at Khalsa College of Engineering and Technology, Amritsar. Her area of interest is Wireless Sensor Network, Autism Spectrum Disorder, IoT, and Wireless Communication. Her research and teaching experience is 15 years and her research findings have been published through more than 60 research papers in referred / indexed journals and international conferences She has attended and presented her research findings in different countries. She is Editorial Board member and Scientific Committee member of various reputed journals and conferences.

Bhanu Prasad Behera has done Engineering from NIT Rourkela, his Masters in Management from Utkal University, Bhubaneswar and obtained the doctorate degree in Management from Berhampur University. He has already published several book chapters and papers in reputed journals. He is currently working at National Institute of Science and Technology, Berhampur.

Aybike Elif Bolcan has graduated from İstanbul University, Faculty of Economics, Labor Economics and Industrial Relations Department. She received her master's degree in 2006 from the Department of Labor Economics, Institute of Social Sciences, Istanbul University with the thesis titled "The Place of Women in Working Life and Women Unemployment in Turkey in the European Union Harmonization Process". She continues her doctoral studies with her thesis titled "Corporate Social Responsibility for Employees: A Field Research". After working as a research assistant at Bahçeşehir University Vocational School between 2006-2009, she was appointed as a lecturer in 2009. She teaches courses about organizational behaviour and human resources management. Since July 2016, she has been serving as the Head of the Department of Foreign Trade. She speaks fluent English and intermediate Spanish.

Renata Čepić is an Associate Professor in the field of pedagogy at the Faculty of Teacher Education, University of Rijeka, where she teaches several courses in the field of pedagogy at the undergraduate and graduate levels. She is also an Adjunct Professor at the Department of Pedagogy at the Faculty of Philosophy, University of Rijeka, where she teaches at the postgraduate doctoral courses. Her research interest is focused on pedagogy with a special interest in general education, in particular in adult education, lifelong learning, learning organisations, and the continuing professional education of teachers/preschool teachers/andragogists.

Ranjit Kumar Dehury, BHMS (Utkal University), MHA (TISS, Mumbai Campus), Ph.D. (IIT, Kharagpur). He has interest in areas of Healthcare Management, Public Health, Global Health Diplomacy, Human, Resource in Health, Strategic Management in Healthcare Organization, Disease Modeling and Healthcare Data Analytics. He has experience of 15 yearrs in various areas like clinical practices, management, consulting and academia.

Ahu Ergen is an Associate Professor at Bahçeşehir University. She studied Business Administration (Betriebswirtschaftslehre) at Marmara University. After graduation, she worked as marketing expert in automotive sector at a multinational company. She holds her PhD. in marketing from Marmara University and joined Bahcesehir University in 2009. She teaches several courses on marketing at undergraduate and graduate levels. Among her research interests are sustainable marketing, consumer behavior, competitive strategies and marketing management. She has book chapters, articles and conference papers published in these fields. She also writes articles about various brand management and marketing topics for the monthly brand magazines.

Suresh K. has completed M.Sc and M.Phil in Physics, M.Ed, M.Phil and Ph.D in Education, M.Sc in Psychology,M.Com (Education Management), and PGDCA. He has four and half years of experience in teaching in colleges of education. Now, he is doing Post Doctoral Research in the Department of Education, Central University of Tamil Nadu, Thiruvarur, Tamil Nadu, India, with the Fellowship of Indian Council of Social Science Research (ICSSR), New Delhi, India. He has published 29 national and international journal, presented 85 papers in national and international level, attended 40 workshops, gave 11 invited lecture at various institutions and received three awards.

Maksuda Khatun is a lecturer of Geography at Armed Police Battalion Public School and College, Bogura, Bangladesh. She has obtained MSc and BSc degree in Geography from Government Azizul Haque College, Bogura. She has several journal publications in the field of qualitative social research.

Vikas Khullar is Ph.D. Scholar at IKG Punjab Technical University, India and also acting as Assistant Professor in the Department of Computer Science and Engineering, at CT Institute of Engineering, Management, & Technology, India. His area of research in Ph. D. is Computer-Assistive Technologies for individuals with Autism Spectrum Disorder. His research and teaching experience is 11 years. His research findings have been published through more than 30 research papers in refereed/indexed journals and international conferences.

Dhananjay Kumar is an Assistant Professor at the Centre for Culture and Development, Vadodara. He has a doctorate in Social Anthropology from the Department of Humanities and Social Sciences, National Institute of Technology, Rourkela, Odisha. He did his post-graduation in Anthropology from the University of Delhi. His academic interests are: the relationships of culture and technology with focus on agrarian studies, traditional knowledge systems, dalit studies and social structure. He has conducted fieldwork among the SCs, OBCs and Tribal communities of India on issues of culture and development. He has authored many articles in professional journals, chapters in edited volumes and co-edited one book. Presently he is working on the social structure of tribal Gujarat.

Rajeev Kumar, Doctoral Researcher at Indian Institute of Technology Kharagpur, availed prestigious Senior Research Fellowship of University Grant Commission, New Delhi. Hold MSW from Tata Institute of Social Sciences, Mumbai, and M.Phil from Central Institute of Psychiatry, Ranchi. Major areas of interests are psychotherapeutic interventions, substance use, mental health and community-epidemiological aspect of HIV/AIDS, children mental health and protection issues and community health issues. Having publications in national and international journals including Taylor and Francis publication group. Mr. Kumar is a member of reviewer board in journals of Sage Publication and Elsevier publication. Mr. Kumar delivered several invited lectures in various state level training programmes, and have taught at the undergraduate and postgraduate level at Indian Institute of Technology Kharagpur. Currently teaching as adjunct faculty at Department of Rural Development and Management, Ramakrishna Mission Vivekananda Universtiy, Ranchi. As a national level master trainer, Mr. Kumar conducted nine week-long training in Jharkhand, West Bengal, and Sikkim states for ongoing multi collaborative National Drug Use Survey sponsored by Ministry of Social Justice and Empowerment, New Delhi. Mr. Kumar has presented several research papers at national and international fora, including International Congress of Psychology, Yokohama, Japan.

Elang M. has completed M.Sc in Mathematics, and M.Ed and M.Phil in Education. He presently doing doctoral research in Department of Education, central University of Education, Thiruvarur, Tamil Nadu, India.

Alberta Mazzola is a certified psychologist and psychotherapist. She graduated in "Dynamic and Clinical Psychology for Person, Organization and Community" and achieved a Diploma in "Psychoanalytic Psychotherapy, Clinical Intervention and Analysis of Demand". She is the founder and director of "Studio Confini. Psychology and psychoanalisys" (Italy), where she actually works, providing psychosocial research-intervention projects for the development of coexistence systems, as well as psychological counselling and psychoanalytic psychoterapy.

Donovan McGrowder holds Bachelor of Science (Honours) and Doctor of Philosophy (PhD) degrees in Biochemistry and Chemistry, and Biochemistry respectively from the University of the West Indies, Mona, Kingston, Jamaica. Dr. McGrowder also holds a Master of Science degree from University of Westminster, London, UK and a Master of Arts in Psychology and Counselling from St. Stephens College, Alberta Canada. He also has post-graduate training and experience in Clinical Biochemistry and Molecular Biology. Dr. McGrowder joined the staff of The University of the West Indies, Mona in 2001 as Research Fellow in the Department of Basic Medical Sciences – Biochemistry Section and was promoted to Lecturer in 2003 and Senior Lecturer in 2009. He is also Consultant of Chemical Pathology at the University Hospital of the West Indies. He is Fellow of the Institute of Biomedical Science, UK, Fellow of the Royal Society of Tropical Medicine and Hygiene, UK, and Member of the Institute of Health Promotion and Education, UK.

Fabian Miller is a Lecturer, Researcher and the Head of Department of Physical Education at The Mico University College; he has participated in research in the Medical field and Sport Science field. He has worked on research in sport services in the CARIFORUM region which aim was to establish regional policies for sport services for the member states involved and to establish sport services as a viable industry in the region. His current research is aimed to establish Biological Passports of College/University Athletes who compete in Sprinting and Long Distance events. Mr. Miller also published peer reviewed journal articles and book chapters. He co-authored the manuscript titled "Prostate Specific Antigen Testing in a Tertiary Teaching Hospital" and co-authored the book chapter titled "Dietary Antioxidants in the Chemoprevention of Prostate Cancer. Mr. Miller is a graduate from G.C Foster College where he completed a Diploma in Education and a Bachelors Degree in Physical Education and Sport, he went on to pursue and complete his Masters of Science in Physical Education at The University of Technology, Jamaica and he is currently a PhD student in Biotechnology, Faculty of Science and Technology, University of the West Indies, Mona. Mr. Miller is a board member of the Social and Human Sciences Advisory Committee of Jamaica National Commission for UNESCO (Period of 2016-2019) and a member of Jamaica Association of Sports Medicine (JASM).

Paul Oppold is a PhD student in the University of Central Florida's School of Modeling, Simulation and Training. Paul joined WEAR Lab as a consultant in 2016. His research interests include wearable technology, workload and how the affordances of computer supported collaborative work (CSCW) enable physically co-located and remote teams to effectively accomplish shared goals. Paul has written extensively about teamwork and community membership in online communities and how hardware and software design characteristics affect individual and team workload and effectiveness.

Lynne Orr has worked in student development for 25 years. She also works at Walden University as a professor in the Higher Education and Adult Learning program, as a chair and mentor with the EdD students. Areas of specialty include:

Career Development, Academic Advising, Assessment, Research, Higher Education, Student Development, and Technology.

Abhijit Pathak is pursuing PhD in the Department of Humanities and Social Sciences at National Institute of Technology, Rourkela, India.

Kathrine Pigeon has her Master's in clinical counseling and an EdS in play therapy, both are from The University of Mississippi. Kathrine has worked with college students targeting personal wellness. Also, she has 9 years experience working as a counselor. Kathrine has worked with both college aged students and elementary school children. She is currently a student at Walden University in the Doctor of Education program with a concentration in college teaching and learning.

Poornima Rajendran is working as an Assistant Professor in the Department of Education, Central University of Tamil Nadu. Her area of interest includes professional competencies of teachers, educational psychology and inclusive education.

Brianna Reyes, BA, is a current William Paterson University MFA candidate pursuing a degree in Creative and Professional Writing. She has dedicated 5 years to serving undergraduate first-year students, regardless of academic discipline, as they transition from high school to college. Areas of specialty include: Student Leadership, Literature, Research, and Technology.

Gitanjali Roy is an Assistant Professor in the Department of Psychology, Faculty of Education and Psychology at The Maharaja Sayajirao University of Baroda (MSUB). She has her doctoral thesis on constructing and testing a trait model of personality in indian psychology. She is a recipient of Dr. Deepak Bhatt Award for Best paper in IAAP-2014 and Sri Satya Pal Malhotra Memorial Award-2017, for Best paper in Indian Journal of Psychology and Education, Vol. 1 & 2, January and July, 2017. She has supervised five Master's dissertation thesis of which four are in the field of Indian psychology. She is a core committee member in Directorate for Student Welfare and Coordinator of the Center of Skill Development and Capacity Building, Management Development Center at The Maharaja Sayajirao University of Baroda (MSUB).

Michael Schwartz is the founder of Wearable Electronics Augmented Reality (WEAR) Lab. His research focuses on the design and usability of wearable devices and alternative interfaces for people with sensory impairments. Michael has a Masters in Psychology from Stephen F Austin University and a Masters in modeling and simulation from the University of Central Florida. He is currently pursuing a PhD in human factors.

Poulomee Shaw is the Founder & Director of Mind's- a Psychologist, Motivational Speaker, Career Strategist and Entrepreneur.She has holding the PgD degree from Rajabajar Science College (Cal), Master degree in Psychology, Mental Health & Counselling Specialist (Cal), Emotional Intelligence Expertise E.I.O.E (IIT Kharagpur). After finishing the Clinical internship from a reputed Govt hospital (IPGMER, SSKM Hospital) – Department of Psychiatry (IOP), she focused her career in research and medical practice. Presently she is working with few research projects and also attached with few corporate hospitals with holding the post of consultant psychologist for last 5 years. Research Interest: Stress, Depression, Anxiety, Post Traumatic Stress Disorder (PTSD), Psycho- oncology, Spiritual aspect in human psychology, Mindfulness.

Harjit Pal Singh is Associate Professor & Head, Department of Electronics and Communication at CT Institute of Engineering, Management and Technology, Jalandhar. His area of interest is Wireless Sensor Network, Autism, IoT, Voice over Internet Protocol, Wireless Communication, Signal processing, Digital Filter Design, and Wireless Sensor Networks. His research and teaching experience is 10 years. His research findings have been published through more than 50 research papers in refereed/indexed journals and international conferences. He is Associate Editor and member of Editorial Board of various reputed journals. He worked as a member of the Scientific Board for different international conferences held in different countries.

Sanja Tatalović Vorkapić, PhD, currently teaches students at the Faculty of Teacher Education, University of Rijeka in: Developmental psychology, Psychology of early learning and teaching, General psychology, Emotional intelligence, Developmental psychopathology, Methodology of quantitative research, and Positive psychology. Her contemporary research interests include biological basis of personality, personality of (pre)school teachers and child personality, contemporary issues from developmental psychopathology and methodology of quantitative research, positive psychology (well-being, optimism, life satisfaction, virtues) and its relationship with other fields through interdisciplinary studies, and also study programs for (pre)school teachers. She has published numerous psychology related articles and has been actively involved within various interdisciplinary research projects. She has awarded as the best scientist in the field of Social Sciences in 2013/2014. year, and as the best teacher in the 2016. year at the University of Rijeka, Croatia.

Dwayne Ricardo Tucker is a senior medical laboratory technologist at the University of the West Indies, Mona, Jamaica since 2010. He holds a Bachelor of Science Degree in Medical Technology from the Northern Caribbean University, Manchester, Jamaica. Dwayne is a 2016 British Chevening scholar who obtained a Master of Science Degree in Oncology in 2017 from the University of Nottingham, United Kingdom. In collaboration with the Caribbean Institute for Health Research, Dwayne contributed to genetics-focused research on prostate cancer survivors of African ancestry during a fellowship at the Fox Chase Cancer Center (FCCC). He is a prospective PhD student at the University of British Columbia in Vancouver, Canada, where he will investigate molecular proteins as potential prognostic and diagnostic tools for prostate cancer. As a member of the African-Caribbean Cancer Consortium (AC3), he hopes to apply the knowledge and skills garnered from his PhD training towards improving prostate cancer prognosis and prevention within the realms of Black men worldwide.

Kurt Vaz is the Administrator in the Department of Pathology at The University of the West Indies, Mona Campus, Kingston Jamaica. He has over fifteen (15) years of experience in clinical laboratory sciences. As a scientist he seeks to make a real difference in biomedical research and always strives to give his utmost best to patient care.

Linda Weekley spent almost thirty years in public education. During that time, she served students with special needs, both academic and behavioral. After retiring seven years ago to spend more time with family and volunteer in the community, she decided to pursue her doctorate in adult education. Today, Linda volunteers as the director of the adult education department at her church, works alongside her husband to offer marriage counseling, and mentors many young women from around the world.

Index

www.ingramcontent.com/pod-product-compliance
Lightning Source LLC
LaVergne TN
LVHW062322300926
849161LV00007B/1535